Public Health in the
People's Republic of China

The Macy Foundation Series
on Medicine and
Public Health in China

Bowers, *Western Medicine in a Chinese Palace: Peking Union Medical College, 1917–1951*

Wegman, Lin, and Purcell, *Public Health in the People's Republic of China*

Sidel and Sidel, *Serve the People: Observations on Medicine in the People's Republic of China*

Bowers and Purcell, *Medicine and Society in China*

Edited by MYRON E. WEGMAN,
TSUNG-YI LIN,
and ELIZABETH F. PURCELL

PUBLIC HEALTH IN THE PEOPLE'S REPUBLIC OF CHINA

Report of a Conference
Sponsored by the
School of Public Health and the
Center for Chinese Studies of the
University of Michigan
and the
Josiah Macy, Jr. Foundation

THE JOSIAH MACY, JR. FOUNDATION
One Rockefeller Plaza, New York, New York 10020

Contents

v

Preface

The Macy conference program goes back to the establishment of the Josiah Macy, Jr. Foundation in 1930. The first conference was convened in the summer of 1931, just one year later, to examine the programs and needs of the American Association of Schools of Social Work. Beginning in the late 1930s and early 1940s the foundation pioneered in the convening of interdisciplinary conferences based on small continuing groups representing a broad spectrum of disciplines.

As Frank Fremont-Smith, the medical director of the foundation, and his staff grew aware of the potential impact of the conference program, the range of topics and the number of scientists involved proliferated. Thus in 1955 the foundation could report that there were nine regular conference groups, with a membership of over 200 scientists from more than 100 health-related institutions. With the retirement of Dr. Fremont-Smith in 1960, the conference program was temporarily halted.

In 1965 the history of the conference program was reviewed and it was reestablished with modifications. Today it is directed toward current health-related issues of regional, national, or global interest, ongoing foundation programs, and fields of potential foundation interest.

Nineteen seventy-two was an especially busy conference year for the Macy Foundation: A total of nine conferences were held on topics ranging from pediatrics in Latin America, to drug abuse in the United States, to public health in the People's Republic of China, the latter held in Ann Arbor in May under the joint sponsorship of the School of Public Health and the Center for Chinese Studies of the University of Michigan.

Why public health in China? First, because our limited observations up until the revolution in 1949 suggested that China suffered from the greatest galaxy of public health problems of any country in the world. Second, because a continuing barrage of reports emanating from Peking since 1949 has described the remarkable accomplishments in public health in the PRC. And, finally, we were eager to build a body of available information on public health in the PRC for dissemination to a wider audience.

A serious limitation on the discussions was the paucity of valid information, even from those who had visited China only months before the conference was held. This lack of intelligence did, however, serve to dramatize the need for scholarly scientific communication with the world's most populous country.

The exchanges that have occurred since the conference, culminating in the visit to the United States of a medical group from the PRC in November 1972, suggest that far brighter days lie ahead.

JOHN Z. BOWERS,
President
Josiah Macy, Jr. Foundation

Introduction

Advances in public health have taken place with increased rapidity in recent years over many areas of the world. Perhaps more than any other field of international interest what one country does in public health has direct and continuing interest for every other country, whether a contiguous neighbor or not. This interest stems as much from what various countries can learn from each other as it does from the danger of communicable disease or environmental contamination.

Reports of accelerated progress in the People's Republic of China thus whetted the desire of health workers in other parts of the world to learn more of the details of the results obtained and the methods utilized. This need was further accentuated by the lack of available systematic publications or scientific communications in the field. With the goal in mind of filling this gap in knowledge the University of Michigan, through its School of Public Health and its Center for Chinese Studies, sponsored jointly with the Josiah Macy, Jr. Foundation a conference on Public Health in the People's Republic of China, which took place in Ann Arbor on May 14 to 17, 1972.

The twenty-nine invited participants included a number of persons with personal experience in China, some quite recent. Although it had been hoped that representatives from the PRC might participate, this did not take place and the conference had to be content with such information as could be obtained from Western visitors, from published information, and from correspondence.

The planning committee decided that the conference could be most productive if it concentrated on those aspects of health organization and group and community interrelationships affecting health progress, rather than on specific medical or surgical techniques. The main subjects are listed in the table of contents. The participants are listed on pages 341–343.

A series of working papers and an annotated bibliography, prepared and distributed beforehand, formed the basis of the discussions. At the conference itself each author introduced his paper in
summary form and the exchange of ideas was spirited and informa-
tive. More than any single conclusion, the conference noted the
absence of firm data on many of the fundamental questions raised.
It is not surprising, then, that the general conclusion was that more
questions had been raised than had been answered. Nevertheless
the assembled expertise was such that there was indeed clarification of many basic points, particularly concerning the combination
of the traditional and the novel, which seems to characterize health
developments in the PRC.

In this publication an attempt has been made to highlight major
points in the introductory notes to each chapter and in the final
chapter on general conclusions. The latter chapter is not to be
interpreted as a general summary but rather as drawing particular
attention to the main considerations of which most note had been
taken. It should be added that the individual papers have in most
instances been modified in the light of the discussion and thus now
reflect in large measure the relevant comments of the other participants.

The sponsors of the conference and the participants hope that
this publication will be a useful reference work and that the obvious
shortcomings will stimulate further attempts to fill the gaps and
extend our knowledge of this most important subject.

MYRON E. WEGMAN
TSUNG-YI LIN

I. Historical Perspectives on the Development of Public Health in China

Introductory Note

In this chapter Arthur M. Kleinman, a medical historian especially interested in the Chinese health care system, and John Z. Bowers, an expert on medical education with broad international experience, discuss the processes of the introduction of public health to China and its subsequent development up to establishment of the People's Republic of China.

Public health, a distinctly Western system of ideas and practices, nurtured entirely within the institutional framework of Western society, found a not too favorable welcome and not very desirable conditions for growth when first introduced to China in the late nineteenth century. China was then at its lowest point of national decline, experiencing serious economic dislocation, social and cultural disintegration, and political fragmentation—the country was plagued by all conceivable human miseries.

The initial phase of health work in China was characterized by a strong foreign interest, and was limited to several port cities with almost no impact on the great majority of the Chinese population, urban or rural, especially the latter. The carry-over from the United States—the major foreign power engaged in health work in China—of the split between medicine and social welfare and of the separation between curative services and preventive work greatly influenced the philosophy of health organization and patterns of training of health personnel. Notable progress in certain areas of medicine and health care were made: for example, the high quality of the medical training program of Peking Union Medical College, the public health training in the First Community Health Center in Peking, and the health component of the Rural Reconstruction Program. Through government and missionary efforts, medical education and curative services spread slowly to other cities. It was concluded, however, that the single

3

important lesson to be learned from the experiences up to the 1930s was that any advance in public health depended on fundamental social and economic reform. Feelings of depression and a sense of futility seemed to afflict many public health workers of that period.

The ensuing period of civil war and the Sino-Japanese War saw the emergence of a new pattern of health care in the Communist-ruled countryside, while the old system, retaining its basic philosophy and character, continued under the Nationalist government. The new public health program under the Communists became an integral and important part of the political and social reconstruction, emphasizing community responsibility for the people's health and hygienic environment. Experiments with free health services, the education and mobilization of the rural masses for health-related activities, and the amalgamation of traditional Chinese and modern (Western) systems of medicine brought forth many grass-roots programs supported enthusiastically by both health workers and the people in general. The foresight of experimenting with the integration of traditional and Western medicine deserves special mention because of its uniqueness in history as well as its contribution to the ensuing program development in the health care system. Although traditional medicine was inadequate in dealing with the public health problems that abounded in China, it had provided illness with socially legitimate meaning and had contributed to the reaffirmation of traditional values and the maintenance of social stability.

It was this new experiment in public health, initiated in Yenan, with its attendant philosophy, methods, and new patterns of health conduct for the people that became the basis for program development of the People's Republic of China after the revolution in 1949.

The Background and Development
of Public Health in China:
An Exploratory Essay

ꕤ

ARTHUR M. KLEINMAN*

The truly immense field encompassed by the somewhat pretentious title of this short paper cannot be covered in any sense of completeness. Nor would attempting such an undertaking be appropriate for the focus and interests of this publication. Rather I propose to describe in a very general way something of the historical and cultural background of our subject: Public Health in the People's Republic of China. This contribution represents, then, neither a history nor an ethnography, but a framework for introducing our topic and raising some of the key issues surrounding it. In any discussion of major aspects of Chinese civilization it must be appreciated that we are entering a very different cultural context and that we are doing so with an implicit Western cultural orientation and tradition.

There is widespread recognition of the tremendous influence of culture upon cognitive and social structures;[1] in China's case, this influence has been described for language, thought, religion, art, science, and medicine.[2-7] We must now develop this same appreciation for public health. Before we turn to Chinese culture and its medical and public health forms, I should point out that examining public health in its Chinese context implies some kind of comparative framework for studying public health activities in different historical and sociocultural settings. Although such a framework has been applied to medicine in general,[8] it has not yet been

* The research upon which this paper is based was conducted during the tenure of a National Science Foundation postdoctoral fellowship in the comparative social study of medicine in the Department of the History of Science, Harvard University, 1970–72; it has benefited also from the author's field experience as a National Institutes of Health research fellow in Taiwan, 1969–70.

5

clearly worked out for public health, and would seem to require a somewhat different approach because of a problem in the history and ethnography of public health itself. While medicine existed as an indigenous cultural system in many and perhaps all societies, to which the origin of modern scientific medicine in the West was merely an addition,[9] albeit an extremely important one, the public health movement *per se* can be viewed only as a discrete and recent product of Western civilization and modern scientific medicine.[10] While we can search for elements of preventive and social medicine in traditional systems of medicine,[11] the comparative study of public health begins with its introduction as a system into other cultures. We should no more speak of public health in ancient China than in ancient Greece or Rome, or, until the end of the nineteenth century in Western Europe or America, when it originated as a system of ideas and practices supported by the germ theory of disease, a statistical approach to disease problems, and quite distinct concerns for and approaches to the social and environmental aspects of illness. This system emanated from the experiences of the industrial revolution and the social and intellectual transformation of European society in the nineteenth century, so that public health developed within the institutional framework of modern Western society. Only later was an organized approach to public health propagated to different cultures, of which China is one of the most important and fascinating examples.

This caution is necessary so that in surveying Chinese culture and traditional Chinese medicine we do not misapply and trivialize the phenomenon of public health, or engage in a semantic dispute and an absurd search for embryonic forms of public health in traditional medicine and social practices. This in no way detracts from the great tradition of Chinese medicine, or denies its preventive and social importance, anymore than it detracts from Hippocratic medicine or traditional African medicine. It does, however, allow us to make sense of the introduction of modern medical science and public health to China, and the ultimate development of a distinctly Chinese form of modern medicine and public health.

Historical and Sociocultural Background

Traditional Chinese *medical systems* are great chapters in world medical history. The plural is used here because, historically, one can discern many systems that differed in varying ways. In this paper I propose to concentrate on two, which I shall call the *high-order* system and the *popular* system.

The high order medical system was embedded in the Confucian and Taoist streams of Chinese culture, and was supported by the sociopolitical structure of traditional Chinese society. It contained both an elaborate theoretical superstructure, as found in classical medical texts such as the *Huang-ti nei-ching*, and an enormously rich empirical substratum, as demonstrsted in the pharmacopoeias, the *Pen T'sao*, and other therapeutic traditions. This tradition, well described elsewhere as a system of ideas and practices,[12] is indeed the only Chinese medical system about which we possess considerable historical information.

We know, for example, that its theoretical structure participated in many of the traditional features of Chinese thought and social organization: an organismic world view in which systematic correspondences were made between the macrocosmic universe and microcosmic man and his inner structure;[13] the *yin-yang* system of polar oppositions, a logical alternative structure in which systematic correspondences and resonant harmonies took the place of the single causal trains of the mechanistic model of Western logic;[14] the radical humanism of traditional Confucian thought;[15] the Taoist pursuit of longevity, "strengtheners" of life, and harmonious integration of human and social elements with nature; the literati tradition and its social forms; and the institutions and social ideology of imperial Chinese society. As a closed theoretical system, high-order Chinese medicine "rationalized" a tremendous body of empirical findings and practices, such as the use of acupuncture and efficacious herbs, many of which were probably derived from folk and popular traditions.[16] Unlike the mind-body dichotomy that held sway in traditional Western medicine, this theoretical structure incorporated a holistic psychosomatic perspective; nor was there an explicit separation between curative and preventive practices. The high-order system of medicine was in contact with other ancient medical traditions, sharing some concepts such as the notions of vital breath and five basic elements. It underwent its own historical changes and interacted with other systems of medicine in traditional Chinese society. We know very little, however, about how this medical system actually functioned.

The role of the traditional Chinese physician supposedly evolved from a shamanistic healer in ancient times to that of the Confucian physician who appears in the late Chou dynasty (700–200 B.C.).[17] A text of this period, the *Chou-li*, suggests that some sort of imperial system of medicine existed in close relation to the emperor and his court, and involved a medical college, medical examinations, and a hierarchy of medical officials, some of whom were responsible for the health of the people. There is uncertainty, however, about how to interpret this document and what the actual medical structure was.[18] Whatever organized state medicine existed was clearly limited to the court, and possibly to the literati and wealthy merchant class.

Not unlike other traditional systems of medicine, this one incorporated a view of illness as disorder; healing was considered to be analogous to the reassertion of sociopolitical order. Thus, *chih*, the Chinese character for healing, also conveyed the idea of good government, management, and stability. The state did indeed accept some responsibility for relief from natural disasters, and during the Sung dynasty this apparently included more general social relief, but probably not in any comprehensive way.[19] While state granaries distributed food during times of famine, this evidently worked more in principal than in fact.[20] Moreover, during the Sung dynasty there were public pharmacies and hospitals for the poor, aged, and incurable; but for the vast mass of people this system of social relief and public medicine evidently had little applicability.[21]

Joseph Needham, who has done so much to make traditional Chinese science and medicine accessible and understandable to the West, has even argued that because high-order traditional medicine existed in a society characterized by bureaucratic feudalism, preventive medical practices were fostered because the prevention of troubles was more highly valued than the recognition and response to existing troubles, including illness.[22] This assertion seems problematic at best. Certainly nothing approaching a coherent system of organized preventive concepts and practices existed, even though isolated examples were to be found. The concept of prevention can indeed be detected at times in traditional Chinese medical ideology, and many preventive practices could be culled from historical records: dietetics, rudimentary sanitation practices, fumigation, personal hygiene, destruction of rabid animals, inoculation against smallpox, at a later date, and much else.[23] But just as the Roman sewer system and preventive aspects of Galenic medicine were *not* part of a real system of public health, neither were the

Chinese practices of drinking boiled water and eating well-cooked food. Removed from their ideological and social contexts and reinterpreted within an alien public health framework, these and other examples cited may have been quite successful as preventive measures.

Unquestionably many aspects of high-order traditional Chinese medicine and its sociopolitical context could be considered as providing a receptive background for the future introduction of public health. Certainly there would seem to be no inherent resistance to public health ideas and practices. For example, in categorizing the causes of disease, and in the process of diagnosis, attention was devoted to environmental and social factors, including climate, family, and personal problems. Much attention was also paid to factors that we now correlate with positive mental health, such as living a harmonious life in balance with nature, sexual hygiene, and spiritual cultivation and discipline. Similarly, the periodic emphasis in Chinese history on collective responsibility among the masses for acts against the social order could be viewed as a foundation for similar responsibility for public health. One could assemble a list of relatively unfavorable factors, including the family-centered orientation of the Confucian ethic and traditional social structure, which probably mitigated against the development of a community-wide concern for health. The historical and sociocultural background is complex and should not be treated simply as a source either of all forward-looking or of all regressive aspects of China's modern condition.

Nonetheless the medical system we have been describing, which some erroneously identify with the whole of traditional Chinese medicine, never extended to include the great body of Chinese peasants. It was *not* in fact a functioning medical system for over 90 per cent of the population, although it greatly influenced local forms of medicine, and in urban areas and amongst the social elite it sometimes formed a functioning part of the popular medical system. Modern ethnographic studies of traditional Chinese cultural areas[24] and certain historical reconstructions of life in traditional China[25] demonstrate that by far the most prevalent system was the low-order folk and popular medical tradition. This system maintained a dynamic interconnection with the theoretical ideology and empirical tradition of the high-order system of traditional medicine, but it incorporated many additional elements and perhaps should be viewed as a clustering of different healing systems. The popular stream is perhaps most notable for its remarkable degree of therapeutic eclecticism, tolerance for all sorts of medical practices and institutions, and syncretism of different medical traditions. Equally as remarkable is the seemingly inordinate amount of general interest that was devoted to medical concerns in traditional Chinese society.

One student of this subject has made a partial list of traditional practitioners that includes soothsayers; geomancers; fortune tellers; specialists in diseases of the eyes, ears, and teeth; herbalists; barbermasseurs; quack doctors; Buddhist and Taoist priest-healers, itinerant drug peddlers; shamans; pharmacists; and traditional doctors.[26] To this could be added members of families, clans, and villages who possessed some sort of special medical expertise. A list of traditional diagnostic and therapeutic forms would be equally as long. Only now are Westerners beginning to understand how these elements and their ideological and social supports fitted together to form a total functioning medical system on the local level of social perception and usage. Such a total structure or medical ethos included not only this varied group of practitioners, but also the attitudes and expectations of patients and the vast body of potential patients who in some way were socialized into this system.

We cannot identify much in the way of prevention in the folk and popular medical systems outside of such practices as the propitiation of disease-producing gods and spirits in healing rituals and activities such as geomancy.

Traditional Chinese medical systems were oriented more toward individual medical care and the personal and family problems engendered by illness. It was probably here that traditional medicine had its greatest effect, particularly when dealing with noninfectious diseases. Epidemics, like surgical problems, but for very different reasons, were beyond its scope.[27] The individual healing function did not extend into areas of social welfare; nor did the system construct a means for delivery of widespread medical care. Instead the orientation was preeminently toward traditional medical care functions: the ordering of disease into a human experience; the classification, explanation, and cognitive management of illness; and healing practices.

The limited evidence we have suggests that public health problems such as famines, floods, uncontrolled epidemics, widespread parasitic infestations, very high childhood mortality rates, and the like were always present, although perhaps not to the same degree as in the nineteenth and early twentieth centuries. In the face of these kinds of problems, neither stream of traditional Chinese medicine was adequate. Nor did the state implement any effective form of social relief. Indeed heavy taxes, forced labor and military service, and a remote and unresponsive governmental structure must have added greatly to the depressed socioeconomic conditions of the peasantry and contributed to the enormous burden of public health problems.

It should be recognized, however, that traditional Chinese medicine, which was clearly efficacious in dealing with certain forms of illness, did function to provide some crucial aspects of medical care, particularly individual and social support at times of great stress. Like most traditional forms of medicine, this system provided illness with socially legitimate meaning, reaffirmed traditional values and behavioral norms, and maintained social stability, while reasserting whatever effective control was available—these critical sociocultural functions of traditional Chinese medicine are by no means to be underemphasized. In addition, it has been argued that traditional medical systems, including Chinese medicine, can be viewed and perhaps evaluated in terms of their important role of cultural adaptation to environmental stress.[28] The evolutionary significance of this function of traditional medical systems for Chinese society may have been considerable.

The Development of Public Health in Modern China

In order to focus upon the development of public health in China we shall make a leap to the last 150 years of Chinese history, the period of modernization, Westernization, and transformation of traditional Chinese society. Beginning in the early nineteenth century and extending up to the present, it led progressively to the opening of China to Western interests, the collapse of the Ch'ing dynasty, the subsequent years of social and political chaos, the Kuomintang interlude, and, eventually, the rise of the People's Republic.

Even before gunboats of the Western powers thrust their way into the Middle Kingdom, the Ch'ing dynasty was undergoing a progressively worsening rural crisis. The Chinese population, for reasons still poorly understood, was increasing at an extraordinary rate, while at the same time there was no substantial increase in usable farmland. Even as late as the period from 1873 to 1933, for example, the population was estimated to have increased by over 30 per cent.[29] The result was a decline in the already marginal standard of rural living, and increasing poverty and social distress. Also present were the largely uncontrolled natural crises: flood, famine, and epidemics. Nor was any significant rural reform and social relief forthcoming from the withering Ch'ing government, which was hardpressed by both the external threat of expansion and exploitation by the Western powers, and the internal threat of social discord and rebellion. What followed was economic dislocation and sociocultural disintegration.

Along with many other aspects of modern Western civilization— mercantile interests, the politics of nation-states, technologies, science, ideas from the nineteenth century liberal tradition, and Christianity—modern medical science and public health were also imported into this rapidly changing and generally depressed socioeconomic, political, and cultural environment.

The missionaries brought modern medicine to China at a time when medical science had hardly advanced and public health had yet to come into existence. Nonetheless, though not an important factor until the end of the nineteenth century, medicine represented one of the early modernizing and Westernizing forces in China. Limited at first to the treaty ports and the care of Westerners, missionary physicians successfully introduced Jennerian vaccination for smallpox,[30] ophthalmological surgery, modern hospitals, clinics, and medical schools. With the opening of China's interior, they began to bring modern medical care services to a few rural areas. For the most part the missionaries' orientation was toward individual illness and curative medicine; but because of the virtual absence of Chinese governmental involvement with social welfare, at a time when the relationship between abysmal socioeconomic conditions and health was becoming obvious, they moved into this area also. By the turn of the century, while China was on the whole becoming receptive to modern medicine,[31] the missionaries' impact on health conditions had not been significant, and modern medicine had failed to become rooted in Chinese society.

In the last quarter of the nineteenth century secular Western interests organized and took control of the Chinese customs service, and via this institution the rudiments of public health—quarantine, sanitation, epidemiological surveys, etc.—were carried into the treaty ports.[32] The reports of medical officers of the Chinese Imperial Customs Service in the 1870s and 1880s reveal just how bad the social and health conditions were in the cities, and suggest that the medical science and the public health system of that time were unable to effect meaningful changes.[33] Western medicine was scarcely more effective than traditional Chinese medicine in treating infectious diseases, and public health, which was just learning the determinants of epidemics, was still unable to control epidemic diseases.

Much of the improvement in European health in the nineteenth century antedated effective therapeutic and hygienic procedures, and was due to the general betterment of socioeconomic conditions.[34] In China, by contrast, conditions were worsening, as was the people's health. By the time of the First China Medical Commission of the Rockefeller Foundation in 1914, it had become obvious that a system of modern scientific medicine had not been adopted in China, nor had it had a notable impact on the country's health problems.[35] Yet it was believed that medical science and technology, if properly applied, would win out regardless of existing social conditions. We now know that the health problems in China at that time will not respond even to sophisticated biomedical technology if the underlying socioeconomic factors remain unchanged.[36] But this hindsight would probably not have been accepted by the fervent early proponents of medical science and public health.

By the time of the fall of the Ch'ing dynasty, foreigners had begun to assume much of the responsibility for public health and social welfare in China. More significantly, modern medicine and public health had become important issues to the Chinese themselves; the slow and painful movement toward a distinctly Chinese form of modern medicine and public health had begun, a movement that was part of the struggle for national development.

After the Ch'ing dynasty suffered a portentous defeat by the Japanese in 1895, and as part of the reform movement of that year, Chinese intellectuals called for government support for and advancement of modern medical science and public health. It was pointed out that Meiji Japan had given state support to modern medicine and had made important advances in public health. China was viewed by reformist elements in its social-elite class as sick and in need of physical and spiritual strengthening.[37] In their search for new sources of wealth and power for their country, Chinese intellectuals became interested in the scientific and technological developments that had originated in the West and that were superior to those of China in so many areas. Similarly, they were actively absorbing such Western intellectual currents as the nineteenth century tradition of English liberalism, social Darwinism, socialism, and the like.[38] Ideas of social welfare and reform were in the air, and the concept of public health fit well into this ideological context.

The first institutional program in public health established by the Chinese government was the Manchurian Plague Prevention Service, set up to control a large epidemic of plague that occurred in Manchuria in 1910. In actuality this body was unable to control the epidemic in Manchuria, although it did prevent its spread to other areas. The real stimulus for and test of this endeavor was international politics.[39] The Chinese government was forced into assuming responsibility for the control of the epidemic by Japanese, Russian, and American interests that threatened to seize Manchuria under the pretext of exerting plague control. Once established, however, the service extended beyond plague prevention into the control of other epidemics, the provision of general hospitals for the care of the poor, and maternal and child health programs. As described in Dr. Bowers's paper, this became one of the central public health institutions in China, along with the Peking Special Health Station and the National Epidemic Prevention Bureau. Public health had finally become part of the construction of a modern Chinese nation.

The almost two decades of social and political chaos that followed the fall of the Ch'ing, until the Nationalist government asserted some measure of control over the nation, mitigated against the construction of a modern system of health. Nor were Westerners able to build a national health service, although they controlled many elements of the inchoate and fragmented modern medical and social welfare systems. For example, Westerners controlled the China International Famine Relief Commission, founded in 1921, which was active in flood control, rural relief, and economic reform, in addition to famine relief and prevention.[40] Missionaries were active in antiopium programs, the YMCA launched an educational campaign in personal and public hygiene,[41] and Christian social reformers were working in rural reconstruction and its health-related aspects.[42] All of these efforts were faced by the paradox that the programs were not rooted in the Chinese sociocultural context that they desired to change, and were adversely affected by the socioeconomic and political conditions within which they operated and which they were unable to alter in any fundamental way. The vicissitudes and ultimate failure of the medical program of Yale-in-China is but one example of this widespread dilemma.[43]

In order to paint a full picture we would have to balance these largely private Western efforts to improve China's social and health conditions with the activities of rampant commercial and political Western interests, often government sponsored, which, for example, sustained the opium market and prostitution while adding to the worsening of living conditions in the urban centers; this other side of the Western effort in China thus contributed to her public health problems.

The situation was further complicated by the polarization of the Western, and subsequently the Chinese, public health movement into scientific and social welfare poles. In the United States the emerging public health system had adopted science as an instrument to aid in the battle against social and environmental aspects of disease, only to become more interested in the scientific side than in social welfare. This separation, which was institutionalized in the professional split between medical and social work spheres of public health, was carried over into China, where parasitology, a basic public health science, rapidly developed as the major direction for the medical research approach to public health. Another aspect of the American public health model that touched China was the separation of preventive medicine from curative medicine. What made John Grant of the Peking Union Medical College so unusual among his medical and public health colleagues both in the United States and in China, as Dr. Bowers suggests, was his attempt to bridge curative and preventive, and scientific and social, approaches in order to create a unified system of medical care that would extend into and alter the desperate health conditions in the regions of urban and rural poverty.

The impact of most of these efforts on the health of China's rural masses was, however, quite small. Unfortunately, this was also the case with public health and social welfare enterprises in the decade of Kuomintang power during the 1930s. The Nanking government no more achieved a functioning national health system than it did a unified state. The same factors working against the latter pre-vented the establishment of the former: persistent economic dis-location, warlordism, political factionalism, corruption, lack of basic social reforms, and civil and foreign wars.[44] If a lesson might be learned from the experiences of the 1930s, it is that any advances in public health depend on fundamental social and economic reforms.

It would be difficult to exaggerate the massive public health prob-lems in China in the twenties and thirties, and the limited re-sources available to deal effectively with them.[45] Although a Minis-try of Health was first organized in Nanking in 1929, it had little baseline epidemiological data, a yearly budget of only $500,000 (Mexican), an organizational structure that existed solely at the top, and a list of Herculean tasks. The League of Nations' medical consultants to China noted that traditional medicine was still the major functioning health care system even in the urban areas; and hospitals and laboratories were mainly in foreign hands.

The Ministry of Health was responsible for only seven major cities; the rest of China, excluding areas controlled by foreign powers, was partitioned into completely independent provincial health administrations. Only a few model health stations were in operation, and no system of public health existed even in most of the urban areas. The league consultants found their Chinese col-leagues overwhelmed with socioeconomic problems for which their scientific training could offer no solutions. Wisely they concluded that the development of public health in China awaited efforts at national reconstruction, and that for the time being limited "model" efforts were all that could be expected.[46]

By 1937, although more health facilities had been established, more health personnel trained, and some programs initiated, the league's public health experts found health conditions barely im-proved. The budgetary allocation for the health sector remained minute, and a system of public health, though detailed in plans, had not yet been achieved. By this time, however, interest had shifted from the national and provincial institutions to a few local projects in rural areas where public health was being implemented as part of efforts, largely private, at rural reconstruction. To the league's consultants this was the most promising development in public health in China, more so than the slowly expanding govern-mental administrative apparatus. They encouraged governmental support for these efforts at providing rural health care, along with social relief, education, and the development of new types of rural medical workers and institutions.[47]

The rural reconstruction movement is a fascinating chapter in modern Chinese history.[48] Although Western missionaries, Chinese Christians, the Nationalist government, and private foundations became active in this promising field, perhaps the best known figure involved was James Yen. Yen organized the Mass Education Movement and established a model center for rural reconstruction at Ting Hsien, where he attempted to attack in an organized community-wide fashion what he felt were the four major problems of rural China: ignorance, poverty, disease, and community disintegration. In place of the feeling of depression and sense of futility that afflicted many public health workers in China, Yen radiated an infectious reforming zeal and enthusiastic dedication that became institutionalized in his center. His program sought not only to educate peasants and to improve their health, but to do so by first alleviating their economic and social plight. Yen recognized that public health had to be integrated into a program of social reform, communicated in a culturally meaningful manner, and made effective at the local level. Yet his center and several other rural projects had great difficulty in attracting physicians and public health personnel, and in engaging the participation of established medical and public health institutions.[49] Nonetheless his work and that of his colleagues, Liang Sou-ming, Chang Fu-liang, and George Shepherd, developed an alternative public health model that differed considerably from the concern of medical institutions in China with training sophisticated physicians and developing biomedical technological solutions. It also differed from the desire of the Ministry of Health for more funds, more *hsien* health centers, and a larger health bureaucracy, and from the interests of the Nationalist government in a national ideological program of spiritual and physical hygiene—the New Life Movement—that was supposed to regenerate Chinese society.

Yen's rural reconstruction paradigm inspired Selskar Gunn of the Rockefeller Foundation, who was greatly impressed by the significance of rural reconstruction as a vehicle for organized, basic, medical and public health advances in China.[50] Gunn reported his observations to the International Health Board of the Rockefeller Foundation, along with his criticism of past programs, and recommended a radical alteration in the foundation's approach to China's health problems. From 1913 to 1933 the Rockefeller Foundation had invested $37 million in medical work in China, an expenditure second only to its investment of $117 million during the same period in health-related fields in the United States. Fully $33 million dollars had been spent to support the Peking Union Medical College, which was transformed into a high caliber medical education, training, and research center.* The enormity of this expenditure can be better understood when compared with the $200 to 300 million roughly estimated as the level of United States government expenditures in China from 1927 to 1937.

In Gunn's report he expressed doubts that PUMC or, for that matter, the foundation's support of graduate and postgraduate medical studies of Chinese in the United States had contributed significantly to public health in China.[51] Indeed he believed that the latter had provided Chinese medical workers with the wrong orientation. Gunn proposed that the foundation should now contribute directly to programs aimed at building a public health base on the economic and social reconstruction of China's rural areas, where unified health programs could be developed at the local level. The outcome of his concern was the formation in 1936 of the North China Council for Rural Reconstruction, whose activities were supported by the Rockefeller Foundation.

Rural reconstruction and its public health aspects succumbed to the Japanese invasion and the Chinese civil war in the same manner as did the government's plans for a national health service. But in light of the subsequent development of public health in the People's Republic of China, the program must be reexamined as a farsighted effort, well ahead of others of the time, to bring public health and medical care into the mainstream of Chinese life. It is remarkable that this program was almost entirely supported by private interests; at most, in 1935–36, the Nationalist government's expenditure for the entire rural sector was well under 4 per cent of the national budget.

In the same period the Chinese Communist Party was also experimenting with public health programs, first in the Kiangsi liberated areas and later in Yenan. Little is known about these early

---

* Editors' Note: All expenditures attributed to the Rockefeller Foundation during this period are approximate.

experiences, save that they were largely organized at local rural levels, involved educational and sanitation programs, and, more importantly, were tied to rural land reform. By the early 1940s the Communists were emphasizing the fostering of community responsibility for hygiene, sanitation, and health programs as part of their ideological campaign.[52] Moreover, some of the enormous energy spent on political and social reconstruction was already being carried over into public health. Cut off by the Kuomintang blockade and by the Japanese from urban areas, modern medical facilities and personnel, and the established public health institutional framework, the CCP experimented with free health services, the amalgamation of traditional and modern systems of medicine, and the education and mobilization of the rural masses for health-related activities.[53] Public health became part of general social change. The local realities of this movement have been vividly described by Hinton and others.[54]

The fledgling medical program in Yenan was aided by a small band of Western physicians who joined Mao Tse-tung and the Eighth Route Army. Most notable were George Hatem (Ma Hai-teh) and Norman Bethune. The former was later to direct the very successful campaign against venereal disease in the PRC.[55] His transformation—from a healer among the whores of Shanghai in the early 1930s to one of the leaders of the public health program that closed the brothels in the PRC and brought venereal disease under control—is a personification of the development of public health work in China.

More than anyone else, however, it was Bethune who became the exemplar of the public health ideal in the PRC. An almost legendary revolutionary, he was a Canadian thoracic surgeon who saw public health in terms of social welfare.[56] Though primarily concerned with aiding the Eighth Route Army in its battles against the invading Japanese Army, via the establishment of forward-area field hospitals, mobile medical units, blood-donor programs, and the surgical treatment of wounds, Bethune also became the medical and public health adviser to some of the liberated areas, where he organized medical teams, sanitation programs, training schools for medical and nursing personnel, the rudiments of a public health structure, and the like. With his Chinese comrades at the front lines, he died in 1939 of septicemia contracted while performing surgery. Almost at once he became a legend, part of a revolutionary ideology that was to have an enormous impact upon China's public health.

Bethune's image is that of a totally dedicated, selfless provider of health care, whose enormous energy and enthusiasm could overcome severe shortages of technological and economic resources. Viewing his professional work as part of a revolutionary social movement that would change the socioeconomic and cultural determinants of illness, Bethune became an ideological model for the Chinese Communists, not only of what revolutionary public health work meant, but of revolutionary efforts in all areas of life. This image represented the special form that public health was to be given in the People's Republic: political enthusiasm and revolutionary fervor to implement mass campaigns against the "four pests," venereal disease, and epidemic and parasitic diseases, and to construct a functioning medical care system for the entire population, rural and urban. [57]

From the birth of the PRC a new direction for public health was suggested: shortly after the new state had come into existence the Central Epidemic Prevention Committee was formed to deal decisively with some of the massive public health problems that followed the long and destructive years of war and sociopolitical crisis. Li Te-ch'uan, for example, who became head of public health in China, had no medical or professional public health background, nor was she a political revolutionary—but she had had considerable experience with social relief. [58] Use would be made of all available scientific and technological inputs into public health, but social welfare, not science, was to be the prime orientation. Public health, now rooted in the new Chinese sociocultural context and its institutions and ideology, would become effective to a degree not believed possible by public health professionals in the 1930s, although it had been anticipated by the advocates of rural reconstruction; moreover, it had assumed a uniquely Chinese form.

Conclusion

Having sketched, in the most general way, an outline of the background to and development of public health in China, it might be valuable to make some broad interpretive comments. Traditional Chinese medical systems were supported by the social and cultural power structure of traditional Chinese society. Even though modern scientific medicine, when introduced during the

nineteenth century, played an important role in China's modernization and thereby helped to transform the social structure, it
failed to tap the traditional sources of cultural power; indeed it
repudiated the sociocultural context of traditional Chinese medicine. On the whole, modern medicine did not succeed very well
during this period.

Among the problems that it faced was an enormous communication barrier that separated two extremely different systems of medical knowledge, values, social forms, and practices—one of which
was alien to and remote from the traditional cultural ethos. This
system was tied to new kinds of sociopolitical and cultural power,
of which gunboats and science were but two intrusive examples.

Modern medical science and, later on, public health entered
China as Western products largely controlled by Western interests.
Only after major social changes had occurred, and the system of
traditional power and interests had been drastically altered, with
modern scientific and Western-oriented sociocultural values replac-
ing traditional Confucian virtues in social importance, did scientific
medicine and public health begin to flourish. They had found new
institutional and ideological supports; they had become significant
in modern China's search for new sources of power and a new
sociocultural, political, and economic order. Public health was
legitimated as an important element in China's modernization, I
would argue, more for these reasons than for its empirical value and
successes, which of course also contributed.

Without fundamental social change it is unlikely that public
health could have succeeded at all. China truly came into possession
of a system of public health only after the "public"—the great
rural mass of impoverished, illiterate, and unhealthy peasants—
had become an important health interest of the system of modern
medical care. The development of a functioning system of public
health for the entire country, and its eventual success in breaking
apart the epidemiological tangle of socioeconomic, cultural, and
major disease problems, required a radical transformation of the
structure of social power in China, as well as a shift in the purposes
and uses of public health.

It should be apparent from this discussion that our understanding of public health in modern China, even prior to the present
era, is still very inadequate. We are in need of an integration of
historical, sociocultural, and epidemiological materials in order to

more fully explore this provocative and very important background. I would again stress that such a fundamental reexamination, although yet to be undertaken in any systematic way, is a prerequisite for our present concern, the foundation for our appreciation of public health in the People's Republic of China. Nor should we fail to note that our subject, with all of its implications for theory, research, and practice, draws us irresistibly into a comparison of medical and public health systems throughout the world, and certainly extends into our own society.

NOTES

1. Contemporary views of culture and the cultural foundation of cognitive and social structures are to be found in the following works: P. Berger and T. Luckman, *The Social Construction of Reality* (New York: Doubleday, 1967); M. Cole, et al., *The Cultural Context of Learning and Thinking* (New York: Basic Books, 1971): pp. 3–25; and A. I. Hallowell, *Culture and Experiences* (New York: Schocken Books, 1967).

2. M. Granet, *La Pensée Chinoise* (Paris: Editions Albin Michel, 1968): pp. 33–53.

3. H. Nakamura, *The Ways of Thinking of Eastern Peoples* (Tokyo: Printing Bureau, Ministry of Finance, 1960): pp. 167–226.

4. H. Maspero, *Melanges posthumes sur les religions et l'histoire de la Chine* (Paris: Presses Universitaires de France, 1967).

5. G. Rowley, *Principles of Chinese Painting* (Princeton: Princeton University Press, 1970).

6. J. Needham, *Science and Civilization in China*, vol. 1 (Cambridge: Cambridge University Press, 1954).

7. P. Huard and M. Wong, *Chinese Medicine* (New York: World University Library, 1968).

8. The comparative study of medicine is discussed and demonstrated in various forms in the following works: C. Leslie, ed., *Toward a Comparative Study of Asian Medical Systems* (Berkeley: University of California Press, 1972); T. Litman and L. Robins, "Comparative Analysis of Health Care Systems—A Sociopolitical Approach." *Social Science Medicine* 5 (1971): 573; F. N. L. Poynter, ed., *Medicine and Culture* (London: Wellcome Institute Publications, 1969); and O. Tempkin, "Comparative Study in the History of Medicine." *Bulletin of the History of Medicine* 42 (1968): 362.

This approach is also discussed in this author's "Toward a Comparative Study of Medical Systems," to be published, and will provide the framework for a conference coordinated by the author, P. Kunstadter, and E. R. Alexander, to be held in the spring of 1973 at the University of Washington, where the focus will be the historical, cultural, and social epidemiological background of Chinese medical systems, as well as other Asian and also African medical systems.

9. R. Shryock, *The Development of Modern Medicine* (New York: Hafner, 1969).

10. T. McKeown, *Medicine in Modern Society* (London: Allen and Unwin, 1965): pp. 39–58; and B. Rosenkrantz, *Medicine and the State* (Cambridge: Harvard University Press, 1972): pp. 1–7.

11. C. Hughes, "Public Health in Non-Literate Societies," in I. Galdston, ed., *Man's Image in Medicine and Anthropology* (New York: International Universities Press, 1963).

12. On the general subject of traditional high-order Chinese medicine see: Huard and Wong, *Chinese Medicine;* Leslie, ed., *Toward a Comparative Study;* Needham and Lu, "Chinese Medicine," in Poynter, ed., *Medicine and Culture;* S. Palos, *The Chinese Art of Healing* (New York: Herder and Herder, 1971); M. Porkert, *Systematic Correspondences in Chinese Medicine* (Cambridge: M.I.T. Press, 1972); N. Sivin, ed., *Chinese Science* (Cambridge: M.I.T. Press, 1972); and I. Veith, "Some Philosophical Concepts of Early Chinese Medicine," *Transactions of the Indian Institute of Culture* 4 (1950).

13. J. Needham, "Poverties and Triumphs of the Chinese Scientific Tradition," in A. Crombie, ed., *Scientific Change* (London: Heinemann, 1963).

14. M. Porkert, *Systematic Correspondences.*

15. J. Wu, "The Paradoxical Situation of Western Philosophy and the Search for Chinese Wisdom," *Inquiry* (Oslo) 14 (1971): 1.

16. W. Cooper and N. Sivin, "Man as a Medicine in Traditional Chinese Medicine," in Sivin, ed., *Chinese Science.*

17. Needham and Lu, "Chinese Medicine," in Poynter, ed., *Medicine and Culture*, p. 257.

18. R. C. Croizier, *Traditional Medicine in Modern China* (Cambridge: Harvard University Press, 1968): pp. 27–28; and J. Needham, "China and the Origin of Qualifying Examinations in Medicine," in J. Needham, *Clerks and Craftsmen in China and the West* (Cambridge: Cambridge University Press, 1970).

19. I. Hsu, "Social Relief during the Sung Dynasty," in E. Sun and J. De Francis, eds., *Bibliography of Chinese Social History* (New Haven: Institute of Far Eastern Languages, Yale University, 1952).

20. See, for example, the description from classical sources of the granary systems in different dynasties, and the account of the severity of some famines and lack of social relief, in T. J. Li, *The Essence of Chinese Civilization* (Princeton: Van Norstrand, 1967): pp. 256–58, and 288–308; and A. Nathan, *A History of the China International Famine Relief Commission* (Cambridge: East Asian Research Center, Harvard University, 1965): p. 2.

21. J. Gernet, *Daily Life in China on the Eve of the Mongol Invasion, 1250–1276* (Stanford: Stanford University Press, 1970): p. 172; and J. Y. Mei, "Public Works and Community Health in Preindustrial China," in *Papers on China from Seminars at Harvard*, vol. 24 (Cambridge: East Asian Research Center, Harvard University, 1971). Mei gives some examples of "medical welfare" in the Sung dynasty, but clearly overemphasizes its extent and effect on community health, about which there is no evidence at all. She also lists some important examples of health-related public works and emphasizes the role of Buddhists in "medical welfare" activities.

22. Needham, "China and the Origin of Qualifying Examinations," in Needham, *Clerks and Craftsmen*, p. 341.

23. Ibid.

24. See, for example, A. J. A. Elliott, *Chinese Spirit-Medium Cults in Singapore* (London: London School of Economics Monographs in Social Anthropology, 1955); B. Gallin, *Hsin Hsing, Taiwan: A Chinese Village in Change* (Berkeley: University of California Press, 1966): pp. 259–66; F. Hsu, *Religion, Science, and Human Crises* (London: Routledge and Paul, 1952); M. Topley, "Chinese Traditional Ideas and the Treatment of Disease: Two Examples from Hong Kong," *Man* 5 (1970): 421; M. Yang, *A Chinese Village: Taitou, Shantung Province* (New York: Columbia University Press, 1965): p. 248.

25. Gernet, *Daily Life in China.*

26. Huard and Wong, *Chinese Medicine.*

27. Hsu, *Religion, Science, and Human Crises.*

28. Cf. F. Dunn, "Traditional Asian Medicine and Cosmopolitan Medicine as Adaptive Systems," in Leslie, ed., *Toward a Comparative Study;* and A. Alland, *Adaptation in Cultural Evolution: An Approach to Medical Anthropology* (New York: Columbia University Press, 1970): p. 41.

29. J. Thomson, *While China Faced West: American Reformers in Nationalist China, 1928–37* (Cambridge: Harvard University Press, 1969): p. 43. A review of some of the historical demographic issues can be found in P. T. Ho, *Studies on the Population of China, 1368–1953* (Cambridge: Harvard University Press, 1959).

30. S. Y. Teng and J. K. Fairbank, *China's Response to the West* (New York: Atheneum, 1963): p. 16.

31. Editorial, *China Medical Missionary Journal* 5 (1891): 137.

32. Jonathan Spence, *To Change China: Western Advisers in China, 1620–1960* (Boston: Little, Brown, 1969): pp. 93–128.

33. "Medical Reports," *Customs Gazette* (Shanghai: Press of the Inspector General of Customs, 1871–83).

34. McKeown, *Medicine in Modern Society.*

35. China Medical Commission of the Rockefeller Foundation, *Medicine in China* (Chicago: University of Chicago Press, 1915).

36. W. McDermott et al., "Health Care Experiment at Many Farms," *Science* 175 (1972): 23.

37. Croizier, *Traditional Medicine,* pp. 59–104.

38. Cf. J. Levenson, *Liang Ch'i-ch'ao and the Mind of Modern China* (Cambridge: Harvard University Press, 1959); and B. Schwartz, *In Search of Wealth and Power: Yen Fu and the West* (Cambridge: Harvard University Press, 1964).

39. C. Nathan, *Plague Prevention and Politics in Manchuria, 1910–31* (Cambridge: Harvard East Asia Monograph, 1967).

40. A Nathan, *A History of the Famine Relief Commission,* pp. 13, 70.

41. S. Garrett, *Social Reformers in Urban China: The Chinese Y.M.C.A., 1895–1926* (Cambridge: Harvard University Press, 1970): pp. 141–48.

42. Thomson, *While China Faced West,* pp. 76–90.

43. Spence, *To Change China,* pp. 161–83.

44. Thomson, *While China Faced West,* pp. 9–17.

45. See, for example, *Proposals of the National Government of the Republic of China for Collaboration with the League of Nations on Health Matters* (Geneva: League of Nations Publications, 1930); *Conference of Far Eastern Countries on Rural Hygiene: Report of China* (Geneva: League of Nations Publications, 1937); and R. Worth,

"Health in Rural China: From Village to Commune," *American Journal of Hygiene* 77 (1963): 228.

46. *Proposals of the National Government.*

47. *Conference of Far Eastern Countries.*

48. Thomson, *While China Faced West*, pp. 122–50.

49. Ibid., p. 117.

50. Ibid., pp. 122–50.

51. Ibid.

52. Mark Selden, *The Yenan Way in Revolutionary China* (Cambridge: Harvard University Press, 1971).

53. Croizier, *Traditional Medicine in Modern China*, pp. 151–57.

54. See, for example, William Hinton, *Fanshen: A Documentary of Revolution in a Chinese Village* (New York: Monthly Review Press, 1966).

55. See Edgar Snow's interview with Dr. George Hatem (Ma Hai-teh) in: E. Snow, *The Other Side of the River* (New York: Random House, 1961).

56. S. Gordon and T. Allen, *The Scalpel, the Sword: The Story of Dr. Norman Bethune* (Boston: Little, Brown, 1952); and Spence, *To Change China*, pp. 216–27.

57. See J. Horn, *Away with all Pests . . . An English Surgeon in People's China* (London: Hamlyn, 1969).

58. D. Klein and A. Clark, *Biographic Dictionary of Chinese Communism, 1921–65* (Cambridge: Harvard University Press, 1971): p. 533.

The History of Public Health
in China to 1937

~
¢

JOHN Z. BOWERS

China was the last great country to accept Western medicine and Western concepts of public health care. It was not until 1910–11 that a devastating epidemic of pneumonic plague in Manchuria, which took 60,000 lives, "laid the foundations for systematic public health in China."[1]

The problems of any underdeveloped country challenged the introduction of public health in China: illiteracy, poverty, a medieval culture, a predominantly rural population, and landlordism. In addition, there were problems specific to China. As the all-powerful Middle Kingdom, China had for centuries scornfully rejected any foreign intercourse. When the Western nations entered China, such wanton acts as the Opium Wars of 1839 to 1842, the Anglo-French seizure of Canton, and the vengeance of the Western powers after the Boxer Rebellion only heightened China's xenophobia. A second problem was the low status of medicine in a country dominated by an abstract Confucian philosophy. A third obstacle was the power and prestige of the indigenous system of medicine. Reverence for the human body made any exploration of human physiology impossible. Due to the use of night-soil as fertilizer, parasitic and enteric diseases were endemic.

Medical Missionaries

The missionary era began when the Jesuits came to the Orient with the Portuguese, who reached Goa in 1511 and made it the seat of their Eastern empire. The Jesuit pioneer, Francis Xavier, the greatest of all missionaries, landed in Kagoshima, Japan, in August 1549. After two frustrating years, but with a mounting affection and respect for the Japanese, Xavier decided to carry Christianity to China, believing that if he succeeded there the

26

Japanese would follow suit. But he died on Shang Ch'uan Island, off the Kwangtung coast, in December 1552, without having reached the mainland.

An Italian Jesuit, Matteo Ricci, who lived in China from 1583 until his death in 1610, was responsible for establishing the Jesuits in Peking as advisors on astronomy, cartography, and mathematics. The first European to prepare a treatise in Chinese on the structure of the human body was a young Swiss Jesuit, Jean Terrenz (also Terrentus, Shreck) who lived in Peking from 1626 to 1630.

Michael Boym, a Polish Jesuit, published the first European work on Chinese botany giving descriptions of plants of medicinal value.[2] He also published the first description for the West of some of the practices of Chinese medicine, in his *Clavis medica ad Chinarum doctrinam de pulsibus.*

As early as A.D. 1000 the Chinese had made efforts to inoculate against smallpox by inserting powdered scabs from patients with the disease into the nostrils of those who had not been afflicted. It was not until 1805 that Alexander Pearson, a surgeon with the East India Company, succeeded in bringing Edward Jenner's vaccination technique to China.

A handful of Protestant medical missionaries from the United Kingdom and the United States came to China in the first half of the nineteenth century, but under the 1842 Treaty of Nanking they were restricted to the five treaty ports of Canton, Amoy, Foochow, Ningpo, and Shanghai, until the Treaty of Tientsin in 1858 made possible an extensive penetration into the empire.

The first medical missionary was Robert Morison from St. Bartholomew's Hospital Medical School in London, who reached Canton on September 4, 1807. His main interests were the salvation of the heathen and the translation of the Bible.

John Livingstone, a surgeon, was the first fully-qualified doctor to practice Western medicine in China when he opened a dispensary in Macao in 1820.

The high incidence of blindness—trachoma, ophthalmia, xerophthalmia, and opacities from smallpox—led to an emphasis on eye diseases by the early doctors.

The most famous medical missionary was the legendary Peter Parker, who had studied medicine and attended lectures in theology at Yale where he was awarded the M.D. degree in 1834. On November 4, 1835, Parker opened the Canton Ophthalmic Hospital at 7 Green Pea Street, better known as "Hog Lane" because of its opium dens, grog shops, and brothels. He performed cataract surgery, principally couching, on scores of patients every day and was the first to train Chinese youths as dispensers and dressers.

In 1838 Parker and Thomas Colledge, a British surgeon, founded the Canton Medical Missionary Society, the first such organization in China. Among its aims were the education of Chinese youths in Western medicine and the promotion of Western medicine among the Chinese. The first significant effort to train Chinese in Western medicine was not launched until 1863, however, when John Glasgow Kerr, who had succeeded Parker in Canton, established a three-year program to train medical apprentices.

The earliest formal program in medical education was established in Tientsin in 1881 by a Scot, John K. MacKenzie. Subsequently other missionary medical schools were established with small classes of up to ten students, and programs based on lectures and demonstrations in Mandarin. Public health education consisted at best of a few lectures in sanitation and hygiene. A survey by James B. Neal in Tsinan in 1897 showed that there were thirty-nine such programs with a total of 462 students and graduates.[3]

As for public health data, Wong and Wu state that in Shanghai "certain death and burial records were kept as far back as 1850," and that "a so-called Nuisance Department was started in the late fifties under a Sanitary Inspector. Its main functions appear to have been scavenging and refuse disposal."[4]

The pioneering research relating to public health in China was carried out by Sir Patrick Manson, the father of tropical medicine. After graduating in medicine in Scotland, Manson had come to China with the Imperial Maritime Customs Service in 1866 and had worked in Formosa and Amoy. In 1879 he demonstrated the nocturnal periodicity of the microfilariae of *Wucheria bancrofti*, and in 1878 proved that microfilaria infected *Culex fatigans* and then underwent development in the mosquito.

After a furlough in England, Manson served for three years as dean of the Hong Kong College of Medicine for Chinese which opened in October 1887. He returned to London in 1890. In 1912 the college of medicine was merged with the newly founded University of Hong Kong and became its Faculty of Medicine.

The Boxer Rebellion in 1900, in which more than 100 Protestant missionaries were slain, focused the eyes of the foreign missionary societies on Peking, the seat of the uprising, as the critical center for their programs. The societies were persuaded that their splintered efforts should be concentrated on denominational mergers for the establishment of carefully selected "union" medical colleges. The first Union Medical College was opened in Peking in 1906 under the sponsorship of three British and three American societies. Other "union" schools developed in Tsinan, Moukden, Hankow, Nanking, Hangchow, Foochow, Canton, and Chengtu.

Three programs in medical education were established under the sponsorship of American universities, the most renowned of which, Yale-in-China, opened in 1908 in Changsha in Hunan Province. It became a cooperative program between the Yale Foreign Missionary Society and the government of Hunan, known as Hsiang-ya—*Hsiang*, the literary name for Hunan, and *ya* from *Yali*, as Yale was termed by the Chinese. Beginning in 1916, however, xenophobic warlords stirred the students to confrontations and the school was closed in 1927.

The Harvard Medical School of China was opened in Shanghai in March 1912. The states of California, Oregon, and Washington were sources of its financial support on the basis that the advancement of public health in the great port city of Shanghai would prevent the transmission of deadly epidemic diseases to the West Coast. (There were 113 deaths from plague in San Francisco between 1900 and 1904, and seventy-eight deaths between 1907 and 1909.) The school was closed in 1917.

A third and more limited effort was that of the Christian Association of the University of Pennsylvania in Canton, and subsequently in Shanghai.

Chinese Foundation for the Promotion of Education and Culture

A far-sighted American beneficance following the Boxer Rebellion gave an important stimulus to the advancement of medicine and public health in China. The original indemnity due the United States as a result of the Boxer Rebellion was $53,348,000, but in 1908 the Congress authorized President Theodore Roosevelt to reduce the bond to $13,655,192 and to remit the balance in favor of China. (The remainder of the indemnity money was remitted in 1924.) With the indemnity funds the Chinese government established scholarships for the education of Chinese youths in American colleges and universities, with special emphasis on science, including medicine, and technology. In 1911, as part of this program, Tsinghua College was founded in Peking as a junior college to prepare students for study in the United States. It later became a full-fledged university. The Chinese Foundation for the Promotion of Education and Culture was established to receive and administer the funds.

Pneumonic Plague

In 1910 Manchuria was China's greatest frontier. Migrant laborers in numbers estimated to be up to 100,000, about 10,000 of whom were amateur trappers, flooded railway boom towns. They were after marmot, *han-t'a*, a woodchuck-like rodent popular as imitation sable and marten in European markets. The marmot was known to be infected with plague, and experienced trappers avoided animals that were sick. The amateur trappers, however, saved every salable animal caught in their traps, and it was only a matter of time until human disease erupted. The first case appeared on October 13, 1910, when a migrant trapper in Manchouli died of pneumonic plague after an illness of three days. The disease spread rapidly, and by January 12, 1911, it had moved as far south as Peking. When the epidemic subsided in March the death toll stood at 60,000.

Meanwhile, the Russians and Japanese, who held extensive railway operations and other interests in Manchuria, threatened to impose by force if necessary their own plague control programs if the Chinese failed to do so. Saoke Alfred Sze (Shih Shao-chi), a graduate of Cornell University, who was counselor and second vice-president in the Ministry of Foreign Affairs in Peking, was instrumental in the organization of a Western-trained Chinese medical team for plague control.* The leader of the team was a Malay Chinese, Wu Lien-teh, who had been born in Penang in 1879 and who had studied medicine at Emmanuel College, Cambridge, and St. Mary's Hospital Medical School in London. Subsequently Wu carried out bacteriological studies at the Institute for Medical Research in Kuala Lumpur. He was serving as vice-director of the Imperial Army Medical College in Tientsin when he was sum-

---

* Alfred Sze was later Chinese ambassador to the Court of St. James and to the United States.

moned to Peking by Alfred Sze in December 1910 and designated
director of the plague-control team.

Wu combined the qualities that were essential for such a mission
—intelligence, a driving capacity for hard work, and supreme self-
confidence. In April 1911 he convened an international plague
conference in Moukden, the first international medical conference
in Chinese history, with delegates from Russia, Austria-Hungary,
the Netherlands, Japan, the United States, Britain, Italy, Mexico,
France, and Germany, including such distinguished bacteriolo-
gists as Shibasaburo Kitasato of Japan, Paul B. Haffkine of Germany, and Richard Strong of the United States.

The most important result of the conference was the recommendation that the Manchurian Plague Prevention Service be established; this was accomplished in October 1912, "the first important native-government regional medical service in Chinese
history run according to principles called 'modern' in the West."[5]*
The director and chief medical officer of the new service was Wu
Lien-teh, who recalled the goals of the program in his autobiography: "It was hoped that such a service might develop into a public
health service for the entire province, and set an example for the
whole of China."[6]

With headquarters in Fuchiatien, the Chinese section of Harbin,
the service operated a farflung network of up to seven hospitals for
the isolation of plague and other communicable disease cases and
for the care of the indigent sick. It conducted programs in health
education, with an emphasis on prevention, and a training school
for paramedical personnel, including dressers, dispensers, and sanitary inspectors. At Fuchiatien there were laboratories for the production of serum and vaccines for plague, cholera, rabies, typhoid,
and scarlet fever, as well as research programs in microbiology.

Vigilance in epidemics was a continuing responsibility: against
cholera in 1919 and 1926; pneumonic plague in 1920–21; and
bubonic plague in 1928–30. In addition to its specific work in the
control of epidemics, the service brought China into active participation in international programs in public health under the auspices of the League of Nations. The dream of the evolution of a
public health service for all of north China was thwarted, however,

---

* Carl F. Nathan, later a medical student at Harvard, prepared an excellent monograph, *Plague Prevention and Politics in Manchuria, 1910–1931*, for his senior honors thesis
at Harvard College.

primarily because of a lack of funds. The Manchurian Plague Prevention Service finally became a casualty of wars—between China and Russia in 1931, and by the Japanese invasion of Manchuria in 1932. But it did establish the importance of public health as a national responsibility, and trained a small cadre of physicians and allied personnel for work in public health in China.

Peking Union Medical College

Medicine in China was a continuing interest of John D. Rockefeller, stimulated in part by his advisor on philanthropy, Frederick T. Gates. In 1909 Rockefeller financed the Oriental Education Commission to study the possibility of establishing programs of higher education in China. Although the commission's report was negative, Gates's interest continued, and when the Rockefeller Foundation was established in the spring of 1913 the advancement of medicine in China became its first program. The First China Medical Commission, representing the foundation, visited China in the spring and summer of 1914 to explore possibilities for a program. Its members included Harry P. Judson, president of the University of Chicago; Francis W. Peabody, professor of medicine at Harvard; and Roger S. Greene, United States consul general in Hankow, whose brother, Jerome D. Greene, was secretary of the foundation.

The principal recommendation was that the foundation should establish a program in medical education in China and that Peking be selected as the place for a Rockefeller-supported medical school. Peking was chosen because it had been the capital continuously since the thirteenth century; it was the educational and cultural center of the country; and it was the site of the best medical school in the country—the Union Medical College. The commission also recommended that medical instruction should be at a standard equal to the best in America or Europe. A second medical school was proposed for Shanghai. Other recommendations included programs in nursing education and postgraduate fellowships for both Chinese and missionary doctors. On November 30, 1914, the trustees of the Rockefeller Foundation voted to implement a program in medicine in China. On July 1, 1915, the China Medical Board (CMB) assumed responsibility for the Union Medical College at a purchase price of $200,000.

The importance of a strong program in public health at Peking

Union Medical College (PUMC) was bolstered when William Welch and Simon Flexner joined Wallace Buttrick, director of the CMB, on the Second China Medical Commission, which visited China in the fall of 1915, for at that time Welch and Flexner were working with Wickliffe Rose, director of the International Health Commission (later the International Health Board) of the Rockefeller Foundation, on a new program to establish schools of public health.* They were completely persuaded of the importance of educating doctors in hygiene and public health and saw this as a major role for PUMC, especially in the prevention and control of communicable diseases.

Welch and Flexner recommended that it would probably be necessary for PUMC to open its own premedical school until premedical education in other selected institutions was upgraded. The Premedical School opened in 1917; the first medical students were enrolled in 1919; and the first graduation ceremonies—for three medical students and one nursing student—were held in June 1924.

The PUMC Nursing School

While plans for a program in medical education were developing, a decision was made to establish a nursing school at PUMC. At that time the care of the sick was exclusively in the hands of a small number of male nurses who were trained in missionary hospitals. Female patients were cared for by the family or by an untrained *amah;* for a woman to handle the body of a male in nursing duties was unthinkable. The nursing school was to meet the same standard of excellence as that of the medical school and to have classes of no more than twenty-five students. Further, the emphasis was to be on education rather than on service, in contrast to practically all United States nursing schools. The first students were enrolled on September 28, 1920. The contributions of PUMC in elevating nursing to a respected position in China were as important as its contributions to medical education.

Education in Public Health

W. W. Peter, secretary of the Council on Health Education in China, began to develop programs in health education for laymen

---

* The first school of public health in the United States was opened at Johns Hopkins in 1918. Subsequent grants totalling over $25 million supported the establishment of schools around the world, including one at Ann Arbor, Michigan.

in Shanghai in 1914. The first significant educational programs in public health in a medical school were established at PUMC by John B. Grant, whose programs were highly innovative and stand as landmarks, not only in China but throughout the Western world.

Grant was born at his father's missionary hospital in Ningpo in 1890. Of Canadian descent, he graduated from Acadia College in Nova Scotia and studied medicine at the University of Michigan. Guided toward public health, in part by his professor at Michigan, Victor C. Vaughan, Grant took graduate work at the new School of Hygiene and Public Health at Johns Hopkins and then joined the International Health Board (IHB) of the Rockefeller Foundation. In 1921 he was assigned to establish a program in public health at PUMC and to represent the IHB in the Far East.

Grant was at least twenty-five years ahead of his time in the public health programs that he launched at PUMC. Today most American medical schools are only beginning to emulate Grant's community-based programs.

At Grant's death in 1962, the Medical Care Section of the American Public Health Association adopted a memorial that read:

> Throughout his long career he has been a towering figure of vision, strength, statesmanship, and leadership in the endless struggle to improve the welfare of mankind through the provision and modernization of health services—in China, India, Europe, the Americas—indeed, the whole world.[7]

When Grant arrived in Peking in 1921 he soon learned that there was essentially no public health base on which to build a program. A so-called public health administration had been established in Canton one year earlier, and Frank Oldt was lecturing on the control of trachoma and hookworm at the Canton Hospital. The impact of the Manchurian Plague Prevention Service was circumscribed. Otherwise the most populous country in the world had no national or municipal public health service. Thus Grant soon found himself in a leadership role in the task of building a national public health service. At the same time he needed to establish strong educational and research ties with PUMC.

While his colleagues on the faculty centered their programs around hospital patients, Grant chose the community. He had no intention of emulating the teaching of public health in the Max von Pettenkofer tradition, with lectures and demonstrations on hygiene and communicable disease control, and only occasional field trips. For Grant the paramount need was to move education in public health out of the medical school and into the community, which would serve as his clinic, his classroom, and his research laboratory.

In 1923 he made an extensive study-tour of China for a first-hand look at existing programs in twelve of the eighteen provinces. Grant judged that while the Manchurian Plague Prevention Service and the Central Epidemic Prevention Bureau, which had been established in Peking in 1919, had potential as health services, he found it difficult to give a succinct account of the state of public health in China. He felt, however, that the work of the National Health Association and of the Council on Health Education had made an impact:

> The birth of a community health conscience has occurred, for there is not a fair sized community visited in a recent tour of twelve of the eighteen provinces which does not possess a group of individuals in various stages of groping toward health efforts. [8]

Grant decided that the initial thrust of his program should be in school hygiene and the establishment of health centers, but he predicted that a tangible advance in public health would take at least ten years. The need for public health services was not recognized by the Chinese bureaucracy—the minimal efforts at sanitation in Peking were relegated to the police department.

In early 1925 Grant persuaded the Peking municipality to join the college in establishing an experimental health station as an educational center in the city—probably the first community center for public health education in any country. The salient points in the cooperative arrangement called for PUMC to contribute 60 per cent, and the city 40 per cent, of the budget; the Department of Public Health at PUMC would nominate the director of the program.

Grant outlined two principal functions for the Peking Special Health Station: to teach preventive medicine and public health to medical and nursing undergraduates and to auxiliaries, and to cooperate with local agencies in demonstration programs in community health practices. Other programs were to include epidemiological investigations and the adaptation of modern public health practices to local conditions. At the beginning there were four divisions: medical services, general sanitation, vital statistics, and communicable diseases; the latter two were subsequently combined. When the full staff had been assembled it included the director and five other physicians, seventeen nurses and nurse midwives, one dental hygienist, one pharmacist, three sanitary inspectors, one secretary, and three clerks.

A study made by the Special Health Station revealed its district to be a true microcosm of the paucity of medical and public health services in urban China. Of the first 1,000 deaths investigated by the staff, 36 per cent had received no medical care whatsoever, and 48 per cent had been treated exclusively by native practitioners; only 16 per cent could be described as having been treated with modern medicine.

The program in maternal and child health was led by a remarkable woman, Marian Yang. A survey of maternal and infant mortality in the special health area gave further evidence of China's problems in public health: the maternal mortality rate was 17.6:1,000 population compared with 3:1,000 in England, 4 in Japan, and 5 in the United States. The infant mortality was 275:1,000 compared with fewer than 75:1,000 in both the United States and England. The principal cause of maternal mortality was puerperal infection; of infant mortality, tetanus neonatorum.

While there were only 500 trained midwives in China, there were estimated to be at least 200,000 untrained midwives. The practices of the untrained women were appalling. The cord was severed with any sharp tool they could find lying about, or, if none were available, with their teeth; to arrest bleeding, the stump of the cord was then covered with dirt, or compressed with a filthy rag. If a woman had difficulty in delivering the baby, as in the deformed pelvis of osteomalacia, the midwife would insert hooks or charcoal tongs into the vagina in an effort to exert traction on the fetus.

The first need, then, in attacking the shockingly high infant and maternal mortality rates, was to train midwives. In 1929 Marian Yang opened the first modern school of midwifery, the North China School of Midwives, under the auspices of the Peking municipal government, in collaboration with the Special Health Station. Here she trained nurses from PUMC in midwifery, and also established special courses to teach untrained midwives sterile procedures and sanitary practices. Upon completion of her training, each midwife was given a basket containing the necessary instruments, medicines, and dressings to enable them to apply the principles and practices they had been taught at the school.

Grant knew that another giant step in public health could be achieved by bringing forth a generation of young people who would understand and adopt the best hygienic and sanitary practices. A school health program emphasizing personal hygiene and health education therefore became a major activity of the Special Health Station. One-third of the 4,000 school children in the area served by the station were examined in the first year the station was opened, and preventive inoculations were given. The most frequent disease diagnosed was trachoma. Other activities included school nursing services, health education, and the establishment of a high level of sanitation through frequent inspections and corrective measures.

The Ministry of Health was established in 1929 by the new Nationalist government and it drew heavily on the personnel of the Special Health Station and PUMC alumni to staff its programs. In the same year the vice-minister of health stated that the importance of the Special Health Station in the development of public health could "hardly be over-estimated." [9]

The Special Health Station was also the base for public health training in the curriculum of the School of Nursing. Each student spent one month working full-time in school health, maternal and child health, and industrial health, and as a visiting nurse.

Twenty-five per cent of the PUMC graduates in both medicine and nursing entered careers in public health through the influence of John Grant and the Special Health Station. With the fall of the Nationalist government in 1949 a number of PUMC graduates moved to Taiwan where they became leaders in developing excellent public health services on the island. Others entered careers in international health and in teaching public health.

Grant's commitment to the team approach in development programs drew his interest in the early thirties to the National Association of the Mass Education Movement, which had been established in 1923 by James Y. C. Yen (Yen Yang-ch'u), a graduate of Yale University who had become stimulated by his work with the Chinese Labor Battalion in World War I. By 1929 the four-fold program of the Mass Education Movement had focused on culture, economics, politics, and public health in the rural districts. Yen opened a rural medical demonstration unit at Ting Hsien, the center of the movement, about 100 miles southwest of Peking, where it pioneered in a community development program based on advanced concepts and practices in medicine and public health education, sociology, and agriculture. The unit at Ting Hsien was also used as a teaching center for PUMC.*

In 1936 Grant left PUMC to devote his full energies to the work of the North China Council for Rural Reconstruction, which was supported by the Rockefeller Foundation.

After the Sino-Japanese War erupted in 1937 all PUMC programs were increasingly compromised; the college was seized by the Japanese on December 8, 1941, and the programs in medical education terminated. The nursing faculty and students made a heroic migration to West China Union University in Chengtu, and the nursing program continued during the war years.

Reopened in October 1947, PUMC was nationalized by the Communist government on January 23, 1951.

Parasitology

Since 1866, when Patrick Manson arrived in China, the country had been of unusual interest to students of parasitology and tropical medicine. The factors contributing to the high incidence of parasitic infection included pollution of food and water with human feces; the ingestion of raw food, especially fish; and unsanitary personal habits, particularly promiscuous defecation. One of the first applicants for an appointment to the faculty at PUMC in 1919 was a young parasitologist, Ernest Carroll Faust. Faust earned his Ph.D. at the University of Illinois, where he taught parasitology from 1912 to 1919. Primarily through his work at Peking, Faust became the great pioneer of American parasitology, in a mold comparable to that of Manson for British science.

In 1920 Faust and his colleagues undertook a series of comprehensive surveys and studies of parasitic diseases in north, central, and south China. Their subjects included healthy and hospitalized humans, as well as mammals, birds, amphibia, fish, molluscs, and arthropods. The numerous reports that flowed from these studies

---

* Other efforts in rural reconstruction, such as the program of the National Council of Churches, followed the comprehensive approach first established by James Yen.

stand today as signal contributions, not only to our information on diseases of China but to our general knowledge of parasitology.

Faust listed malaria, amebiasis, and kala-azar as the most important protozoan diseases; the leading helminthic diseases were oriental schistosomiasis, clonorchiasis, fasciolopsiasis, hookworm, and filariasis.

Schistosomiasis

Fifty years after he had initiated his studies in Peking, and at the twilight of his brilliant career, Faust looked back to the studies he had made with Henry E. Meleney on *Schistosoma japonicum* as his most important research contribution.

The studies were collected in a massive monograph in 1924, and in his prefatory note Faust cited Meleney as the first scientist to identify the molluscan host, *Oncomelania hupensis*.[10] Further research showed it to be the intermediate host throughout the vast Yangtze flood area in central China. The schistosomiasis problem in 1924 was of such magnitude that 100 million people were endangered by the disease.

Faust and Meleny reported the first detailed information on the morphology, biology, and life history of *Schistosoma japonicum*. In dogs that had been experimentally infected, eggs appeared in the feces as early as twenty-nine days after infection.

The route of the infected larvae, cercariae, from the skin to the lungs was known to be by way of the lymphatics. The principal manifestations of the disease, however, consisted of involvement of the liver and the intestinal tract; the route from the lungs to the abdominal viscera was not known. Faust and Meleney showed that after the cercariae reach the lungs they enter the pulmonary veins, pass to the arterial circulation, and are then deposited in the gastrointestinal capillaries and the portal veins. The blood of patients with schistosomiasis was found to have a high serum-globulin level that could be used in screening for the disease and in specific diagnosis.

While molluscicides and other measures were proving effective in controlling *Schistosoma japonicum* in Japan, Faust and Meleney recognized that such relatively advanced approaches would not be practicable in China because of the vastness of the problem. Instead they recommended a three-pronged, more fundamental approach—

control of feces disposal; avoidance of wading in ponds and other freshwater areas; and intensive therapy for proven cases.

Clonorchiasis

Clonorchiasis, caused by the Chinese or Oriental liver fluke, *Clonorchis sinensis* (Cobbold), was the "most important of the fluke infections in China" because of its high incidence in dogs, horses, cats, and other mammals.[11] The incidence of the disease in humans was confined almost exclusively to Kwangtung and Swatow in south China, where it was widely prevalent. For example, 50 per cent of the sailors from south China who were imprisoned in Hamburg by the Germans in World War I showed *Clonorchis sinensis* eggs in their stools, as did a group of Chinese who were examined while in quarantine at San Francisco at about the same time. On the other hand, the prevalence of human infection in north China was less than 1 per cent, although nearly one-third of the dogs and cats in the north were infected.

The principal studies on clonorchiasis were carried out by Faust and a young Chinese graduate of the Faculty of Medicine at Edinburgh, Khaw Oo-kek, who joined the faculty of PUMC in 1925. Faust and Khaw showed that almost every freshwater fish in south China was capable of serving as the second intermediate host. Raw fish was a popular delicacy in the south, and the fish, heavily contaminated with *Clonorchis*, usually came from commercial ponds that had been fertilized with human feces. Thus the problems in controlling the disease were enormous. Faust and Khaw recommended the avoidance of native dishes and of raw fish as the best means of prevention.

Fasciolopsiasis

Fasciolopsis buski, a giant liver fluke found in central and south China as far north as the Yangtze valley, had a specially high frequency in Chekiang and Kwangtung, two coastal provinces south of Shanghai. Faust estimated that 5 per cent of the population in these provinces had the fluke, although only a small percentage showed symptoms. While the hog was the most frequent reservoir, Faust found the dogs also to be an important source. With guidance from Faust, C. H. Barlow and Claude Henon worked out the life cycle of *Fasciolopsis buski*. After passage from a hog, man, or dog, it enters a snail which then encysts on a variety of aquatic plants, especially water chestnuts, water bamboo, and the water caltrop (*Trapa natans*). In humans the parasites usually attach to the mucous membrane of the duodenum or jejunum where they produce inflammation, ulceration, and abscess formation. The infection responds promptly to hexylresorcinol, tetrachlorethylene, or stilbazium oxide.

Kala-azar

Visceral leishmaniasis, also known as kala-azar, was primarily a disease of children and adolescents in north China. Charles W. Young, who was in charge of the Kala-azar Field Studies Unit at PUMC, showed that the disease was confined to the region north of the Yangtze, and Faust suggested that it had been introduced by way of the northwest trade routes. Young found that 70 per cent of the cases were in persons under twenty years of age.[12]

The Leishman-Donovan bodies could be most readily demonstrated through smears and cultures taken from punctures of the greatly enlarged spleen; similar preparations from the peripheral blood were less frequently diagnostic. Splenic puncture was a dangerous procedure, however, because of the possibility of bleeding from the tense and congested organ; sternal puncture therefore became the preferred method.

Another approach to the diagnosis of kala-azar came from the studies of Sia Ho-p'ing (Richard), of the Department of Medicine, and Wu Hsien, head of biochemistry, at PUMC. They showed that the striking increase in blood globulin levels could be applied as a diagnostic procedure through existing precipitation-flocculation tests, especially Ray's hemolysis test; positive reactions were also elicited in malaria, tuberculosis, schistosomiasis, and trypanosomiasis. In addition, Sia and Wu found a marked increase in the total serum protein in active cases of kala-azar.

The ability to reproduce a human disease in an experimental animal is an important research tool, especially in studies of pathogenesis and treatment. In 1924, Young and Jocelyn Smyly demonstrated that kala-azar could be reproduced in both the striped hamster, *Cricetulus griseus*, and the giant hamster, *C. triton*. Henry Meleney then undertook a series of studies on the histopathology of kala-azar in the hamster. He found that the fundamental and specific tissue reaction is the production of a large mononuclear phagocytic cell, variously known as a clasmatocyte, an endothelial leukocyte, or a macrophage.

James R. Cash, who was appointed head of pathology at PUMC

in 1924, and Hu Cheng-hsiang identified large concentrations of Leishman-Donovan bodies in the pigmented, granulomatous patches that develop in the skin and subcutaneous tissues of hamsters. They suggested that the disease might be transmitted through these infected lesions. Later, Claude Forkner of the Department of Medicine and Samuel Zia of bacteriology collaborated in a study that isolated the causative organism from nasal secretions and from the tonsils, and proposed that the disease could also be transmitted through droplets from the mouth or nose.

Amebiasis

In 1924 John F. Kessel, associate in parasitology at PUMC, made a survey of amebic disease in China. Although both amebic dysentery and liver abscesses could be found throughout the country, there were regional differences, with a high incidence in the central Yangtze valley and in Wuchang Province. Kessel and Faust found that in tropical and semitropical south China, clinical disease with acute dysentery or abscess was more frequent, while in the north there was a higher proportion of carriers. They were also impressed with the relatively high incidence of amebic disease in foreigners, whose resistance did not approach that of the Chinese.

The remarkable tolerance of the human tissues to *Entamoeba histolytica* was demonstrated by Faust's finding that although 50 per cent of the patients in one mission hospital had *Entamoeba histolytica* in their stools, only 15 per cent had dysentery. Similar studies by other investigators showed that such symptomless carriers may discharge 35 million parasites daily. But the problem in controlling the disease was demonstrated by the fact that 35 per cent of the individuals harboring the ameba had no clinical manifestation and thus could disseminate the parasite uncontrollably.

Hookworm

The massive hookworm problems in China attracted the attention of the International Health Board of the Rockefeller Foundation, which was studying the disease on a worldwide basis. In 1923 and again in 1924 the foundation sent out the China Hookworm Commission led by William W. Cort of the Johns Hopkins School of Hygiene and Public Health who had studied hookworm in the West Indies for the board. The commission was organized as a joint study by the foundation and PUMC, with John Grant representing the medical college; the report of their studies was published in 1926.[13]

The commission found that hookworm was as massive a challenge in central and south China as it was in India. The central issue was the ancient, organized system of soil pollution and fertilization with human feces in the rural areas. While stool examinations in Peking showed that as high as 28 per cent of the specimens contained the parasite, clinical disease seldom occurred because of the relatively rigorous nature of the climate. Hookworm flourished in more tropical climates lying between 36° north latitude and 30° south latitude.

The commission found the incidence of hookworm disease to be especially high among the millions of adults and children engaged in sericulture. Human feces was the prime fertilizer for the mulberry trees whose leaves were used to feed the silkworms, and the hookworm larvae easily pierced the skin of the barefooted, barelegged workers harvesting the leaves during the rainy season. On the other hand, hookworm did not represent a hazard for the millions who toiled in the rice paddies, although they too were exposed to night soil, because as soon as the rice fields had been fertilized they were flooded, and the eggs could not develop when covered with water.

Because of the dimensions of the hookworm problem in sericulture, the commission realized that they were up against an almost insoluble challenge. The use of human feces for fertilization was an economic necessity—more than 24 million tons were used each year; it was an essential part of the Chinese culture that could not be abandoned. Beyond identifying the unique nature of the problem, and urging adequate therapy for proven cases, there was little else the Cort Commission could recommend.

Malaria

In 1926 Faust reported that malaria was found throughout south and central China—from the extreme south to as far north as Peking, and from the east coast to the western boundary of Szechuan Province; it was most severe in the south and progressively less so toward the north. There were major areas where the prevalence of malaria was as high as 90–100 per cent.

Although in 1926 blackwater fever was virtually unknown, it later became a problem in Peking, particularly among opium addicts; highly virulent strains of the parasite were passed from addict to addict through hypodermic needles.

National Reconstruction: League of Nations

The advancement of public health as a part of the national reconstruction movement in China, through a cooperative effort with the Nationalist government, was a major interest of the League of Nations. In 1933 the great Yugoslav public health leader, Andrija Stampar, came to Shanghai as the expert representative of the League of Nations, to be "at the disposal of the Chinese government in connection with the plan of technical co-operation with the League of Nations in national reconstruction."[14] Stampar spent three years in China, visiting provinces throughout the country and cooperating with J. Heng Liu and James Yen in developing an integrated public health program through a National Economic Council, with land reform as its primary objective. Stampar's major recommendation on public health was the establishment of a network of health centers with programs in school health, control of epidemics, and dispensary services.

In 1936 Stampar prepared an extensive report on the status of the land reform program, which he found had made relatively little progress. He was especially concerned that because of social grievances, including exploitation by landlords, the peasants who represented 90 per cent of the population would ignore public health programs. In conclusion he appraises some of the problems of public health:

> Successful health work is not possible where the standard of living falls below the level of tolerable existence. . . . The prevalence of most diseases is due to bad water supply, unhygienic housing conditions, ignorance, and poverty of the population. Public health policy must be intimately connected with a programme for general social improvement. Education is important, since, unless the farmer can read pamphlets, and is given a rudimentary scientific attitude, it is very difficult to reach him by propaganda.[15]

The programs to improve public health in China were dependent to a large degree upon a stable nation. The ascendancy of the Kuomintang in 1928 had given promise of the development of a national unification that would make a comprehensive nationwide public health program possible. But in 1937, when the efforts of

J. Heng Liu, James Yen, John Grant, and Andrija Stampar might have begun to produce enduring results, the full-scale war between Japan and China erupted, beginning with the Marco Polo Bridge incident outside Peking on July 7.

With the conclusion of hostilities in 1945, China was soon involved in the conflict between the Nationalists and the Communists which culminated in the surrender of the Nationalists in 1949.

Thus we can designate 1937 as the year when the history of public health in China entered a phase in which progress was largely replaced by major hostilities that continued until 1950.

NOTES

1. Wong K. Chimin and Wu Lien-teh, *History of Chinese Medicine: Being a Chronicle of Medical Happenings in China from Ancient Times to the Present Period* (Tientsin: Tientsin Press, 1932).

2. Michael Boym, S.J., *Flora Sinensis, ou Traité des fleurs, des fruits, des plantes et des animaux particuliers de la Chine* (Vienna, 1656).

3. Wong and Wu, *History of Chinese Medicine*.

4. Ibid.

5. Carl F. Nathan, *Plague Prevention and Politics in Manchuria, 1910–1931* (Cambridge: Harvard East Asia Monograph, 1967): p. 5.

6. Wu Lien-teh, *Plague Fighter: Autobiography of a Chinese Physician* (Cambridge, England: W. Heffer, 1959): p. 376.

7. Conrad Seipp, ed., *Health Care for the Community: Selected Papers of Dr. John Grant*, American Journal of Hygiene Monographic Series No. 21 (Baltimore: Johns Hopkins Press, 1963): p. vii.

8. PUMC Weekly Newsletter, May 1, 1923.

9. Mary E. Ferguson, *China Medical Board and Peking Union Medical College: A Chronicle of Fruitful Collaboration, 1914–1951* (New York: China Medical Board of New York, 1970): p. 58.

10. Ernest Carroll Faust and Henry E. Meleney, *Studies on Schistosomiasis Japonica, With a Supplement on the Molluscan Hosts of the Human Blood Fluke in China and Japan, and Species Liable to Be Confused with Them, by Nelson Annandale*, American Journal of Hygiene Monographic Series No. 3 (Baltimore: Johns Hopkins Press, 1924): p. iii.

11. E. C. Faust, "Parasitic Infections and Human Disease in China," *Archives of Pathology and Laboratory Medicine* 2 (1926): 223–40.

12. C. W. Young, "Kala-azar in China," *Chinese Medical Journal* 37, no. 10 (October 1923): 797–822.

13. W. W. Cort, J. B. Grant, and N. R. Stoll, *Researches on Hookworm in China*, American Journal of Hygiene Monograph Series No. 7 (Baltimore: Johns Hopkins Press, October 1926).

14. M. D. Grmek, ed., *Serving the Cause of Public Health: Selected Papers of Andrija Stampar* (Zagreb, 1966): p. 37.

15. Andrija Stampar, "Health and Social Conditions in China," *Bulletin of League of Nations* 5 (1936): 1091–1126.

II. Organization of Public Health Services: Policy and Strategy

Introductory Note

An often-stated goal of nearly all less-developed countries (LDCs) is the development of an adequate, integrated program of preventive and curative health in both rural and urban areas. What is compelling about China is that the hope of realizing this goal may not be as illusory as it is in many other comparable countries. In this section, Ezra F. Vogel and Peter S. Heller focus on key elements of China's strategy in the health sector. Dr. Vogel, a sociologist at Harvard University, presents an overview of the reorganization of the Chinese medical system after 1949. Dr. Heller, an economist at the University of Michigan, examines China's strategy for the delivery of preventive and curative health services.

To attain this goal, an effective health strategy must overcome several bottlenecks endemic to many countries; specifically: (1) shortages of financial and skilled manpower resources; (2) the absence of viable technological and organizational alternatives to the conventional systems of medical care delivery observed in most Western countries; (3) the absence of an organizational structure through which to implement a health sector policy; and (4) the powerful political resistance to any meaningful rectification of the imbalance in medical facilities between the urban and rural areas. In the evolution of China's health system one can observe attempts to overcome each of these obstacles.

First, shortages of both medical manpower and financial resources often prove to be limiting factors to the establishment of an extended curative health system. The Chinese attacked these shortages by the innovative use of existing medical technology required to treat specific health problems, and by an expansion in the training programs for different categories of medical personnel. Key to the former was the integration of the traditional and modern medical systems. The rural population in particular has considerable confidence in traditional practices when they are complemented by a referral or combined system that does not attempt the management of illnesses through Western medical technology alone.

Concomitant with a sharp expansion in enrollments, training programs for modern medical personnel have been shortened and their content focused on the essential elements of a medical education. The curriculum is sensitive to the medical needs of the rural areas and the problems of prevention and treatment in a rural environment. In order to provide a first level of low-cost curative and preventive care, training programs for new categories of paramedical manpower such as "barefoot doctors" have recently been begun. This should sharply increase the curative system's capacity in the rural areas.

Second, to compensate for the lack of ordinary systems for delivery of curative care, beginning as far back as 1950 the Chinese began devoting considerable attention to the role of preventive health programs in both urban and rural areas—programs of mass inoculation, environmental sanitation, health education, and nutrition. Many observers attribute much of the improvement in China's morbidity and mortality statistics to the effectiveness of these programs.

Third, a byproduct of China's overall development strategy has been the elaboration of a compliance system, with an organizational correlate, to motivate health sector action by the mass of the population. This system has not relied exclusively on remunerative rewards. China's ability to call forth voluntary health work and to change individual behavior with respect to personal or food hygiene is of crucial importance in understanding the operational mechanism underlying its health sector strategy and the probability that this can be transplanted to other countries.

Finally, despite recent political pressure to force a reallocation of medical personnel from the urban to the rural areas, the central government's responsibility is limited to support of mobile medical teams, training programs, advanced medical care, and medical research. Hence the innovative restructuring of the medical care delivery system has been of crucial importance, providing a medical technology that is both potentially efficacious and within the financial means of the relatively poor rural areas.

Organization of
Health Services

§

EZRA F. VOGEL*

The basic components of the Chinese health program are hardly unique to the People's Republic of China. Public health programs to extend sanitation, control pests, and provide inoculations to prevent communicable diseases are basic to any developing country. Wide use is made of paramedical personnel to perform midwifery, give inoculations, and distribute medications in countries without an ample supply of fully trained doctors. State initiative in extending health care is found not only in Communist countries but in many capitalist countries. What is unique to China is the solid organizational base that combines these specific programs into an effective overall effort capable of rapidly extending public health and medical coverage in a country not yet industrialized.

At the center of the organization at each level is the Chinese Communist Party, with a loyal membership prepared to supervise and implement programs enunciated by higher levels. Paralleling the party structure at each level is a government structure ready to carry out the more complex administrative tasks under the direction of the corresponding party unit. Below the national level of party and state organization is the province, the special district, and the county or large municipality. Within large municipalities there are, in turn, districts, wards, and neighborhood committees; within the county there are smaller cities, towns, and communes; and within the communes there are brigades and production teams. It is this responsive, well-organized leadership at each level that makes the organizational structure effective.

What follows is a brief overview of the reorganization of the medical care system after the Communists came to power in 1949.

---

* Dr. Vogel was unable to attend the conference.

After describing the basic rationalization of health organization, I shall treat three specific organizational problems: the modernization of traditional medicine, the extension of public health services, and the creation of medical facilities in more remote areas.

Rationalization of Health Organization

The Chinese Communists took over an existing Ministry of Public Health that had already enunciated enlightened programs to develop more modern hospitals, more effective sanitation, and medical training. Under the Nationalists, however, the ministry had lacked an organizational base for implementing health programs on a broad basis throughout the country. Beginning in 1949 public health officials began to expand the staff of the ministry in Peking in a variety of specialties, and to increase the number and size of lower-level health administrative units under the ministry's aegis.

The title of the ministry, "public health," reflected the overall orientation of China's health program, an orientation appropriate to a country that had not yet dealt with many of the more basic public health problems. Although the ministry supervised the establishment of higher medical training, research, and hospitals, its predominant orientation was toward establishing the basic breakthroughs in sanitation, maternal and child health care, and inoculation against and control of communicable diseases. The generation of Mao Tse-tung, preoccupied with the question of how to increase national strength, felt that national strength depended on the cultivation of individual health, and that the most basic breakthroughs in improving physical health and extending longevity lay in the extension of the basic public health services.

At each level of government down to the county level, a branch of government concerned with public health was established where it had not already existed under the Nationalists. These branches of public health—departments at the provincial level, bureaus at the county or large municipal level, and sections at the district level—became the instruments through which the new public health program was organized.

Many of the problems of health organization confronting the Chinese in 1949 were comparable to those confronting medicine in the United States at the time of the Flexner Report of 1911. Many medical practitioners in China had acquired their knowledge through apprenticeships to other practitioners, and had been through no standardized training or certification procedures. In rural areas, midwives without training were delivering babies, and a variety of sorcerers, faith healers, and magicians were still giving medical advice. Much advice was also given by druggists who made use of herbs and special potions passed on through tradition and with a folklore about usage that had not yet been subjected to scientific testing. Many medical practitioners had begun their practice as druggists, moving to medical practice as they acquired a bigger clientele.

The problem of establishing standardization and certification was complicated by the fact that even those formal training programs that existed varied widely in quality and organization. Because of the disruptions from 1937 to 1949 caused by World War II and the civil war, the amount of medical training provided even within a single institution varied almost from year to year.

In rationalizing higher education in the early 1950s the Chinese used a major metropolitan area as the unit for reorganization. All the faculties in a given field at the various universities in that area were combined into a single specialized institution. All the education departments of major institutions in Peking were combined, for example, to form a single University of Education. Similarly, the medical departments of all the universities in a given metropolitan area were combined into one or two major medical schools. This made it possible for the government to establish an organization more responsive to new directions than the old leadership would have been. By combining all trained personnel in the various fields of medicine, new medical schools could provide better training in the various specialties, with a better coordinated and fuller program than was possible in the smaller programs. Higher medical training was offered primarily in four-year medical schools which the student entered after secondary school. Therefore, even doctors produced after 1949 lacked a liberal arts background comparable to that of an American physician. In some medical schools the course of training was longer than four years; in other areas there were briefer, three-year programs.

Doctors from the major east coast urban medical centers were recruited to help establish medical schools in most of the inland provinces that had had no first class schools, and to standardize the curriculum with materials from the better developed east coast institutions. Many of the syllabi produced by specialists working at the latter institutions were mimeographed and distributed as the basic texts in those schools and, with minor modifications, in the other medical schools also. Some of the new teaching materials were imported from the Soviet Union and translated into Chinese.

Because there were few existing training centers for ancillary professions and paramedical personnel, several new institutions were created at various levels of government. Better educated medical personnel in provincial capitals assisted special districts in establishing their own training courses for ancillary and paramedical personnel, and special districts in turn assisted counties in establishing their programs. Many of these courses for nurses, public health worker, sanitation workers, and midwives were brief, intensive, three- to six-month training programs that were only gradually regularized into ordinary school programs.

In the early 1950s, under the supervision of the public health bureaus at the municipal and county levels, a socialist transformation of medical practice took place analogous to that of economic institutions. Larger hospitals and clinics were run by the government from the time the Communists came to power. Other moderately large institutions were brought under governmental management, while smaller clinics were formed as cooperatives and doctors from private practice were brought into them.

In the course of selecting doctors who would be allowed to take part in the newly established or expanded medical centers, judgments had to be made about qualifications. Although there were no standardized tests, the public health bureaus investigated the qualifications of various doctors and brought into the hospitals and clinics only those with a certain measure of competence. Older doctors with a moderate degree of competence were retired early; younger doctors with very limited competence were given special training programs or supervision on the job to develop a higher level of skill.

The selection of doctors to participate in these medical institutions was in effect a kind of certification of their skill level. Nonetheless some doctors who were accepted into these practices initially were in essence on trial. Those who did not prove to have enough adaptability, flexibility, and skill were dropped. In the course of raising standards many doctors from smaller, lower-level institutions were sent for brief periods to higher-level hospitals and clinics for special training. A doctor at a small county hospital, for example, could go to a special district-level hospital, receive more advanced training, and return to his post at the county hospital. As new graduates of medical institutions were produced, they too could be sent out to lower-level institutions to lead the development and expansion of medical services and to provide further guidance for raising the quality of those institutions.

Similar selection procedures were used for ancillary and paramedical personnel. For example, old midwives who proved inflexible were dismissed, younger midwives capable of learning new skills were given three- to six-month training courses at higher administrative levels, and young women were given midwife training to take the place of older midwives who were retired prematurely.

Although efforts were made to recruit doctors from peasant and worker families, most trained medical personnel in 1949 had depended in large part on family support to complete medical training and were not therefore from poorer social classes. Even after 1949 medicine was one of the safer fields for children of bourgeois and landlord families to enter; their political attitudes were less likely to interfere with their work because a certain amount of humanitarian concern could be safely assumed. Even most students who had completed secondary schools in the 1950s were from families of some means, and medical schools anxious to train large numbers of medical practitioners had no choice but to accept these students.

By 1956, when the socialist transformation was essentially completed, most fully qualified doctors were therefore working at set salaries in state hospitals or clinics as part of team practices. At lower levels, doctors with less training were engaged in kinds of group cooperative practices that were, however, bounded by regulations set by the government. Because of these regulations, doctors in the cooperative institutions generally did not earn as much as those in the larger state hospitals and clinics.

A small group of less competent rural herbalists and old fashioned practitioners were still allowed to practice, but they were not licensed and if they charged large fees they were subject to prosecution. Because medical expenses at the state and cooperative institutions were very low, the remaining private practitioners without certification and sanction could not be competitive, and their incomes were far less. Their practices were gradually reduced, although not entirely eliminated in remote areas where the more superstitious elderly people still chose to consult them.

The state gradually acquired control over the collection, manufacture, and distribution of drugs, and the public health bureaus supervised their distribution. In large part, drugs were distributed through hospitals and clinics under the direction of medical specialists. By 1956 China had therefore achieved the basic reorganization of public health and medical practice, medical education, and the allocation of drugs. The municipal and county bureaus that had led this transformation continued to supervise most of the hospitals and clinics, although medical schools, training hospitals, and the largest medical facilities were administered through higher levels of organizations.

The Modernization of Traditional Medicine

When Western medicine spread to non-Western areas, in most countries traditional medical practices were of such a primitive level that they could not survive the onslaught of more advanced, scientific Western medical technology. In a number of countries traditional medicine was somewhat more developed and an effort was made to preserve and refine traditional practices. The most sophisticated non-Western medical practices were to be found in China, and traditional practices were thus more viable in the modern age than in any other country. As Ralph Croizier has shown, the special emphasis on traditional medicine in China both prior to World War II and in the late 1950s was related to a strong nationalist effort to find sources of pride in the Chinese tradition.[1] It was precisely at the time of the reaction against Russian dominance in the late 1950s that traditional medicine was given special support, just as Chinese tradition and Chinese techniques in general were given greater relative support than the emulation of international socialist practices.

Many traditional medical practices undoubtedly had an element of scientific validity, although in the 1950s these were still often intertangled with metaphysical explanations, superstitious beliefs, and a variety of magical and even harmful practices. Although the Chinese were emphasizing traditional medicine as a matter of national pride, they were simultaneously modernizing and casting it in a mold resembling Western medical practice.

Communist administrators supervised the collection of all traditional herbalist remedies and drugs, and those traditional practitioners who were reluctant to share their secrets were criticized for their selfish capitalist thinking. Once the millions of remedies were collected, an effort was made to sort out those that were effective from those that were not. The means used to make this distinction were Western scientific laboratory tests and, as they were completed, very often the effective elements in traditional medicine were no longer administered as roots or brews but as extracts in the form of pills and inoculations, as in Western medicine.

Acupuncture, which had had a very wide following, even among the Western-educated elite, for curing certain kinds of illnesses began to wane as a medical treatment in the early 1950s when it did not stand up in laboratory or clinical experiments. Acupuncture underwent a revival, however, when it was discovered through similar experimentation that it could be very effective in relieving pain and that it had great utility as an anesthetic for surgery.

Chinese medical information was no longer passed on through the traditional apprenticeship but was taught in regular classrooms with textbooks modeled after modern Western medical training. Chinese medicine was no longer dispensed in traditional druggist settings, but in hospitals and clinics organized along Western lines. In short, while traditional medicine had maintained its nationalist appeal, its organization and rationale were distinctly Western.

Most doctors now receive primary training in either Western or traditional medicine, and many clinics and hospitals still distinguish between practitioners so trained. The relationship between these two kinds of practitioners has been relatively easy, similar to the relationship between different medical specialists in the United States. Traditional doctors in a given clinic or hospital are generally considered to have special skills that they can use on patients with certain problems; those trained in Western medicine have other skills. Patients are generally given their choice of Chinese or Western practitioners; many rural patients who feel more comfortable with older, more rustic traditional practitioners generally choose to consult them. On the whole the distinctions between traditional and Western practices have declined over time as traditional practices have been modernized and as the effective techniques acquired by either group are taken over and shared by doctors trained in other orientations. It would not be surprising if, in the not too distant future, the Western and traditional Chinese medical training systems continue to lose their distinctiveness and essentially become assimilated.

Extension of Public Health Services
to Remote Areas

When the Communists came to power they were confronted with a number of basic problems of sanitation, nutrition, communicable diseases, and maternal and child care that had long since been largely resolved in more advanced countries. Since the fighting with the Kuomintang continued well into 1950, and the fighting in Korea began before the fighting with the Kuomintang had subsided, the government was able to make use of the patriotic appeal to launch its initial public health measures. Fear of the enemy's use of biological warfare was widely publicized and used as a vehicle for arousing the population to take basic sanitation measures and to receive inoculations against the most serious communicable diseases. By the mid-1950s, when the government's administrative organizational base was fairly well established, it was used as a means for carrying out systematic sanitation and inoculation programs. In January 1956, just as the agricultural collectivization was basically completed and provided an effective organizational base in the countryside, the Chinese carried out an impressive and successful blitz campaign against the four pests—mosquitoes, flies, rats, and bedbugs. Since basic public health measures of sanitation and inoculation are relatively simple and do not require complex skill levels, an effective organizational structure with good publicity enabled the Chinese to make tremendous advances in the field of public health in relatively short order. Villagers could easily be rounded up for inoculations, and urban neighborhood and rural cooperative organizations were very effective structures for carrying out sanitation measures. In short, the close collaboration between public health and other administrative units provided an impressive combination in making the basic public health breakthroughs of the 1950s.

Extension of Medical Services

Unlike the extension of basic public health measures, the extension of quality medical services requires a high level of skill, and the Chinese have not advanced nearly as rapidly on this front. Throughout the 1950s and 1960s continuous efforts were made to train larger numbers of quality medical personnel and deploy them to more remote areas. The criticisms of the Liu Shao-ch'i line in the medical field during the Cultural Revolution, however, made it very clear that as of the late 1960s distribution of quality health care in the countryside was still a serious problem. In the wake of the Cultural Revolution, and in the absence of greater numbers of quality doctors, the government has made renewed efforts to train lower level personnel—the barefoot doctors (ch'ih chiao i sheng)—who will provide medical service in the interim decades until more quality medical personnel can be trained in larger urban medical schools.

Nonetheless the organizational capacity is sufficiently great that there are some medical facilities available at all organizational levels down through the commune. When contrasted to recent reports of the widespread lack of any medical care for much of the population in developing countries, this in itself is a major achievement.

There are many facets to the difficulty of extending high-quality medical care to the remote areas of the countryside. Transportation in these areas, especially in mountainous regions, is very inadequate: in many places there are no roads or waterways connecting the population with medical centers. A sick patient may have to be carried by porters some distance to get to any hospital, and this inhibits rural patients from going to medical centers. As yet, quality medical personnel in rural hospitals simply do not have the time to make frequent visits to the more remote areas in their administrative units. The result is that many patients in these regions do not in fact receive any professional medical attention. There is a current effort to establish small hospitals in most communes, which have an average population of 8,000 to 10,000, but this goal is far from being achieved; the transportation problems in some communes are sufficiently difficult so that not everyone in the administrative area covered by a commune is serviced by its hospital.

Not only are there few competent doctors at the commune level, but the supply of basic diagnostic machinery and of various kinds of expensive drugs is very limited. Because the supply of modern drugs is still limited even in larger urban centers, drugs are in effect rationed to each clinic and hospital, and doctors must make decisions about which cases are sufficiently serious and promising for the scarce supply of quality drugs to be utilized.

Another problem inhibiting the distribution of quality services is the fact that the state is not yet affluent enough to guarantee social services, including medical services, for everyone in the society. Over 80 per cent of the people receive their income not on the basis of a set salary but on the basis of their cooperative organization's profits. Profits are calculated after the cooperative—rural production team, handicraft cooperative, or service cooperative— sells its products to the state or on state-supervised markets and expenses are deducted. Employees of the state on a set salary— either the Communist Party, the state administrative structure, state factories, state teaching institutions, or other state-run enterprises—are provided with a welfare package that includes payment for medical care. For the remaining 80+ per cent of the population, patients and their families are expected to bear the cost of medical services and the cost of drugs. Since incomes in the countryside are still relatively low compared to urban incomes, many peasants have been inhibited from using medical services and drugs because of the expense, even though it is quite minimal. The regime's effort, especially since the Cultural Revolution, has been to get the commune production teams and the brigades to develop a savings fund that can be used to pay the medical expenses of their members. Although no precise data is available to outsiders on the size and number of production teams, it is clear that there is a wide variation in their ability to set aside a large enough fund to cover all their members so that they need not feel inhibited about going to medical clinics because of the cost.

Although China has had a consistent policy since 1949 of deploying more trained doctors to the rural areas, even with the government's tremendous organizational capacity, it is not a monolithic state and there are many imperfections that prevent more highly trained doctors from going to the countryside. At the present stage of development the cities can still use far more doctors than they now have and urban units often make great efforts to retain individual doctors. Since most doctors would prefer to work in better medical centers in urban areas than in remote areas with less adequate facilities, they are glad to cooperate. Criticisms expressed during the Cultural Revolution reveal that, despite policies to the contrary, many medical units in the cities did make an effort to keep medical personnel rather than reassign them to lower levels and more remote areas. AnElissa Lucas has traced all reported cases in the Chinese press and on the radio in which doctors have been sent from the city to the countryside and has found that overwhelmingly they were not sent great distances from major urban areas.[2] In other words there is still a concentration of greater medical talent in areas closest to the large cities.

Despite its organizational capacities, China is not a monolithic country and therefore must make continuous efforts to send more medical personnel to the countryside. In the medical field the repudiation of the Liu Shao-ch'i line was utilized at each level as a vehicle for criticizing doctors and medical administrators who stood in the way of the reassignment of more medical personnel, and there is no question that such efforts and campaigns will continue.

In short, the People's Republic of China is making a vigorous effort to extend higher quality medical services to more remote areas, but, as with her industrialization, this movement is still at a very early stage. In the interim, the government is establishing clinics with less trained personnel to provide the most basic medical services. It is an organizational triumph that has made this program as effective as it is.

NOTES

1. Ralph C. Croizier, "Chinese Communist Attitudes Toward Traditional Medicine," *Asia* 5 (Spring 1966).

2. AnElissa Lucas, "Legitimate Criticism or Cultural Revolution Rhetoric? An Analysis of Mao's Indictments Against the Ministry of Public Health," unpublished manuscript (Harvard University: 1970).

The Strategy of
Health-Sector Planning

PETER S. HELLER*

In no other country has the role of health as both a means and an end of economic development been trumpeted so loudly and consistently as in the People's Republic of China. Yet health programs in other countries of the underdeveloped world have failed to effectively deliver health services to a large proportion of the population or to control many infectious and parasitic diseases for which well-developed preventive measures exist.[1]

Two questions emerge immediately. First, what was the strategy underlying China's health programs, and its role within the context of China's overall development program? Second, what has been the impact of these programs on the health of the Chinese people? Our focus shall be primarily on the first question.

Between 1949 and 1965 China's health policy paralleled that of many less-developed countries (LDCs) in terms of its bias in allocating both medical manpower and financial resources to the urban sector, rather than to the rural areas where the bulk of the Chinese population is concentrated, as is the case in many other LDCs. Shortages of both financial and medical manpower resources in these areas has created critical barriers to the development of a rural health network in most LDCs. How have the Chinese attacked this problem?

The Policy Environment of Health

The Chinese emphasis on health reflected both an awareness of its political significance for the maintenance and development of popular support for the regime, and a belief in its crucial role in

* The author is grateful for the encouragement and perceptive criticism and suggestions of Dean Myron Wegman and Professors Alexander Eckstein, Tsung-yi Lin, Robert Worth, Robert Dernberger, and Robert Grosse; and to the Center for Research on Economic Development of the University of Michigan for its financial support.

facilitating and expanding the productivity of the economy. Better health is an end of development in and of itself. Reduction in child and maternal mortality, expansion of available health delivery services, and control of mass infectious diseases were important benefits to be expected from a revolutionary government. These benefits are "consumption goods" that must receive some attention, regardless of whether they also have some developmental impact.

The Chinese have placed equal stress on the importance of health as a component of their economic policies. Repeatedly in the statements of China's leadership one hears that "the firm guide of health work is to proceed from production, coordinate closely with production, and serve production."[2] Similarly, in the context of a China with a high dependent population under the age of fifteen, a

> . . . policy of health first is connected with our long range national interest and our national health. A student begins school at age seven and graduates after age twenty. If, during such a long period of time, attention is not given to his health it will affect the physical condition of the entire nation.[3]

Indeed one often finds a castigation of the so-called "dangerous bourgeois" view that health should be supplied only for health's sake.[4]

Yet the implications for policy of the linkages between health and economic development are vague. Should one divert investible resources from industry or agriculture to health? One may assert that investments in health lead to an expansion in an individual's lifetime productive capacity, or ultimately have positive effects on slowing the rate of population growth through reductions in child mortality, or reduce the consumption losses implied by early deaths. Nutritional programs may prevent irreversible brain damage and losses in individual productivity. Since the validity of these assertions and the magnitude of the purported linkages are still unproved for both health and economic planners, it is difficult to assert that the Chinese have explicitly or implicitly allocated resources to health strictly on a cost-benefit basis.[5]

Similarly, should the public sector at the provincial or central governmental level financially ensure an adequate level of health services to the population? In most LDCs virtually all rural health services, and a substantial proportion of urban services, are delivered within the public sector. This mix of private and public sector responsibilities is not based on any firm theoretical delineation of the "public" and "private" components of health as a "commodity." Health has both investment and consumption characteristics and is of importance both to individuals and society.

It is a "public good" in the sense that man is in the transmission cycle of many infectious and parasitic-borne diseases. Thus an individual's actions and his personal health may affect the health and the utility of others. Likewise, society may derive social benefits, or prevent social losses, from the provision of better health for its members. Yet health is also a private good in that it is "consumed" by the individual, yields in large part its utility to the consumer, and is to a high degree not shared jointly with others. This justifies the individual's absorption of a certain proportion of the costs of providing better health. Society collectively absorbs a share of the costs in order to insure a socially adequate level of consumption of health services.

In most LDCs the commitment by the government to assure a minimal level of health facilities to the population becomes transformed into a financial commitment to bear the costs of these services. The effect is to place a substantial financial burden on the government's recurrent budget, and to ensure that the budgetary constraint limits the possibility for an expansion of such health services.

A problem confronting any policymaker is the determination of what constitutes "delivery" of this consumption good, "health." Is it manifested through popular feeling that immediate health needs have been satisfied? Is it manifested by a perception that the health of oneself and one's children is improved? Is the economic payoff to increments in the quality or quantity of health services greater where economic change is more apparent, viz. the urban-industrial centers? In the agricultural sector, where there may be a surplus of labor, does it really matter in terms of economic development whether an individual peasant's productive capacity is improved? Given the massive relative size of China's peasantry, and the limited financial and health resources available, would not a rural-oriented, egalitarian strategy spread these resources so thin as to vitiate any economic impact, while prejudicing high quality care for urban centers?

Should one emphasize the provision of maternal-child health care and nutrition programs, or the elimination of parasitic diseases and curative services to reduce losses in work activity among active workers? What role should the commune or production team play relative to the central government in the financing and implementation of health programs?

The answers to some of these questions hinge on several critical assumptions about the role of health in the production of human capital that are not readily verifiable. Moreover the political weights attached to each group and, perhaps as important, the way in which the peasants and workers perceive the utility of health, crucially determine the relative allocative priorities of the political decision maker. If the mass of peasantry attach a high utility to the consumption of health, that is, to the availability of basic services, whether or not they receive sophisticated services, then regardless of the economic impact this may provide support for an "egalitarian" health policy.

Since 1949 one can observe a conflict, still not fully resolved, within Chinese policy-making circles as to the relative emphasis to be placed on the urban versus rural sectors, the proletariat versus the peasantry. The emphasis can be seen to vary over the last twenty years, paralleling the relative balance between agriculture and industry in national economic policy. The position of the pendulum has decisively affected the observed policies, primarily through its effect on the allocation of limited budgetary and manpower resources between the two sectors. Indeed the cyclical recurrence of tightness of budgetary constraints upon agriculture crucially shaped the feasible range of health policies in that sector.

Since the Cultural Revolution the stated emphasis of policy has been oriented towards the rural peasantry. Mao has stated that the goal of health policy should be

> to satisfy the medical need of the broad peasant masses and to change the public health appearance of the rural areas, as well as to provide material conditions for building the new socialist countryside.
> The peasant is the forerunner of the Chinese worker, the main factor of China's industrial market, the source of the Chinese army, the backbone force of China's democratic politics, and a major target of Chinese cultural movement. [6]

Policy Setting: 1949

In 1949 one facet of China's underdevelopment was the range and severity of the diseases that afflicted its population. Communicable diseases such as smallpox, tuberculosis, typhoid fever, shigellosis, kala-azar, schistosomiasis, and many others decimated the population.

The Japanese occupation and the civil war had disrupted agricultural and industrial production, causing extensive food shortages and consequent malnutrition beyond previous levels. China's infant mortality rate in 1949 ranged upwards of 200:1,000; even in Peking it was 117.6:1,000.[7] The crude mortality rate was at 25–30:1,000. Worth has estimated that 30 per cent of Chinese children died before the age of five.[8] The maternal mortality rate was at 2–3 per cent.

At the time of the revolution China's medical resources were meager in contrast to the medical needs of the population. Health facilities were staggeringly few: There were only 2,580 hospitals, with 84,000 beds, approximately 30 per cent of which were either privately or foreign owned. At least 70 per cent of these facilities were said to be in urban areas. Nationally there were approximately 6,550 persons per hospital bed; in the rural areas the ratio rose to 19,600.[9] The average *hsien*, comprising about 300,000 people, had only seven health "institutes," each averaging 7.8 beds. There were fewer than 400 health centers in rural China. C. Y. Cheng's paper on health manpower in this volume (p. 139) indicates that by any Western standards there were tremendous shortages of personnel at all levels, particularly in the rural areas. It is clear that there was negligible capacity to rapidly attack China's health problems with any substantive impact. To add to these constraints, China was heavily dependent on imports for the bulk of its modern pharmaceutical needs.

Policy Constraints

Despite the emphasis attached to an expanded health program by Chinese leaders, the magnitude of any effort in the health sector was severely constrained by two factors that are similar to those found in other LDCs. First, China was not a wealthy country: its per capita income in 1950 was approximately U.S. $50, and by 1966 it was no more than $130.[10] Second, the character of China's health effort was constrained by the limited priority attached to health relative to other competing sectors in the central government's development program, and by the allocation of this health budget between the urban and rural sectors.

Since there are no published statistics on the level of government expenditures in the health sector, one must fall back on secondary estimates (Table 1). During the period prior to 1966 not more than 16 per cent of central government resources were spent on "culture, education, science, social welfare, and public health." It is reasonable to assume that the first three accounted for the largest proportion—certainly above 75 per cent—because this sector included ever-mounting expenditures on nuclear research.

On the other hand, this may be an underestimate of the total social resources allocated to health. First, while a certain number of military or agricultural projects with health components may have been financed by the central government, they were probably not significant. Second, we have omitted expenditures made at the non-central-government level; we can obtain a crude estimate of the importance of this omission by examining the level of capital investments in health in the total economy (Table 1). Even if we were to assume that the ratio of capital investments to recurrent outlays was 10 per cent, which seems extremely low, in 1958 the level of total outlays on health would have been no more than 1,210 million *yüan*. If the level had risen at the same rate as total state outlays in the "health and other" sector, total health expenditures in 1966 would still have been less than 1,810 million *yüan*. As a proportion of the GNP in 1966 this would have been no more than 1.2 per cent;[11] as a proportion of state expenditures, health accounted for no more than 4 per cent. Table 2 lists comparable statistics for a set of other LDCs.

Assuming the above statistics are not severely underestimated, China's health allocations are not significantly above average— China has not supported its policy emphasis with unusually high expenditure per capita. Indeed it has been argued that one important motive for the decentralization of rural health services arising during the Cultural Revolution was to shift the cost of providing services from the central government to the communes.[12-14]

The gross inequalities between urban and rural areas in most LDCs were similarly observed in China prior to 1966. The formal structure of curative health facilities resembled a pyramid, with local dispensaries and health centers feeding into larger hospitals. Yet the distribution of these health institutions and the level and quality of their equipment, facilities, and personnel were highly skewed towards the urban areas, the apex of the pyramid. In the

Table 1. Allocation of Central Government Resources

(in million *yüan*).

Expenditure Category	Ratio—1954/57 %	Final Accounts				Estimates	
		1958	Ratio %	1959	Ratio %	1966	Ratio %
National economic construction	50–52	262.7	64.1	321.7	61.1	184.0	46.0
Culture, education, science, social welfare, and public health	15–16	43.5	10.6	58.6	11.1	64.1	16.0
National defense		50.0	12.2	58.0	11.0	85.0	21.3
Administrative expenses		22.7	5.6	29.0	5.5	22.0	5.5
Debts and foreign aid		11.8	2.9	13.2	2.5	20.0	5.0
Other		18.9	4.6	47.2	8.9	25.0	6.2
Total		409.6	100.0	527.7	100.0	400.0	100.0

Source: People's Republic of China, State Statistical Bureau, *Ten Great Years* (Peking: Foreign Languages Press, 1960); and Union Research Institute, *Communist China 1966* 1 (March 1968).

Table 2. Approximate Level of Government Expenditures on Health in Some Less Developed Countries

	GNP Per Capita— 1965 (in U.S. Dollars)	Government Health Expenditures as a Percentage of:		Government Health Expenditures per Capita — 1963–64 (in U.S. Dollars)
		General Government Expenditures (1963–64) %	GNP (1963–64) %	
Indonesia	99	2.8	0.23	0.20
Nigeria	83	12.0	0.62	0.50
Thailand	126	3.4	0.5	0.60
Malawi	40	5.8	1.6	0.64
Sudan	95	4.8	1.07	1.02
Guatemala	300	9.1	0.78	2.36
Senegal	170	6.6	2.4	3.47
Colombia	277	11.0	1.26	3.5
Jamaica	460	11.0	2.08	9.6
Kenya	85	6.0	1.3	1.1
Tanzania	70	9.2	1.3	0.90
People's Republic of China (1966)	85–100	≥4.0	>1.2	≥0.99

Source: Combined from John Bryant, *Health and the Developing World* (Ithaca: Cornell University Press, 1969); International Bank for Reconstruction and Development, *World Tables 1968*, Mimeographed (Washington, D. C., 1970); and People's Republic of China, State Statistical Bureau, *Ten Great Years* (Peking: Foreign Languages Press, 1960).

rural areas accessibility to curative services was more a function of proximity and individual financial capacity than degree of medical need. Prior to 1958 only in the maternal-child health area can one find any modern medical curative programs geared to the rural areas. Not until 1965 do we find any blossoming of the commune curative health systems that began in 1958.

In some provinces upwards of 80 per cent of total government health expenditures were allocated to urban hospitals and clinics. This is further shown by the nature of the central government's budgetary responsibilities in the health sector, which encompass the financing of: (1) hospitals at the county level and, in large and medium cities, at the district level; (2) medical educational facilities; and (3) the manufacture and distribution of medical equipment, drugs, and supplies.[15]

Omitted are the costs for the bulk of preventive health campaigns, and for basic medical units in urban and rural areas. In the rural areas these were financed, if at all, at the commune or district level, and were obtained from "after-state tax" disposable income. This probably means that the financing of health was at best proportional, if not regressive.

This differential is further substantiated by C. Y. Cheng's study on medical manpower in this volume. From his statistics we have estimated the number of doctors per capita in the urban and rural areas, using the oft-quoted assertion that 60 to 80 per cent of China's medical manpower is located in the urban areas. The resulting ratios of doctors to population range from 1:7,640 to 1:15,400 in the rural areas, to 1:680 to 1:890 in the urban areas; in Kwantung Province the ratios range from 1:600 in Canton to 1:10,000 in the rural sector.[16]

In the formal structure of China's health policies we therefore find that the level of state resources allocated to health, and its distribution between urban and rural areas, would not appear favorable for the implementation of anything more than a skeletal rural health program. Yet throughout the postrevolution period, and increasingly after 1958, one observes a set of significant adaptations to this formal structure, based on the government's ability to mobilize and allocate effectively additional resources for health purposes. Prior to 1958 these adaptations occurred primarily on the preventive level; thereafter, an alternative strategy for curative health care began to emerge, which snowballed only after 1965.

Preventive Health Strategy: 1949–65

Prior to the Cultural Revolution the most significant innovations in China's health strategy occurred in the area of preventive health. There were two central elements to their policies. First, the Chinese were able to mobilize additional human resources for their preventive health program in what might be termed a "surplus labor absorption" strategy. Second, and more central, these resources were used directly in effective preventive health measures. This prevented any bottlenecks to a large-scale preventive health program arising from shortages of trained public health personnel.

To carry out this policy only minimal allocations were needed from the state budget; the chief burden could be transferred to the commune and individual levels. On the other hand, adaptations were needed among a much wider target group than would be true for organizational changes in institutions that fall more traditionally within the health sector. A mechanism capable of inducing an adequate level of individual and communal participation in health programs, often termed "moral" as opposed to "material" incentives, needed to be developed.

There were four specific components of China's preventive health program. First, the Chinese began to develop a basic preventive health infrastructure throughout the country, although it was more elaborate in the urban areas. The basic underpinning for this policy was provided by the state's investment in facilities to train a core of professional public health workers, and in a network of epidemic prevention centers located principally in the urban areas. These centers disseminated information on the means of containing the spread of infectious diseases, and managed mass immunization campaigns. With the elaboration of decentralized curative health networks in municipal areas—hospitals, work clinics, dispensaries— virtually all urban children were routinely immunized against smallpox, tuberculosis, and diphtheria.[17] In the rural areas, particularly in the principal villages, comparable institutions were far more skeletal and only childhood immunizations received the degree of financing from the state necessary to make the program moderately successful; the rural immunization rate was probably half that of the urban areas.

In certain cities there was evidence of active maternal and child health programs at the district level that sought out children and mothers rather than let the provision of health be dependent on parental initiative. Some centers were said to combine curative and preventive work, systematically providing check-ups to children under age seven, and offering health education and family planning guidance to mothers. Whether these district and street health centers were available in all urban areas is not clear.[18]

This institutional infrastructure was complemented by extensive state investment in urban sewage systems and water supplies. Sewage treatment plants were set up, tapwater availability was expanded, and regular garbage collections were instituted. This engendered rural medical problems in that urban human waste was often transported for use in agriculture, which resulted in the transmission of various infectious diseases.[19] Such state-financed investment was not made in the rural areas, where it occurred far more gradually, if at all, and was dependent upon local and eventually communal financing.

Second, one observes the use of continuous social pressure to induce changes in individual behavior and attitudes toward personal hygiene, environmental sanitation, and nutrition.[20] Whether these behavioral changes occurred in the rural areas prior to 1965 is more uncertain. The relative difference in the success at the urban and rural levels was likely to be a function of the differential quality of curative health networks that existed prior to 1965. These provided a vehicle for health education that was particularly necessary among relatively uneducated workers or peasantry to insure that the linkage between a given set of individual actions and its effect on personal health was clearly understood.

Third, mass mobilizations of the labor force in short intensive campaign periods and the use of peasant public health teams provided both the resources and inputs critical to the program's success. In both rural and urban areas, however, prior to 1965 this preventive work through mass mobilization distinguished the Chinese experience from other LDCs. Throughout the period there were reports of short bursts of frenzied activity, lasting anywhere from a week to a month, against the various "villains" of health. Initially this involved mass immunization campaigns against smallpox and cholera. The patriotic campaigns against the purported American chemical-biological warfare during the Korean war involved mass extermination campaigns against the four pests—bedbugs, flies, mosquitoes, and rats—with extensive publicity given to the numbers killed. In virtually all areas of China mass sanitation campaigns to dispose of garbage and manure and to clean the streets and homes appear to have been regular occurrences.[21-23] These action campaigns were extended to the repairing of water channels and road surfaces in order to destroy the breeding grounds of mosquitoes and flies.[24,25]

The campaigns also involved the use of what Salaff calls "community action and self-help" in mass *curative* services designed to attack one point in the transmission cycle of certain infectious and parasitic diseases.[26] At various times, medical teams were sent from the urban areas to train corps of medical workers drawn from the peasantry and proletariat in simple diagnostic and treatment methods and control procedures for a limited number of diseases. This approach was initially developed for an antisyphilis program, but such techniques have more recently been used in campaigns against schistosomiasis.[27,28]

A byproduct of these campaigns was the transmission of health information to the Chinese population. Salaff states that this approach had an "unknown, but undoubtedly great, influence on depressing the incidence of all diseases."[29] This is a critical prerequisite for any attempt to induce changes in individual behavior and attitudes toward disease problems.

There is both a political and an economic rationale to the use of mass action campaigns on so large a scale as was manifest in China. Mass campaigns for health purposes are politically safe vehicles for engendering popular support for collective social action and united effort. The same medical teams that lead the population in health campaigns or provide mass immunizations are in a crucial position to stress and disseminate the ideological message of the regime because they already have the trust of the people.

The Chinese consciously attempted to integrate the realization of health and agricultural objectives in the hope of economizing on the resources devoted to both sectors. For example, one aspect of the antischistosomiasis campaign was mass action work in developing irrigation networks and expanding cultivable farm acreage.[30] In the process of digging new irrigation canals and filling existing snail-infested canals, the snails that serve as the intermediate hosts could be uprooted and buried. Throughout the entire farming season, repeated emphasis was placed on increasing the consciousness of the peasantry to eliminate the snails.[31] Similarly,

various localities have mobilized half a million laboring people and
some 200 tractors; thirty-one conservancy projects for elimination of
snails have been started successfully.[32]

To the extent that this effort was focused on periods when there
was a slackening in the level of agricultural work, it proved a relatively costless means of taking such preventive health action. To
the extent it was combined with agricultural efforts, its cost was
further reduced, thus effectively providing a productive outlet for
surplus labor. The use of mass campaigns and community effort
provided a model for the latter reforms implemented after 1965,
both in preventive and curative health measures.

Furthermore, the emphasis on self-reliance and social mobilization as key ethics of socialist public health policy implies a strategy
of resource allocation different from that commonly observed in
the health policies of most LDCs. First, the Chinese government
has emphasized that the primary burden of financing health measures must be borne out of the disposable incomes of those directly
benefiting from them: the rural communes, production brigades,
and production teams. Although the central government clearly
subsidizes elements of the health program, this is not the budgetary
constraint that fixes the level of the program. Both an ability at
the local level to mobilize resources and the availability of resource
allocational options are required to show the people enough health
output to assure continued popular support for the resource burden.
If the cost of public health programs proves high to the peasantry
they will be less willing to pay the price.

This mode of resource mobilization is a classic strategy involving the organization of "surplus" labor. What is crucial in the
Chinese strategy is less the fact that it is heavily labor intensive,
which it obviously is, than that: (1) it implies a transfer of the burden of health activities to those whom it directly affects; and (2)
the Chinese have found the institutional and organizational keys
that allow them to use a labor-intensive strategy where so many
other LDCs have tried and failed.[33]

The extent to which "surplus" is an appropriate term is unclear
since either the individual or the society will usually bear some of
the cost of this activity. Three examples may be cited: (1) If the
peasant's marginal productivity is not zero during the period in
which he is mobilized for health purposes, the commune clearly

faces a trade-off between present agricultural output and the output of health improvement, even though the latter may have dynamic implications for the former; (2) in slack seasons it involves a trade-off by the individual of the utility derived from leisuretime and that derived from his own improved health and that of his family and the community because of his actions; this may require the individual to recognize that his peers are similarly engaged; and (3) when the health input is realized by an individual's reorganization of the way he meets certain basic physiological needs, such as cooking fish rather than eating it raw, and defecating in a latrine rather than in a field. The cost is the lost utility arising from the period of adjustment to new habits. Of the three possible sources of surplus, only the first involves an explicit trade-off in output; the latter two clearly add to output.

In all three cases the resources are *not only mobilized* but *directly used for health purposes.* An alternative option might be to utilize these resources to generate a marketable output, the revenues from which could then be used to purchase specialized health sector inputs. In most LDCs the latter option is often adopted because the possibility of the former has not been recognized.

The Chinese strategy of self-reliance rests on the assumption that there are a range of health actions that can be taken by individuals or by rudimentarily trained personnel whose primary occupational focus lies outside the health sector. As can be seen in Table 3, many of the fundamental actions required to bring about a dramatic improvement in the health status of a rural peasant population require only a small input from advanced health sector personnel. Many of the major causes of mortality and morbidity at the time of the revolution could be dealt with on a preventive level, with only a minimal level of curative health infrastructure—health centers, hospitals, laboratories, and pharmaceutical supplies. They require improved environmental sanitation, changes in individual behavior with respect to personal hygiene and nutrition, control of certain disease-bearing insects or animals such as dogs, rats, fleas, bedbugs, and mosquitoes, a supply of simple drugs, and the minimal competence necessary to give mass inoculations. As a resource allocational strategy, concentration on mass preventive measures circumvents specialized manpower constraints by rationing their use to managerial and pedagogical purposes.

There is no intention to minimize the role played by the organ-

Table 3.   Selected Major Diseases in China in 1949,
and Chief Means of Attack

Smallpox	Vaccination
Diphtheria	Immunization
Tetanus	Immunization; maternal hygiene
Tuberculosis	Immunization; social improvement; case finding; and chemotherapy
Venereal disease	Social improvement; chemotherapy
Cholera	Environmental sanitation and personal hygiene
Typhoid fever	"
Shigellosis	"
Intestinal parasitism	"
Schistosomiasis	"
Typhus	"
Malaria	Eliminate breeding; kill infected mosquitoes; chemoprophylaxis and therapy

Some Other Problems:

Malnutrition	
Maternal and infant mortality	Social improvement; education; trained
Heart diseases	personnel; and professional facilities
Cancer	
Mental diseases	

ized health sector, for it provides the critical input of an informational transmission mechanism to the peasantry. Most individuals in any society are ignorant of the "technology" of personal health, particularly if it involves the presence of parasitic organisms. This ignorance may inhibit an individual from allocating individual labor and financial resources in a manner that would rationally be in his and his family's self-interest. The individual's behavior must be predicated on his maintaining confidence that such activities are socially and personally significant. Over the long run the organized health sector must convince the people, through visible results, that the technology has tangible benefits.

Promotion of this type of "self-reliance" strategy is predicated on the ability to induce basic changes in an individual's allocation of labor, leisure, and financial resources. A factor of obviously critical importance is the mechanism by which the Chinese were able to mobilize these campaigns (see Robert Chin's paper in this volume, p. 113). Winckler and Skinner noted a cycle in the choice of instruments used for inducing social action.[34] At various points in the cycle there was coercion, mass exhortation and propaganda, and remuneration. The relative emphasis on each of these in the health sector was critically determined by the target group involved. For example, one might have expected that a high degree of coercive pressure was required to achieve the resettlement of large numbers of medical professionals in the rural areas in the late 1960s, as well as for mass agricultural actions.

In concluding this section it should be noted that this type of preventive health strategy is inherently *limited* in its potential impact on the critical disease problems of a community. As one controls the major infectious diseases, the importance of trained personnel, sophisticated drugs, and proper facilities becomes more important—and more costly. Indeed the basic success of these preventive health programs will shift the central health problems to those for which these health sector inputs do become critical. One must point out, however, that success of the preventive health strategy may itself be limited by the degree of development of the curative health infrastructure.

Structural Changes in the Rural Curative Health Strategy

Despite the apparent inequality in allocation of state health funds between the urban and rural areas, the Chinese were nevertheless able to mount a substantial rural preventive health program. The budgetary inequality became most evident with respect to curative health services. Both in terms of manpower and budgetary resources, substantial inequalities on a per capita basis existed prior to 1965, and were not offset by any substantial, sustained effort by the commune to mobilize resources for these services. Indeed such an effort was not likely to have had a major impact given the high cost of curative services prior to the Cultural Revolution. What marks the Cultural Revolution is its impact on lowering this cost and increasing the financial feasibility of such services in rural areas.

The inadequacy of rural health services became apparent during the Cultural Revolution. As mobile medical teams from the urban areas returned from brief stints in the countryside, forums were held to evaluate their experiences. These meetings were peppered with descriptions of the neglect of curative health services for the peasantry. They indicated extreme shortages of funds, equipment, personnel, facilities, and, equally important, an ignorance of the appropriate technology of medical care for use under such constrained circumstances.

For example, the average *hsien* of 300,000 people usually had no more than one major hospital with 100 to 200 beds. Furthermore, even though many communes constructed health centers during the Great Leap Forward, the level and quality of care was often extremely poor, and medical equipment to perform routine examinations was often lacking. Many examinations necessitated long journeys to the *hsien* hospital, journeys often rewarded by possible exacerbations of a patient's illness, loss of working time, and lengthy delays in obtaining both treatment and drugs. Such rewards often proved inadequate to induce people to seek them.[35] Most health centers had inadequate inpatient facilities; chronic understaffing and low quality personnel were common; and many had no doctors. Although most medical graduates were obligated to spend several years in the rural areas, this had only minor impact because of the magnitude of the need and the infrequency of any mobile medical work within the *hsien*. Moreover the most skilled medical graduates were usually sent to the urban areas, and the needs of the urban hospitals were sufficient to attract doctors after their stints in the rural areas.

Medical and pharmaceutical supplies were often unavailable, and even Chinese herbal drugs were frequently in short supply.[36] Many production brigades and teams were not readily accessible even to the commune health center, and this could not be offset, given the limited number of personnel;[37] home visits were infrequent and usually limited to maternity cases.

Perhaps as important as the shortage of funds and services was a basic ignorance of the most efficient and inexpensive means of organizing and treating the health needs of the rural population. An expansion in the level of budgetary support by the government was not likely. The high cost of modern forms of medical technology and medical care organization, in terms of budgetary costs and specialized manpower, was brought home to Chinese health planners after the initial forays of the mobile medical teams.

The modern or "Western" medical educational system transmits a "decision process" for doctors that emphasizes the importance of increasing the probability of the correct diagnosis of a patient's illness by requiring complementary inputs to attain an ever-increasing degree of certainty. Although the normal medical doctor's experience and degree of perception allows for shortcuts and rationalizations of diagnostic and therapeutic procedures, there exists a basic hesitation to synthesize this ability in a way that can be used by lesser-trained personnel. Hence the basic specialization of medical function with low potential for substitutability remains.

Application of this technology under severe budgetary constraints and shortages of these personnel inputs is inherently limited in extent. Modern medical technology would be described by economists as a "fixed-coefficient" technology. For a given output of inpatient and outpatient services it conventionally requires capital, as well as pharmaceutical and specialized personnel inputs organized in a fairly determinate structure.[38] Any substantive improvement in rural health care would thus require technological and organizational adaptations so that these input requirements might be drastically lowered, with as small a loss in the quality of health service as possible. In December 1965 Chinese Minister of Health Ch'in Hsin Chung stated that "we know very little about . . . the way to find medicines and apparatuses which are economical and convenient to use and yield good results."[39]

The absence of curative services engendered both political and economic problems while presenting obstacles to the successful implementation of preventive health policies. As they began to prove successful, the changes in the characteristics of China's disease problems made the absence of curative services more critically apparent. Many childhood diseases went untreated, and the drop in infant mortality allowed more to survive with one or another illness. A critical factor was that unavailability of basic curative services was politically detrimental to the continuing support of the regime by the peasantry. The economic objectives attributed to health policies, whether real or fictitious, were similarly unlikely to be realized in the absence of available medical care.

We define "curative" services in terms of personnel with a basic level of specialization in medical science. This does *not* imply that their health activities are wholly restricted to treatment, for indeed many preventive health measures, particularly for childhood diseases, must be delivered within the framework of curative institutions or by their personnel. This not only relates to their capacity to deliver curative services, but to their ability to work with the target group to help them become receptive to health education:

> It is essential to combine therapeutic and prophylactic measures to emphasize early diagnosis and early treatment at the nearest clinics. Either prevention without treatment or treatment without prevention would be an imperfect method of practice. The chief concern of the parents is the cure of their children's diseases. Once this is obtained, they would be glad to accept suggestions on prophylactic measures and to propagate them consciously among the inhabitants.[40]

The deficiency in the quality of the medical network in China meant that continuous health pressures could not be maintained. Reports during the Cultural Revolution that family health workers and barefoot doctors were fighting "the habit of paying no attention to health work" indicates that a spotlessly clean rural society did not yet exist:

> In the countryside, it has become a new fashion to pay attention to public health, eliminate diseases, do away with all fetishes and superstitions, and change old customs and habits.[41]

The post-1965 reforms in rural curative health care were aimed at remedying this deficiency in curative services.

The Cultural Revolution and its aftermath were frontal attacks on two primary causes of the dysfunctionality of modern medical science in the rural curative health system: (1) The unwillingness of the practitioners of modern medical technology to adapt and compromise this technology, and the organizations within which it is delivered, to the reality of curative services in inadequately equipped and staffed rural health institutions; and (2) the bias in medical and organizational research toward new modes of treatment of more advanced medical problems in a well-equipped setting. The effect of the first was to constrain health planners to a narrow range of options as to the form and substance of the health delivery system. The lag in organizational research on rural health problems retarded the development of those alternative options that could have relieved the inflexibilities of the existing system. The primary characteristic, or potential effect, of the Chinese adaptations since the mid-1960s has been to increase the number of viable policy options open to health planners.

The Rationalization of Medical Technology in China:
The Role of Traditional Medicine and Its Practitioners

Thus far little attention has been paid to the role of the traditional Chinese medical system, a key element in rural curative health services, particularly before 1965. Very quickly after Liberation the critical policy decision was made to support *chung-i*, traditional medicine, as an integral part of the health program. As early as 1944 the Communists had abandoned their previous rejection of traditional medicine as "pre-modern."[42,43] The shortage of Western medical personnel, coupled with the deep-rooted confidence of the peasantry in the efficacy of Chinese medicine, made this decision inevitable:

> Chinese medicine is still the principal strength on which the great masses of our people depend in overcoming disease and maintaining health.[44]

and:

> If traditional Chinese medicine were to be prominently held up by the party as being equal to Western medicine, and used as part of the government medical services, the already existing faith in it should serve as a powerful force to the political advantage of the party and a step forward in healing the cultural wounds of the Chinese people.[45]

An equally important factor was that this was not merely a transitional decision; it would be accompanied by an expansion in the stock of Chinese medical practitioners through the establishment of separate colleges of Chinese medicine. This may have been related to logistical difficulties in training enough Western doctors within ten or twenty years.

The scientific merits of Chinese medicine thus received a political legitimacy that was further reinforced by the establishment of several research institutes in Chinese medicine. Yet throughout the period only partial rapprochement occurred between the two systems, government attempts at integration notwithstanding. As of 1966, Western medical doctors were enrolled in programs of Chinese medicine in order to provide a core of researchers familiar with both systems and capable of providing a firm scientific ground for the yet inexplicable efficacy of acupuncture and of many Chinese herbal cures. The success of this early integrative effort is unclear. The vice-minister of health reported that:

There are some young ones who study Chinese medicine but there are few specialists and professors who do so; there are some practitioners who study it, but there are few among theoreticians; there are people who make a cursory enquiry, but there are few who make a prolonged and systematic study.[46-49]

Although traditional medical practitioners were increasingly "integrated" within the institutional apparatus, this proved to be more of a bureaucratic than a scientific merger. Patients were theoretically given freedom of choice as to which door of the health center they could enter, but this choice was often moot, particularly in rural areas. Moreover, as long as a screen existed between the two technologies neither would benefit from the other, and the result would be an inefficient two-track system of health.

An evaluation of Chinese government policy prior to the Cultural Revolution would therefore have to conclude that traditional medicine's role was more a reflection of its political inviolability and of the lack of any alternative in the rural areas than a component of an evolving unified health system. As put by Ho Cheng, former minister of health, traditional medicine's importance in many eyes

> originated from a temporary viewpoint and for the sake of meeting the present emergency [in the belief] that Western medicine would ultimately replace Chinese medicine.[50]

Although the stock of traditional practitioners in the rural areas was large relative to that of modern doctors, both were primarily concentrated in the major villages. As with the commune health centers, inaccessibility often limited their outreach to the community. Moreover, the price of their services often outstripped the capacity of most peasants' incomes.

Likewise, Chinese medicine as practiced was not sufficient to treat the entire range of rural disease problems. It is quite clear that despite the shakiness of their theoretical underpinnings there were many illnesses for which the use of acupuncture, moxibustion, and traditional herbs could be quite efficacious.[51] Yet the effectiveness of different medical practitioners and the herbs and treatments they prescribed were undoubtedly subject to considerable variation, which was not reduced by the secrecy of individual practitioners that inhibited any free flow of medical information to the body of practitioners at large. To assert that the rural areas were served by a stock of such practitioners does not therefore relate to the breadth and character of the medical services offered.

The Cultural Revolution appears to have accelerated markedly the evolution of an integrative process between the two systems. One observes greater interaction between the two types of medical practitioners at the mobile medical team and health center level. Short training courses in certain areas of modern medicine are offered to rural practitioners by visiting mobile medical teams. At the health centers emphasis is placed on joint diagnosis and treatment, and this effectively offers the traditional doctor further on-the-job training in modern medical procedures. One purported reason for the increased consultative arrangements derives from the political insecurity of both types of practitioners. Because of the ability of patients to file complaints with local party secretaries, one way of spreading the risk is through consultation. [52]

One would expect this increased interaction to have an impact on the quality of medical manpower in the rural areas, and on the suitability of the technology chosen for particular health problems. Encouraging greater examination and research into Chinese medicine and increasing the interaction between the two types of practitioners should lead to the identification of those elements of traditional medicine that can be substituted for comparable modern treatment, with substantial savings in costs. The recognized effect of acupuncture as an anesthetic and for the treatment of certain diseases is an obvious example of a technology that is more practical in a rural setting.

Similarly, a wide range of traditional herbs may have an impact on certain diseases; to the extent that these may be easily cultivated and prepared by commune members, this may be a less expensive and more accessible form of treatment than modern pharmaceuticals. [53,54] Emphasis is placed on Mao's dictum to "inherit and develop the motherland's medical legacy," which is interpreted to mean discarding what proves useless and developing what is effective, regardless of whether the mechanism that explains the effectiveness is known. By encouraging the private and communal cultivation and collection of herbs, the health centers' external financing requirements and dependence on subsidies are effectively lowered, while their capacity to afford other health services is potentially increased. [55] At the brigade level, 85 per cent of prescriptions are for herbal drugs; at the production team level virtually all prescriptions are for traditional herbs.

This interaction contributes to an upgrading of the quality and versatility of traditional practitioners, and to an increase in the efficiency with which they interact with modern rural health services. As their diagnostic capacity and their awareness of the limitations of traditional medicines improve, they will operate more effectively as curative agents and channel the more complicated disease problems to the communal health center:

> The correct attitude toward Chinese doctors should be to ascertain that the unification of Chinese doctors is a long-term policy . . . *because* it is a powerful force in the public health enterprise of our country. In fact, more than half of the urban populace and practically the entire peasantry of our country is still dependent on the existing several hundreds of thousands of Chinese doctors for treatment.[56]

By joint treatment, the traditional doctor also becomes a vehicle for the introduction of modern curative techniques and health education against which there are often many superstitions and taboos. Indeed one could argue that even if partial reliance on traditional medicine is at the expense of better health for a given bundle of resources, its value lies in crucially facilitating the dissemination of modern forms of medical care.

Implementation of this policy has not been without certain strains. The intensified use of herbs was often excessive and not based on scientific tests of effectiveness. When combined with the hasty expansion in the number of barefoot doctors and People's Liberation Army corpsmen, and with quick "cookbook" courses in acupuncture and herbal medicine, there was unquestionable resistance to these curative services in many areas. Chinese medicine is not applicable in all instances, and the experimentation with new herbs often proved unsuccessful. Reports of herbs insufficiently baked or processed, and incorrect applications of acupuncture treatments, have not been uncommon.[57,58]

> The "barefoot doctors" usually treat their patients with medicinal herbs. However, reportedly the patients do not always trust them and have doubts about the efficacy of wild herbs in the treatment of illness.[59]

Conversely, many groups, particularly in urban areas, still reject all traditional medical practices as "unscientific" and "pre-modern."[60,61] Hence it is clear that there are limits to the rate at which integration of the two systems of medicine can be paced to gain general acceptance by some social groups.

Motivating Technological Change:
Medical Technology and Income Distribution

At present, the set of methods of examination and treatment in hospitals is basically unsuitable for the countryside. The method of training doctors is also for the cities. But China has over 500 million people who are peasants.[62]

A second policy development emerging from the Cultural Revolution was a focusing of medical research and the medical school curriculum on the problems of effective delivery of mass health services. On the one hand this represented an attempt to reorient the direction of technological change in both medical science and medical care organization.

In the terminology of economists this argues for technological research and for new criteria that embody: (1) change in output objectives, viz., the prevention and treatment of common rural diseases as opposed to urban illnesses; and (2) a new set of factor price criteria reflecting the high cost of capital and skilled labor inputs. Such adaptations refer not only to new medical science developments that are strictly technological, but to what might be considered organizational adaptations.

On the other hand this development was an attempt to move toward a reallocation of health inputs, within the framework of existing medical knowledge, and toward a new output mix as between the urban and rural sectors. Beyond the need for a reallocation of medical inputs as *between* the rural and urban sectors, it required innovations in existing medical care technology organization and education that involved: (1) rationalization of existing medical knowledge and the priorities in its transmission; (2) a reconsideration of the basis for the functional delineation of responsibilities as between different levels of medical personnel; and (3) a reorganization of the process of health delivery within existing rural health institutions.

The first policy was manifested in an attempt to pressure urban physicians into focusing their research efforts on the problems of the rural areas and to ensure that medical students were oriented to service in these areas. These policies were an attempt to remedy what the Maoists view as the dysfunctional perspectives engendered by the modern medical educational system.

The modern doctor undergoes a rigorous period of training in the most advanced areas of medical knowledge, utilizing the sophisticated medical equipment available in most medical schools. In the absence of complementary capital inputs, these technologies become inapplicable. Hence the doctor immediately has a basic professional resistance to practicing in areas where there are inadequate medical facilities. Adaptation to the rural environment requires a compromise with the standards of quality with which a Western-trained physician is professionally imbued. The character of training required for service without sophisticated resources also differs, in that the doctor must be capable of making quick diagnoses without the benefit of a battery of laboratory tests or diagnostic equipment.

Deep-seated resistance to any delegation of responsibility to nonprofessional practitioners, whether or not traditional doctors, is inherent in the training process. Reliance on Western-trained doctors as the core of a rural medical program can thus immediately narrow the range of allocative options, for they cannot render quality service in sufficient quantity. The policy trade-off is between the benefit from expanded coverage, that is, a greater number of patients treated, as against a lower probability of correct diagnosis and treatment for any given patient.

Similarly, the medical education process induces motivations that are inconsistent with a mass perspective. The technical expertise inherent in the profession, the long periods of schooling, and explicit specialization of functions lead to an elite approach that makes it difficult to communicate easily with the uneducated. As in Western societies, this impels the urban-trained physicians not to settle in rural areas. An outgrowth of the urban-oriented perspective is a paucity of research on the ways in which Western medical techniques can be applied outside the context of well-equipped urban hospitals.

A primary motive for urging doctors to settle in the rural areas of China was to force them to develop a greater awareness of both the character of the disease problems found there and the primitive condition under which such diseases must inevitably be treated. This might be considered an expansion of their awareness of factor price ratios and budget constraints. Mobile medical teams from the urban areas were of necessity forced to devise new techniques based on their rural experiences. Often this involved no more than an exploration into the areas of medical procedure that could be modified without substantial damage to the success of the treatment. Examples of "alternative" technologies included: substituting grass sheds for sterilized rooms; simple tables for operating tables; willow tree branches for swab sticks; kerosene lamps and flashlights where electricity was unavailable; and distilling spring water.

Similarly, research was focused on ascertaining the pathogenic characteristics of the common rural diseases. Ideological factors also motivated greater contact with the peasants and their life styles as a way to weaken the doctors' narrow, elitist class orientation.

A second set of policies attempted to prevent the present generation of medical students from developing the types of dysfunctional medical competence that had characterized their elders. A restructuring of the medical curriculum appears to have occurred, with increased emphasis on clinical work and a shortening of the length of formal courses. The policy statement of the June 26th Commune of Shantung Medical College best exemplifies the reformers' arguments. It involved: (1) the integration of the medical school and teaching hospitals with nearby nursing schools; (2) the establishment of rural branches; (3) the merger of preventive, modern, and traditional medicine; (4) a change in the class composition of the student body, with increased emphasis on peasant youth recruitment and their return to rural areas; and (5) reduction in training from five to three years.[63] Medical and pharmaceutical courses were shortened by half, and an expanded part of the training was to be taken with mobile medical units. Whether these reforms have been instituted in all the country's medical schools is not clear.

Implicit in Chinese policy is a theoretical perspective on the way technology and class interest interact. For example, one could view these policies narrowly, as an attempt to expand available technologies in a labor-intensive direction, and to increase the capacity of the medical educational plant to produce physicians who are able and willing to use different techniques at existing wage rates. The goal appears to be to expand the capacity of the health system, at a given budgetary level, to handle the magnitude of rural health problems by reducing the average cost of treatment.[64,65]

Yet this policy shift is not without cost. If there is a reduction in the quality of medical education or of the student body, many advanced modern technologies will be neglected and the professional competence of Chinese medical personnel weakened. This would presumably be reflected in a deterioration in the quality of available medical care. Similarly, the reorientation of research will retard the development of Chinese research relative to that of the West.[66] Whether it is necessary to bear this cost depends on whether it is possible to continue to train modern-style physicians at *past* levels of quality and still ensure that they make the adaptations necessary to deliver the desired quality of medical services. Recent Chinese policies suggest a rejection of this possibility. Although more rigorous and better quality training *will* allow a physician to make the adaptations to rural conditions with a *smaller* loss of quality, the training will also instill in him a value system that substantially resists making such compromises or settling in rural areas under present conditions of poverty. The technology implicit in the medical education process cannot be separated from the range of income distributional outcomes that this technology renders probable. If one rejects the distributional effects of high quality training, one must accept a less rigorous, more practical educational process. The best that can be hoped for of the *current* stock of urban physicians is some resettlement and a more detailed focus on developing new cures for the health problems of the rural areas. On the other hand, an emphasis on seeking medical students with peasant roots reflects an attempt to ensure that their perspective will be correctly focused.

> To make health work strike root in rural areas, greatest attention must be paid to the training of rural medicine workers not detached from agricultural production . . . of desirable family background, ideologically sound, having certain cultural levels . . . *not* detached from production, [they] live among masses, can easily perform mass work.[67]

Future medical graduates will thus be able to deal better with rural medical problems.

What remains to be evaluated is the advisability of trading off quantity for quality in the training of modern doctors. This was only one aspect of a larger trade-off between quality and quantity in the delivery of health services implicit in the entire range of technological and organizational changes proposed after the Cultural Revolution. Yet the issue of optimization of resource utilization must be separated from optimization of output. Given the status quo it is extremely difficult to judge scientifically whether a greater quantity of lower quality medical services will have a positive or negative impact on either the Chinese economy or the health status of the bulk of the population.* The policy chosen also reflects income distributional issues subject to the broader mandates of political and ideological policy. Given a decision on this larger issue we must then judge alternative organizational strategies in terms of their relative impact on policy objectives.

Even with a quantity-oriented goal system there remain important arguments *against* a dilution of the quality of medical graduates. The "individualistic" argument was aptly expressed at the Canton forum of mobile medical teams that had returned from the rural areas. They argued that

> without proper medical instruments and equipment, teaching and study cannot be carried out, and at most you will reach a level equivalent to part-time rural medical workers and you will not be counted as university graduates when you finish your studies.[68]

Moreover, to the extent that a policy of quality dilution is adopted in all of the nation's medical schools it will have serious dynamic implications for the future quality of the Chinese medical system. In the same way that the success of past preventive policies led to their present insufficiency, the success of present curative policies may lead to greater requirements for sophisticated medical expertise. Hence the Chinese should be concerned with the impact of present policies on their future options. In a quantity-oriented system, with a broad base of semiskilled health workers at the first

---

* For those more versed in economic terminology, one can specify the following functional relationships that reflect the nature of the quality-quantity trade-off in political and economic terms. First, let health $= f$ (quality of health care, x_1, x_2, x_3, . . . x_n) where x_1, . . . x_n are a range of possible environmental and physical factors. Let cost $= g$ (quality of health care, y_1, y_2, . . . y_n). Let individual productivity $= h$ (health, z_1, z_2 . . . z_n). Let us hold all vectors x, y, z fixed. If h', $f' > 0$ and h'', $f'' < 0$, and $g' > 0$, $g'' > 0$, then for a given cost it might be important, in terms of productivity, to provide a greater quantity of low quality health than vice versa. If there is a diminishing marginal utility to better health, this is reinforced from a political point of view. If, however, different groups have different vectors of associated factors, particularly the level of capital equipment in h( ), the economic argument is weakened.

level of treatment, it may be crucial to have high quality modern doctors at the apex for treatment, education, and management.

The significance of this trade-off also depends on the character of the rationalizing process in medical education. If it involves no more than a trimming of the truly superfluous or marginal elements, then the loss in qualitative effect may be small. Furthermore, the Maoists have argued that "one must solve the problem as to what purpose one should raise one's skill," and the "M.D.'s should not remain in urban areas to 'add flowers to embroidery'."[69] Finally, to the extent that the previous arguments on the negative ideological impact of a high quality education are correct, they may provide further support for the "quantity" arguments.

Organizational Adaptations: Resource Reallocation between Urban and Rural Areas

There were two phases to the reallocation of urban medical personnel to the rural areas. The publication of Mao's famous directive to right the urban-rural imbalance[70] led initially to the formation of mobile medical teams, ideally composed of a representative cross section of urban medical personnel. These toured the rural areas for one to three months and were expected to remedy the deficiencies in rural curative and preventive care while correcting their own ideological perspectives, both as to class interest and medical focus. Base camps were set up for one or two weeks in the major villages of a county. While some team members held clinics and training sessions for barefoot doctors and family medical workers, the others traveled to outlying towns for two- to three-day clinics. The doctors were also expected to assist the health departments of each commune in the operation and development of their "cooperative medical service."[71]

At the same time it was hoped that the doctors would receive ideological education from the peasants and party cadres, thus involving them in "serious class struggle" and effecting a "revolutionization" in their ranks.[72] At any one time it was expected that one-third of urban medical personnel would be moved to the rural areas. Both Western-trained and traditional doctors were presumably included in these teams and training sessions involved the interchange of basic techniques of both types of medicine (see the next section of this paper).[73]

For example, a reported 1,000 doctors, nurses, pharmacists, and chemists left Shantung; fifty medical workers left Hupeh; 150 doctors and nurses left Shanghai; 3,000 doctors left Szechuan. Overall, in 1965, 165,000 city doctors and other medical personnel were reported to have formed 10,000 mobile medical teams that went to the rural area.[74] As a component of the strategies of aiding the rural areas and reorienting the medical workers, this undoubtedly required both ideological and coercive pressures, due to the relatively elitist composition of most of the mobile teams.

The resistance of the medical educational system to these assignments may be gleaned from the nature of the criticisms directed at them as late as 1970 by students at various medical colleges.[75] The resistance proved particularly deep, extending to the vested urban party interests. It became apparent that the proposed mobilization of one-third of urban medical workers was often unrealized in many rural areas of China. Lower-level personnel were often promoted to the rank of "doctors," the least competent doctors were often assigned to the teams, and the length of rural stay was often shortened in order to prevent the deterioration of the urban medical corps. Moreover the effectiveness of the tours in terms of their various objectives was often vitiated by their short duration. In one month "we cannot even see clearly the places; we cannot accomplish the rural health work . . . Three months is better, but doesn't help us much in ideological reform."[76]

By 1967 there had been a shift in policy geared toward the gradual resettlement of one-third of urban medical personnel. Over the last several years there have been many reports of large numbers of physicians being forced to settle permanently in rural areas.[77,78] Although such resettlement does seem to be occurring, a lack of statistics prevents any assertion on either the magnitude, extensiveness, or degree of permanency of this change. The permanent settlement policy is undoubtedly aimed specifically at new medical graduates, so that over time there may be a gradual convergence to an optimal distribution. The major rationale for the emphasis on admitting medical cadres from the peasantry into medical schools is a reflection of the difficulties and resistance encountered in transferring urban-oriented personnel.[79]

Negatively, the reallocation policy *may* have affected the quality of urban health services, depending on which health services were reduced and on the substitutions in paramedical staffing that were made within and between urban health institutions. In some cases the policy has led to urban training courses comparable to those in rural areas in order to replenish the stock of health workers. In Shanghai, for example, industrial workers were given short courses in medicine in order to replace health workers transferred to the communes. In 1969 there were reports of shortages of urban doctors and personnel, which led to: (1) a reduction in services and the level of care in hospitals, sanitoria, rest homes, and special clinics; and (2) an increased sharing of responsibility by medical personnel —nurses doing diagnoses and giving treatment, workers performing nursing functions, etc.[80]

The Reorganization of the Delivery System of Rural Curative Health Services

Perhaps the most important set of policy innovations that occurred after 1965 related to the expansion in financing and physical accessibility of curative services in the rural areas. They constituted an attempt to expand rapidly the supply of medical manpower to, and the facilities in, these areas. For their success they had to overcome several critical bottlenecks. First, there was a supply bottleneck in terms of the capacity of medical manpower training institutions to accelerate their production of medical auxiliaries. Second, the manpower had to be effectively integrated within the existing health system in order to assure a more effective rationing of skilled medical resources. Third, additional resources were required to finance both the construction of basic-level health stations and, more important, their operating costs.

Prior to 1965 the provision of rural health services was fragmented among the commune health centers, the *hsien* hospitals, private clinics, and traditional medical practitioners. The *hsien* hospitals were at the top of the health pyramid. In size they ranged from thirty to 300 beds, and they usually had the equipment and staff to handle more advanced medical problems. Their staff generally included specialists in internal medicine, obstetrics, preventive medicine, pediatrics, traditional Chinese medicine, pharmacology, and radiology.[81,82]

Theoretically the *hsien* hospital served two primary functions. Since it was usually located in the major population center of the *hsien* it provided outpatient services for the community. Second, and more important, it served as the final medical referral point for the entire *hsien* population. One would therefore expect inpatient services to have been rationed to those individuals with illnesses requiring the sophisticated medical skills available only at this level. Yet this rationing could occur successfully only if there existed a set of local curative health institutions with sufficient capacity to absorb a large proportion of the basic demand for health services. Such a primary health care system was nonexistent until 1958.

Prior to 1958 access to curative services was not a function of the degree of medical need, but more of financial status and physical proximity to the *hsien* hospital's outpatient clinic. Hence the pool of patients that reached the outpatient clinic was not subject to a rationing process. This was compounded by the congestion at the clinics arising from their incapacity to process the existing level of demand. The inaccessibility problem was not affected by the presence of traditional practitioners in that they also tended to be located in the major villages and their fees were often prohibitively expensive.

At the time of the Great Leap Forward the commune health systems emerged in a flurry of capital construction and communization. Health centers and "medical rooms" were constructed at the commune and production brigade levels, respectively. The former became the focal point of most curative services for the commune's population, while the latter served primarily as a first-aid clinic. The health center was usually staffed by a graduate of a regular medical school and one or two "middle doctors," graduates of medical secondary schools and comparable to the medical auxiliaries found in many LDCs, and several untrained nurses who served effectively as apprentices to the doctors.[83]

Often the commune established a cooperative medical system to finance the health center's activities, and it was this system that provided the model for those adopted after 1965. Access to this health system was available to nearly all commune members. Each individual paid annual dues of 1 to 3 *yüan*, and a matching contribution of 10 *fen* was paid by his production brigade's collective welfare fund. In addition, a token registration fee of 5 *fen* was often required for each visit. In most instances these fees covered all treatment and medicine.

Those in serious illness [would] stay in [the] hospital and 60 per cent of the charge for medicine would be paid from the brigade account.

> For those who suffer from chronic ailments and frequently using medicine, 50 per cent of the charge for medicine is to be paid by themselves. [84]

Thus the system was potentially self-financing at the commune level, which could imply that the government was able to shift the fiscal burden of these costs downward.

By 1965 the commune health systems were still inadequate to deal with the basic problem of the unavailability of curative health services in the rural areas. Many communes had either not constructed primary health centers or had not provided sufficient financial support to sustain them. In 1961 Vice-Minister of Health Hu Yun-pei noted that:

> The organization of public health in the villages is the general wish of all commune members. It is hoped that this system will be gradually introduced, and that each locality will take positive measures in this direction. [85]

Even in those communes with fully operative centers, their outreach was primarily localized to the immediate commune village area. At the production brigade and team levels, health services were often inaccessible. Long distances proved to be sufficient deterrents for many peasants in the outlying areas of the commune. Lengthy queues, inadequate equipment, and shortages of drugs were additional obstacles to the effective diagnosis and treatment of those who did seek out these services. The lack of any formal screening process at the health center level further exacerbated the basic shortage of trained personnel.

The resulting output of services did not therefore meet the most important medical problems. Trained personnel often found their time poorly spent in screening cases that could have been dealt with by less skilled personnel. The physical inaccessibility of the system implied that many sick peasants never reached the health center. The same type of congestion and inefficiency in the allocation of skilled medical resources observed at the *hsien* hospital level was also to be found at the commune level.

There were four primary aspects to the post-1965 new curative health policy: (1) further decentralization of health institutions at the family, production team, and production brigade levels; (2) use of mobile medical teams to provide a linkage mechanism with these institutions and the health center; (3) reorganization of the delivery process *within* the commune health center; and (4) rapid expansion in the capacity to train a corps of semiskilled medical personnel—the so-called barefoot or peasant doctor—to staff these new facilities. Also involved were policies relating to the cultivation of traditional herbs, the increasing integration of traditional and Western practitioners, and the merger of curative and preventive activities. These changes were introduced on an experimental basis in 1966, and by 1968 they had become a firmly established policy. As reported by Radio Yunnan in July 1969: "The system should now be established in places which have not yet adopted it."[86]

The core of the reforms lay in the establishment of brigade health stations and "red medical" (herbal) rooms at the production brigade and team levels, respectively. The former now became the primary curative unit in the new rural medical system, with the latter serving as a first-aid dispensary. Each health station was to be staffed by at least two part-time peasant doctors and two midwives. Thus for a large proportion of the commune's population the health center was transformed from a primary to a secondary referral institution. The brigade health stations were expected to be readily available screening mechanisms to screen out cases that could be handled quickly and easily by semiskilled medical personnel. Moreover, by locating them at the grass-roots level, peasant doctors would be in a position both physically and socially to actively identify those in medical need who were reluctant to utilize the health service. They could also serve as instruments for social control and education with respect to various preventive activities, family planning, nutrition, and environmental sanitation. "Peasant doctors," for example, would receive training in the insertion of intrauterine devices.

The rationale for this should be apparent. By adding an additional base of medical services, a preliminary screening and treatment mechanism was created. Simultaneously, scarce medical resources could be rationed to those with medical problems for which no lower-cost or lesser-skilled substitute existed. The bulk of curative problems could for the first time be diagnosed and treated. One could not argue that the "quality" of health care was negatively affected by these peasant doctors, because for many peasants they represented the first set of curative services that had ever been effectively available. Those for whom access had not previously been a problem were not legally bound to consult the peasant doctor first. Indeed the peasant doctor's services were contingent on the general support of his production brigade.

The success of this strategy hinged on: (1) whether the Chinese could in a short period of time create a corps of medical workers capable of meeting a large proportion of the rural population's curative needs; and (2) whether the peasant doctors could gain the confidence of the population. They had to be able to distinguish those diseases that could and could not be treated at the brigade level. For the former their treatment had to be relatively effective; for the latter they had to assure that the referral process would actually operate. The training process had thus to provide the peasant doctor with a basic core of skills necessary to satisfy both objectives. The confidence factor would yield a critical momentum that could either support or undermine the viability of the decentralized program. Conversely, a narrow capacity to treat problems would not prevent congestion at a higher referral level.

The creation of this corps of medical manpower was fundamentally intertwined with many of the policies of the Cultural Revolution discussed earlier. Some urban doctors on mobile medical teams were expected to double as medical educators. They were to develop on-the-job training courses that would, within the span of three or four months, provide a basic core of relevant medical skills to a group of secondary school peasant youths chosen by individual production brigades. Thus the process of training was initially distinct from ongoing medical training institutes, and was integrated as much as possible with the actual process of rural health delivery. The course regimen has been aptly described by Joshua Horn:

> For the first two weeks they studied anatomy and physiology, dissected pigs, and attended lectures illustrated by models and lantern slides. After this introductory course they learned the elements of bacteriology and pathology in the mornings and clinical medicine and hygiene in the afternoons. They learnt to identify germs in contaminated water and to recognize the eggs of worm parasites in excreta. They learnt how to make drinking water safe, how to treat nightsoil, how to sterilize needles and syringes, and how to give injections. They learnt how infectious diseases are spread and how to diagnose them. They accompanied their teacher-doctors on their rounds, learnt the use of the stethoscope, how to take a medical history, how to diagnose common diseases, and how to detect the signs of serious ill-

ness. They examined patients who came to the clinic and discussed their findings with the doctor in charge. They concentrated on a few diseases commonly seen in the neighborhood, and on the use and dosage of some forty drugs. They memorized fifty acupuncture points and the symptom complexes which they control, and they practiced the technique of acupuncture. Each student was issued with a well illustrated book specially written for peasant doctors. [87]

The barefoot doctor's first period of training was therefore intended to provide the minimum threshold of skills required to perform curative services effectively. In subsequent years he or she would be able to return to these training "clinics" in order to obtain a more thorough theoretical underpinning for his curative skills. For example, Horn notes that

> . . . last year, they studied anatomy and physiology as a whole in a short, concentrated, superficial course. This year, they are re-studying it in relation to diseases of particular organs . . . last year they studied only commonly seen diseases, but this year they systematically study all the diseases of particular organs. [88]

It should be noted that the content and duration of these courses exhibited considerable variability throughout China, particularly in the period directly after the Cultural Revolution. [89-91] Some reports indicated that peasant doctors were being trained at medical secondary schools or at separate joint farming-study departments within the medical colleges. [92,93] They were aided by medical handbooks on the uses of herbs and on the symptoms and treatment of a range of common diseases.

The cost of training was minimized by scheduling the courses during the slack season in agriculture, thereby not impinging on the size of the brigade's work force. The cost of teaching personnel was lowered by combining the teaching and curative responsibilities of the mobile medical teams as much as possible. Clinical teaching occurred at the commune health center. The trainees and the community provided the labor to construct primitive dormitory facilities.

The risks involved in sole reliance on this corps of hastily trained personnel were lowered through the elaboration of a linkage mechanism between the peasant doctor in the field, the trained professional medical personnel at the commune health center, and the urban mobile medical teams. Brigade health stations were linked by telephone to the commune health center, ensuring both a viable backup system for critical cases and the provision of guidance to the peasant doctors. Mobile medical teams made regular visits to each production brigade, thus providing an additional source of medical education to the peasant doctor.

This type of organizational structure struck at the goal of integrating agricultural production and health. At the brigade level the peasant doctor divided his time between agriculture and medicine; often he was fully employed in agriculture and performed his medical duties in his free time. For this reason the "political" criteria underlying the brigade's choice of those who were to be trained as barefoot doctors reflected their degree of social dedication and communal spirit. If the peasant doctor found that he required more time for his medical duties, his brigade allocated work points for this service. What is important is that these were indeed peasant doctors engaged at least part time in agricultural activities. Their training periods were spaced over several years and occurred during the slack agricultural periods, so that the cost to the brigade of preparing these medical personnel was not excessive. Where work points were allocated, this reflected a communal decision that could be changed if it was felt that the peasant doctor's services were not sufficient or that he was unqualified. At the production team level, family health workers were full-time agricultural workers. Hence these reforms represented a net addition of health services at the commune level, with the financial burden clearly thrust upon the brigade collectively, rather than on the commune, *hsien*, or state.[94]

The brigade health rooms were constructed with brigade funds, although abandoned buildings were frequently repaired to serve this function. The continued emphasis on the use of traditional herbs likewise implies that only a minimal amount of health supplies need be purchased externally.[95] Similarly, emphasis was placed upon treating diseases at the point where costs were minimal, given the differential cost of treatment at the health center, brigade room, and hospital. The fiscal burden for treating minor ailments was therefore transferred to the brigade level, thus expanding the level of resources the total community expended on health.

An "antiregularization" campaign has been waged to prevent commune hospitals from becoming mirror images of the county and urban hospitals, reflecting more efficient allocation of staff resources and greater responsiveness to the needs of the peasantry.[96] The campaign manifested itself in a reduction in specialization, a simplification of bureaucratic procedures, economies in laboratory work, and more mobile medical activities. At the Chin Yuan *hsien* hospital, for example, the five windows for registration, medical histories, cost estimations, payments, and dispensing of medications were merged into two; likewise the departments of internal medicine, surgery, pediatrics, gynecology, and the "five organs" were merged into internal medicine, surgery, and gynecology-obstetrics.[97] The pressure toward rationalization may also have been motivated by the abuses observed in the earlier system, such as multiple visits to both Chinese and Western-type doctors, overuse of drugs, etc.[98]

Perspectives on Curative Health Reforms in Rural China

There is considerable theoretical attraction to the basic thrust of the changes made in the rural curative health system. Given the apparent resource bottlenecks to providing these services within the existing technological framework, one observes a search for ways to expand the substitutability of less costly methods of providing a given health output. By rationing access to more expensive and better qualified personnel on the basis of relative need, and by creating new categories of health manpower, one may reduce the quantity of highly qualified medical personnel from that which has been *applied* to the minimum *required* for a particular medical problem. Less urgent problems are caught at an earlier stage by health workers with a level of competence sufficient to treat them. Congestion at the health center level is lessened, and the capacity of the overall system is enlarged. The cost rises with the possible "misdiagnosed case" that is not properly channeled to the higher level, and the increased "time" cost to the seriously ill patient who must be reexamined several times.

Likewise, innovations or adaptations in equipment and drugs required may prevent them from serving as bottlenecks to the use of lesser-skilled personnel. Again the question becomes one of expanding the capacity of the health system, reducing queueing and congestion, and economizing on skilled resources at the cost of a loss in the quality of health care.

The second attractive adaptation is an economical use of the state's budgetary resources allocated to those health programs—curative, preventive, and research—for which there is limited effective substitutability of private for public action. Hence the state must either be actively involved or assure that the private sector—the communes—can adequately meet the level of demand. The role of the state involves: (1) provision of inputs to the lower levels —production of Western medicines, and training of certain types of health personnel; (2) the fostering of research in new medical technologies; (3) implementation of mass preventive campaigns for which interregional coordination is necessary; and (4) provision of more advanced curative services. By shifting the burden of basic health provision and financing to the private sector, the state may allocate more of its scarce budgetary resources to those health programs with broad national benefits.

What remains unclear is whether these substitutions are occurring and whether they are technologically feasible, effective, and socially acceptable. For example, in those rural areas where physical or financial obstacles prevented access to the communal health center for anything but major illnesses, the availability of the barefoot doctor was probably a positive change. If he proved ineffective there was minimal loss relative to the status quo. But in areas where the health center outpatient department was accessible, did one find that the barefoot doctor was ignored and ineffective? The reports emerging seem to indicate that this was not a problem.[99] Have the Chinese developed a mechanism to ration access to health center personnel? What effect does a lack of confidence in the barefoot doctor have on the peasants' acceptance of other preventive, health-related actions proposed by the political cadres and the government?

What is the proper strategy in developing a cadre of minimally skilled medical corpsmen who will be accepted by the rural masses? The Chinese opted for a rapid buildup with an upgrading according to skill over time through on-the-job clinical experience and two- to three-month classes annually. The cost is that the corps of barefoot doctors may often be insufficiently trained *initially*, which breeds a resistance by the masses that may be difficult to overcome at a later stage. The alternative strategy, the slow development of cadres with a specified standard of competence, trades off the provision of health care at the present time for a higher probability of popular acceptance.

What is the nature of the interaction between the medical cadres and the skilled medical personnel at the health center level? How are their activities functionally delineated? Are the barefoot doctors competent enough to know the limitations of their training and the points at which referral is critical? Is there adequate potential at the apex of the system to receive the referral flow? The lower the level of skill at the base, the less impact the decentralization will have on reducing congestion at the apex. Further, the extensive reliance on traditional medicine, primarily for budgetary reasons, means that there are limits to the range of disease problems that the barefoot doctors can treat. Certain preventive and curative actions by necessity require Western drugs or Western medical skills. Are these nonsubstitutable inputs being supplied through the mechanism of mobile medical teams?

For the Western scholar these unanswered questions are at the heart of any final evaluation of the desirability of transferring the Chinese adaptations to other LDCs.

The Chinese Gift to LDC Health Planners: An Existence Theorem

Beyond curiosity, a major motivation for this study was to determine whether the Chinese have developed a viable, alternative health strategy of immediate relevance to other LDCs. What fresh insights into the problems of health delivery and disease prevention may be gleaned from the Chinese experiment? While we do believe that the Chinese have utilized a basically different strategy—its uniqueness being left unsettled—its transferability is far less clear.

There are three primary characteristics of the Chinese strategy. First, there is an extensive and successful reliance on a variety of measures, voluntary or coercive, for inducing social and individual behavioral actions in support of national policies, including health. The strategy not only increases the level of social resources allocated to health but provides an efficient means of striking at some of the roots of China's disease problems. These instruments appear to be a fundamental aspect of the *overall* process of development in China; whether they can be applied *piecemeal* for health alone remains unclear.

Complementary to this is the degree of priority attached to "red" over "expert," and the willingness to maintain this dominance by coercion. It seems probable that the Chinese will be able to fundamentally reorient the technicians toward adapting their technology to the "for whom" of the health problem. In most LDCs the insufficiency of resources for an adequate program, under the existing technology of health delivery, is obvious. Yet the ability of the system to compromise on this technology is thwarted by the attitude of its practitioners. This is not to argue that the Chinese alternative is wholly successful; the probability is much higher that it will evolve towards a more effective solution.

Second, problems have arisen in China from an unbalanced strategy with respect to preventive and curative health services. The insufficiency of resources for the latter in the rural sector weakened the impact of the fundamentally innovative reforms on the preventive level. The Cultural Revolution in health reflected an attempt to remedy this imbalance, to provide the complement of curative services. The implication is that, in the absence of an ability to make adaptations on the curative level, other LDCs will find there are limits to the impact of preventive measures on the health status of their populations.

On the other hand, if in 1950 the Chinese had attacked their curative health problems with the zeal of the post-1965 period, it is not clear whether this would have had as much of a substantive impact. It may have required the earlier period of preventive health action as a precondition for the delivery of these services with an *effective* impact. It would always have had some impact, but whether it would have been no more than a "finger in the dike" effect is not clear.

Third, the Chinese were blessed with a medical legacy at a demonstrated level of effectiveness, and a substantial stock of practitioners to deliver it. Although there are limits to its applicability, there existed a large stock of "medical" manpower in which the masses had a high degree of confidence. The "modern medicine demonstration" effect had not yet permeated the value system of the mass of the peasantry so as to render these practitioners suspect and untrustworthy. Moreover, the pharmaceutical base of the traditional technology was relatively inexpensive and did not constrain the operation of the system. This is not a wholly unique legacy, in that most LDCs are "blessed" with comparable groups of practitioners. Are their technologies viable, and can they be incorporated as instruments of an integrated health delivery system? If not, China's traditional technology could conceivably be exported to other LDCs. Its acceptability by the masses and by the Western health care system is more questionable.

The curative adaptations are no less transferable. Indeed the theoretical role of the "medical auxiliary" in East Africa and other areas is remarkably similar to that of the barefoot doctor. Handbooks on the diagnosis and treatment of the common diseases are equally available. What often constrains these other systems is the mode of financing the health service and the training costs of the medical auxiliary. These financially constrain both the capacity of the system to expand its stock of nonmedical personnel and its ability to support their recurrent cost requirements. By pushing for a cooperative, self-financing medical system that draws on part-time agricultural effort, the financial barrier has been mitigated in China. By emphasizing a gradual upgrading of quality and extensive on-the-job training, the cost of preparation has been lessened.

A final reflection that emerges from this study is that the capacity to introduce severe "shocks" into the operational system is critically important. Such shocks can prevent ossification of the system and insure that it remains responsive to the needs on which its existence is predicated. The post-1965 reforms in health were attempts at effecting such a jolt to a health system that was inappropriate to the needs of the mass of the population. This type of periodic jolt has substantial short-run costs and is susceptible to substantial resistances. It may be what is necessary, however, to prevent the system from deviating from the optimal path. To insist that this is indeed a prerequisite to a structural reform of health policies in an LDC is perhaps to be overly pessimistic. While many adaptations of details can be transferred without the need for a "jolt," to exert major structural changes in such key areas as budgetary and skilled manpower allocations may indeed require such "jolts" to the system.

NOTES

1. John Bryant, *Health and the Developing World* (Ithaca: Cornell University Press, 1969): pp. 1–55.

2. Chang K'ai, "Health Work Makes Big Strides in the Service of Industrial and Agricultural Production," *Kuang-ming Jih-pao* (October 6, 1964), in *Joint Publications Research Service* no. 28543 (January 29, 1965).

3. Feng P'ei-chih, "The Dialectic Relationship of Ethics, Intelligence, and Health," *Kuang-ming Jih-pao*, in *Joint Publications Research Service*, no. 33312 (December 14, 1965).

4. Marie Sieh, "Medicine in China: Wealth for the State," *Current Scene* III, no. 5–6 (October 15–November 1, 1964).

5. S. Rifkin and R. Kaplinsky, "Health Strategy and Development Planning: Lessons from the People's Republic of China" (University of Sussex, Science Policy Research Unit, December 1971).

6. "Strengthen Medical and Health Work in the Rural Areas," *Union Research Service* 40, no. 19 (September 3, 1965): 273–86.

7. Janet Salaff, "Social Mobilization and Public Health in Communist China," in Kingsley Davis, ed., *Essays in Comparative Demography* (Berkeley: University of California Press, in press): p. 15.

8. R. M. Worth, "Health in Rural China: From Village to Commune," *American Journal of Hygiene* 77, no. 3 (May 1963): 228–39.

9. People's Republic of China, State Statistical Bureau, *Ten Great Years* (Peking: Foreign Languages Press, 1960): p. 8.

10. A. G. Ashbrook, "China: Economic Policies and Economic Results, 1949–71," in *People's Republic of China: An Economic Assessment*, Joint Economic Committee, United States Congress (Washington, D. C.: Government Printing Office, 1972).

11. International Bank for Reconstruction and Development, *World Tables 1968*, Mimeographed (Washington, D. C., 1970).

12. "Public Health Developments—Continued Focus on the Farms," *Current Scene* XII, no. 24 (December 15, 1969): 1–12.

13. "Medicine in the Villages," *China News Analysis* no. 602 (March 4, 1966).

14. "The Mao-Liu Controversy over Rural Public Health," *Current Scene* VII, no. 2 (June 15, 1969).

15. Chang Tze-k'uan, "The Development of Hospital Services in China," *Chinese Medical Journal* 84 (June 1965): 412–16.

16. "Canton Forum of Medical Personnel on Tour in Rural Areas," *Union Research Service* 49, no. 22 (December 15, 1967): 289–303.

17. "Health Work Makes Big Strides in the Service of Industrial and Agricultural Production," and "Minister of Health Reports on China's 15 Years of Achievements in Health Activities," *Joint Publications Research Service* no. 28543 (January 29, 1965): 25–46.

18. "An Experimental Study on the Organization of Urban Child Health Sources," *Chinese Medical Journal* 84, no. 9 (September 1965): 563–70.

19. Leo A. Orleans and Richard P. Suttmeier, "The Mao Ethic and Environmental Quality," *Science* 170, no. 3963 (December 11, 1970): 1173–76.

20. Salaff, "Social Mobilization and Public Health."

21. "Public Health Developments."

22. "Recent Developments in Medicine and Public Health Work," *Union Research Service* 32, no. 11 (August 6, 1963).

23. Li T. C., "Ten Years of Public Health Work in New China," *Chinese Medical Journal* 79 (December 1959): 483–88.

24. "Recent Developments in Medicine."

25. Worth, "Health in Rural China."

26. Salaff, "Social Mobilization and Public Health."

27. Ralph Andreano, "Farewell to the God of Plague: The Economic Impact of Parasitic Disease (Schistosomiasis) in Mainland China," *Health Economics Research Center, Research Report No. 3* (University of Wisconsin: Department of Economics, 1972).

28. ————, "More on the God of the Plague: Schistosomiasis in Mainland China," *Health Economics Research Center, Research Report No. 7* (University of Wisconsin: Department of Economics, 1972).

29. Salaff, "Social Mobilization and Public Health."

30. C. S. Den, "Success of Patriotic Health Movement for 1958," *Journal of Microbiology, Epidemiology, and Immunobiology* 30, no. 10 (October 1959): 17–22.

31. "Schistosomiasis under Control in Fukien Province," *Joint Publications Research Service* no. 39411 (January 4, 1967): 137.

32. "The Elimination of Schistosomiasis," *Union Research Service* 62, no. 3 (January 8, 1971): 30–44.

33. Rifkin and Kaplinsky, "Health Strategy and Development Planning."

34. G. William Skinner and Edwin A. Winckler, "Compliance Succession in Rural Communist China: A Cyclical Theory," in Amitai Etzioni, ed., *Complex Organizations, A Sociological Reader*, 2nd ed. (New York: Prentice-Hall, 1969).

35. "Canton Forum of Medical Personnel."

36. "Health," *China News Analysis* no. 365 (March 24, 1961).

37. "Canton Forum of Medical Personnel."

38. Bryant, *Health and the Developing World.*

39. "Mao's Revolution in Public Health," *Current Scene* VI, no. 7 (May 1, 1968): 5.

40. "An Experimental Study on Child Health Sources."

41. "The Elimination of Schistosomiasis."

42. John Z. Bowers, "Medicine in Mainland China: Red and Rural," *Current Scene* VIII, no. 12 (June 15, 1970).

43. Ralph C. Croizier, *Traditional Medicine in Modern China* (Cambridge: Harvard University Press, 1968).

44. "5,000 Western Doctors Will Systematically Study Chinese Medicine This Year," *Union Research Service* 3, no. 20 (June 8, 1956): 277–78.

45. R. M. Worth, "Strategy of Change in the People's Republic of China: The Rural Health Center," in Daniel Lerner and Wilbur Schramm, eds., *Communication and Change in the Developing Countries* (Honolulu: East-West Center, 1967).

46. "Health."

47. "Training in Medicine," *China News Analysis* no. 577 (August 20, 1965): 6–7.

48. "5,000 Western Doctors Will Study."

49. "Medical Services in the Countryside," *Union Research Service* 58, no. 21 (March 13, 1970): 294–309.

50. Ho Cheng, "Examination of My Mistaken Thinking in Health Work," *Union Research Service* 3, no. 30 (June 9, 1956): 280–86.

51. Stephen Palos, *The Chinese Art of Healing* (New York: Herder and Herder, 1972).

52. Worth, "Strategy of Change."

53. "Develop Rural Medicine and Health Services from the Viewpoint of War Preparedness," *Selections from China Mainland Magazines* no. 5 (September 8 and 15, 1970): 689–90.

54. "Medical Services in the Countryside."

55. *Selections from China Mainland Magazines* no. 21 (March 13, 1970): 294–309.

56. "5,000 Western Doctors Will Study."

57. "Medical Service in Rural Areas: Party Policy on Traditional Medicine Reviewed," and other articles on traditional medicine, *Joint Publications Research Service* no. 43903 (January 8, 1968): 160–77.

58. "Chinese Traditional Medicine and Western Traditional Medicine," *Union Research Service* 63, no. 25 (June 25, 1971): 341–55.

59. "Medical Personnel Work and Train 'Bare-Foot' Doctors in the Countryside," *Union Research Service* 61, no. 26 (December 29, 1970): 349–62.

60. Croizier, *Traditional Medicine in Modern China.*

61. "PLA Medical Health Units Serve Rural Areas," *Federal Broadcast Information Service* (June 26, 1969): B1–3.

62. "Canton Forum of Medical Personnel."

63. Janet Salaff, "China's Medicine: Physician Heal Thyself," *Far Eastern Economic Review* 62, no. 44 (October 31, 1968): 292.

64. Bowers, "Medicine in Mainland China."

65. "Medical Service in Rural Areas."

66. "Mao's Revolution in Public Health."

67. "Strengthen Medical and Health Work."

68. "Public Health System in Yunnan Improves," *Federal Broadcast Information Service* (June 25, 1969): E1–2.

69. "Senior Medical Personnel and Popular Physicians Go to the Countryside," *Union Research Service*, 38, no. 23 (March 19, 1965): 340–58.

70. "Mao's Revolution in Public Health."

71. "Public Health System in Yunnan Improves."

72. "Senior Medical Personnel Go to the Countryside."

73. Bowers, "Medicine in Mainland China."

74. *Joint Publications Research Service* (Articles on health) no. 37161 (August 22, 1966): 124–30.

75. "Barefoot Doctors Become Surgeons," *Joint Publications Research Service* no. 52613 (March 12, 1971): 11–12.

76. "Canton Forum of Medical Personnel."

77. "Medical Personnel to Settle Down in the Countryside," *Union Research Service* 54, no. 4 (January 14, 1969): 46–60.

78. "Health for the Millions," *China News Analysis* no. 738 (January 3, 1969).

79. "Mao's Revolution in Public Health."

80. "Public Health Developments."

81. "Health Work Makes Big Strides."

82. Chang, "The Development of Hospital Services."

83. Sieh, "Medicine in China."

84. "Cooperative Medical Services in the Countryside," *Union Research Service* 54, no. 5 (January 17, 1969): 61–74.

85. "Health."

86. "Public Health Developments."

87. Joshua S. Horn, *Away with All Pests . . . An English Surgeon in People's China* (New York: Monthly Review Press, 1969): 129–43.

88. Ibid.

89. E. G. Dimond, "Inside Look at Chinese Medicine," *American Medical Newsletter* 14, no. 1 (October 11, 1971).

90. "Medical Teacher Has to Rewrite His Teaching Materials," *Joint Publications Research Service* no. 51724 (November 5, 1970): 21–22.

91. "Health for the Millions."

92. "The Trend of Medical Education," *Joint Publications Research Service* no. 51280 (August 31, 1970): 14–16.

93. "China Directs Its Medical Service to the Five Hundred Million Peasants," *Joint Publications Research Service* no. 35144 (April 22, 1966): 74–76.

94. "Public Health Developments.

95. "Medical Health Units Serve Rural Areas in Hsinhua," *Federal Broadcast Information Service* (June 26, 1969): D1.

96. "Socialist Rural Hospitals Need This Kind of Regularization," *Joint Publications Research Service* no. 33484 (December 27, 1965): 5–9.

97. "Strengthen Medical and Health Work."

98. "The Abuse of Free Medical Service," *Union Research Service* 38, no. 14 (February 16, 1967): 208–25.

99. Horn, *Away with All Pests.*

III. Participation of the People

Introductory Note

Robert Chin, a social psychologist, and Ruth Sidel, a psychiatric social worker, discuss the behavior of the Chinese people and their role in participating in public health programs.

The people—peasants and workers—hitherto regarded as ignorant, dirty, disease-ridden, passive consumers of health care programs provided by elite professionals, have reportedly been transformed into "New Men" who are vivacious, clean, healthy, active participants, capable of decision making in the implementation of health measures. Their participation in health matters is a variety of moral and political conduct, and they accept their new role and destiny with pride, enthusiasm, and a strong sense of responsibility to their fellow countrymen.

This change has been brought about as an integral part of a social revolutionary master plan systematically designed and carefully executed, employing political methods based on Mao Tsetung's ideology. This political indoctrination involves the change of an individual's cognitive-perceptive patterns, and of his rational inference and synthesis, leading to the formation of "correct" concepts and theories about himself and his relation to the surrounding world. Thus in the health field a New Man is expected to acquire a capacity to perceive causal dynamics and outcomes as essential for prevention, to acquire skills and a common framework for problem solving as necessary for "mass line" operation (the conviction that the ordinary people possess great strength and wisdom and that when their initiative is given full play they can accomplish miracles), and to raise individual consciousness and world outlook in which the New Man is the major source or a responsible change agent of the revolutionary processes. The evolution of a barefoot doctor or a "health worker" in the commune or the production brigade is predicated on the fact that every individual is considered an active health agent, actually or potentially capable of taking care of health measures for himself and others in the community. Such workers not only complement the lack or shortage of trained health professionals, they function as the mainstay of health practice and the conscience in the community. It is this total mobilization of the inner and outer resources of the New Man that has made the health achievements possible. In addition to the role of the mass and that of the indigenous health worker, the individual patient is given a key role in the promotion of his health and his recovery from disease.

Two major forces seem to provide positive reinforcement of the people's health conduct. First, it is imbedded in the whole framework of change and intermeshed with all aspects of social, cultural, and political conduct. Second, the contrast between the past (prerevolution) and the present (postrevolution) conditions serves as a constant reminder to motivate the people for such change.

The Changing Health Conduct of the "New Man"

M

ROBERT CHIN*

Health conduct in China is improving in astounding leaps, resulting in unprecedented qualitative and quantitative achievements. How these outcomes are being accomplished is the topic of this paper. An understanding of the processes may point the way to improving health systems and health behavior elsewhere.

In China health behavior is more accurately described as health conduct. The older connotation in English of the word "conduct," meaning moral behavior, is appropriate here because health acts are "political." For China and the "New Man" no act is devoid of political factors, which define the purposes and direction of the society. Thus health conduct is moral-political conduct laced together by the cognition, ideologies, actions, and spirit of the socialist state and of the socialist citizen.

This paper will deal with three aspects of health conduct in China:

1. What are the implicit criteria used by Chinese leadership for assessing success or failure in the health conduct of the New Man?

2. What is the model of the utilization of knowledge—the process of dissemination, utilization, and change?

3. What forces are mobilized to push toward an increase in health conduct, in terms of both quality and quantity?

Criteria of Evaluation of Health Conduct

There appear to be four evaluation criteria for health conduct: (1) medical-health outcomes; (2) the individual's acquisition of knowledge about diseases and health; (3) improvements in health

* Assistance in preparing this paper was given by Rance Lee, lecturer in sociology at the Chinese University of Hong Kong.

care organization as consistent with societal and political factors; and (4) the individual's consciousness and world outlook. These four criteria are seen as interrelated, and conflicts between them are not considered major contradictions. In fact, viewed as ends, the achievement of one facilitates the others, although at any given time one or another of them may receive primary focus. Each also serve as means to the others as ends. Of the four criteria I have chosen the last one to discuss at some length. A few brief words will suffice to define the others.

1. The medical-health outcomes reflect how well the *tasks* or missions of preventive or curative activities are accomplished: indices of disease eradication, statistics of injections given, or number of treatments and operations. To accomplish these the masses are mobilized, specialists are reorganized, knowledge is put to sophisticated application, and networks of social organization, including various levels of party and army units, are pressed into service. While no sharp distinctions are maintained, there are evaluations of techniques and outcomes of modern and traditional medicine for preventive, curative, and rehabilitative functions. Combination treatments are more frequent. (In traditional China, food and herbs overlapped with each other as nutriment for preventive and rehabilitative values, and to a much lesser extent for curative values.)

2. The second criteria for evaluation is the amount and quality of information about health, whether it be an illness and its treatment, public health diseases, or personal hygiene. There are concerted efforts to study illnesses and diseases. Hence instead of being at the passive receiving end of the transmission belt of information, the individual undertakes active study of the political roots, the physical aspects of the problem, the conduct needed for solution, and his individual responsibility in health problems. He learns not only about diseases but about cases of successes or innovative problem solving. Patients and victims of social-political factors study their own medical or health problem and curative health conduct.

3. The third criteria for evaluating health conduct is its congruence to the organized goals and the sociopolitical factors of the society. Similar to changes in educational and other institutions, programs in the health field also stress the large mass of citizenry in the countryside—service to the people. Resources are spread out as far as possible and benefits are intended to be equal-

ized for all. The program for adaptation of new conduct leading to desired family size is influenced by other factors of society.

4. Raising individual consciousness and world outlook comes via reading, understanding, and applying Chairman Mao's thought. The manifest content acquired through such study is the moral-political message encapsulated in slogans and epigrams. In addition the individual acquires a desired cognitive structure that facilitates the implementation of correct health conduct. Thus individual or collective acts of health conduct, no matter how small, are elevated to the highest moral and political plane and infused with meaning central to the person and to the fate of China itself. This means that carrying out correct health conduct is not a mere act of compliance with orders from above, or even a voluntaristic, rational, and internalized act of health conduct—health conduct is a high-order political act. Such is the way some individuals have defined their own behavior to outside observers.

Chairman Mao very early pointed to the necessity of moving from cognition-perception through rational inference and synthesis to the formation of correct concepts and theories. What is involved in this? We propose to deal with three features of the cognitive structures, or mental framework, of the New Man: common vocabulary; perceived causal dynamics; and a problem-solving structure and skill.

The first feature is the establishment of a common set of terms— a common language or set of metaphors through which perceptions are formed. Examples of a new activist vocabulary in health conduct include terms borrowed from military campaigns: "know your enemy," "paper tiger," "fight, attack the weak points, and then pick only the battles that can be won." These terms are being adopted not only by special health workers but by patients and by the masses; they help build a common definition of the situation, or clarify a situation in which a common definition has not yet been achieved.

The activist counterattack vocabulary forces the concept of "men-over-nature" to be immediately present in the people's perceptions, and indeed in the statement of the health problem. It would seem that diagnosis is diagnosis-for-intervention in place of, first, diagnosis, and then work out a strategy of action.

The second feature of the cognitive structure is the emphasis on perceiving causal dynamics and outcomes. The New Man is seeing

events as deterministic; man and nature are both causal and outcomes in a chain of causes. Yet with determinism there is alter-
ability. Outcomes of events can be changed by intervening in one
or another of the preceding causes. And there are no artificially
placed limits on the interventions that can change outcomes, except
the limited investment of human energy, temporary ignorance,
the wrong political stand, and analysis of reality.

Preventive intervention in health is heavily dependent on notions
of causes. The adopters of new practices have to have a conviction
or an empirical demonstratuon of the chain of causes. Techniques
and treatments, whether modern or traditional, and mass actions
in public health have been adopted with a scientific-empirical
approach. Politics is brought to bear on how man and his intentions
are also part of the causal links in health and medical conduct. In
health practices, as in other areas, intention and responsibility are
allocated and/or attributed for successful and unsuccessful outcomes.

An important key to understanding conduct in China is this
relationship between intention and responsibility for effects. Let us
quote extensively from Chairman Mao Tse-tung on this question.
At the Yenan Forum on Literature and Art in 1942,[1] he first cited
a "muddled idea" of a writer and then went on to correct it:

> "It is not a question of stand; my class stand is correct, my intentions
> are good and I understand all right, but I am not good at expressing
> myself and so the effect turns out bad."
> I have already talked about the dialectical materialist view of motive
> and effect. Now I want to ask, is not the question of effect one of stand?
> A person who acts solely by motive and does not inquire what effect
> his action will have is like a doctor who merely writes prescriptions but
> does not care how many patients die of them. Or take a political party
> which merely makes declarations but does not care whether they are
> carried out. It may well be asked, is this a correct stand? And is the
> intention here good? Of course mistakes may occur even though the
> effect has been taken into account beforehand, but is the intention
> good when one continues in the same old rut after facts have proved
> that effect is bad? In judging a party or a doctor we must look at prac-
> tice, at the effect.

Or, in another section of the same discussion:

> How can we tell the good from the bad by the motive (the subjective
> intention) or by the effect (social practice)? Idealists stress motive and

ignore effect, while mechanical materialists stress effect and ignore motive. In contradistinction to both, we dialectical materialists insist on the unity of motive and effect. The motive of serving the masses is inseparably linked with the effect of winning their approval and bene-fiting them. In examining the subjective intention of a writer or artist, that is, whether his motive is correct and good, we do not judge by his declarations, but by the effect of his actions (mainly his works) on the masses in society. The criterion for judging subjective intention or motive is social practice and its effect.

The sequence used by the New Man is as follows: See whether the consequences of acts are good or bad, then evaluate the motive, and indeed at times determine what the motive or intention really was in terms of the outcome. The ideal sequence is that good intentions lead to a good outcome. The other possible sequences are: incorrect intentions lead to a good outcome, a bad outcome-good intentions lead to a bad outcome, and bad intentions lead to a bad outcome. All these are incorrect conduct.

Thus it is that performance of health conduct is always to be accompanied by the examination of the intention, that is, the active consciousness of the actor in light of the effects (social practice).

For the poor and lower-middle peasants especially, it is necessary to learn a common language, a cognitive framework of a dynamic sequence, and evaluation of effects and intentions. For preventive work in public health a rational etiology and a science of causes are being built into the consciousness of these groups.

The third feature in the cognitive systems is the crucial indi-vidual skill and a common framework for problem solving as nec-essary for successful operation of the mass line and maintenance of centralism in health conduct. Mass line covers several processes: Renewed energies are mustered, and immense problems are tackled in a self-reliant way. Blended with the mass line are elements of technical knowledge and specialized competency. In the Great Leap period, the mass line meant the organizing of large numbers of individuals to undertake highly technical tasks that were partly broken down into separate components. The mass line also meant releasing the skills and aptitudes of large masses of workers and peasants. In the period since the beginning of the movement toward the countryside the emphasis has been on learning from the peasants in the mass line. The poor and lower-middle peasants are known to be familiar with local concrete conditions, and have good judgments and correct interests in mind. The expert medical specialist surrenders his total authority—to become a member of a team that includes the patient. The poor and lower-middle peasant does not possess technical information about special topics, disease etiology, or preventive and curative activities, but he is in the position of making judgments about means and ends as they impinge on the local people and as they affect the welfare of socialist China. Most importantly the peasant and health specialist must use problem-solving skills to create mutually satisfying and effective solutions.

In developing the new cognitions and cognitive structure of the New Man there are elements similar to those of "sensitivity training"—the face-to-face working together of a group, taking time out to look mutually at *how* they are working together, becoming sensitive to the needs and perceptions of others, and learning from this process. The health worker and the poor and lower-middle peasant work together in the countryside and engage in mutual learning. Under the mass line one must listen to the peasant, develop problem-solving skills, learn decision-making processes, and adopt a general orientation to the strategy and tactics of change. For the peasants, being involved in change and being explicit about the change processes rest upon the foundation of a uniform vocabulary, perception of the dynamics of causes, including those of failure, and a special concentration on the self as the major source and on the change processes. His methodological skills are to blend in his own values and local knowledge with those of the experts in order to solve a problem.

Given the nature of health problems and the possible attendant anxieties on the part of individuals, we have no evidence that particularized attention is given to any overdependency by peasants on the expert—the doctor, surgeon, or other medical specialist who "know" and can "solve" or treat. This dependency may be counteracted by the intensive concern about sending the specialized medical professional into the countryside to experience the life of the peasants. This is his "sensitivity training" for empathy, for role taking, and for ascertaining his effect. His vocabulary, dynamics, and experiences in change processes become oriented towards innovation and progress, a sense of movement, change, and improvement. These methodological processes, anchored in ideology and in practice, are in constant contrast to the terrible past sufferings of the poor and lower-middle peasants.

The specialist in health work also widens his problem-solving skills by considering *people* and their conditions of life as the backbone of the country. "Sensitivity" processes are involved in the new experiential contact with the poor peasant and his mode of living. Doctors, nurses, and other health workers once concentrated in urban areas now have new existential knowledge *of*, which goes beyond knowledge *about*, peasants. Feelings, sentiments, and sensitivities are acquired and incorporated; there is a personal identification with particular persons and their individual lives. The mass of peasants become *people*. As such, the health worker's *effective* problem-solving skills become improved as he takes people as well as local conditions into account in using his technical knowledge for improving life conditions. The fact is that there is reciprocal learning on the part of the peasants and others when they work together on problem solving and decision making, and in learning to make use of each other's resources and concerns. This is an important common feature added to the cognitive structures of people from different layers.

These four criteria are not explicitly stated by the leadership in China. They are inferences on my part based on the fact that the leadership appears to act as though it had these four criteria in mind. The common language, perceived causal dynamics, and problem-solving cognitions are not unique to health and medical sectors.

Innovation and Modification in Knowledge Utilization

Changing the health conduct of the New Man in China requires the dissemination and utilization of technical knowledge and the coordination of the roles involved for an everimproving system. There is modification and/or elaboration of the procedures for utilization of knowledge.

First, there has been conscious adaptation of the basic stock of modern and traditional medical knowledge, not only for China as a whole but region by region and locality by locality. During the Great Leap period, local investigators initiated developmental research, such as procedures for efficient mass screening, to find those cases that needed special attention. These involved great numbers of persons undertaking large-scale screening. Developmental research is also being carried on, for example, in the evaluation of treatment programs of modern and traditional medicine.

Second, the innovation of new practices tends to come from the clinic, hospital, commune, or brigade—the unit that is the responsive and responsible system for new ideas and evaluated techniques and treatments—with the individual health worker still initiating innovations on an ad hoc basis.

Third, the most important modification in the model of knowledge utilization is the position of the consumer—the poor and lower-middle peasant and the worker. He is no longer the passive target of services. His cooperative and voluntary services are required for massive health projects. The whole viewpoint of the ideology makes him an actual partner, if not the pivotal person and the leader, in the making of New China. He is the main beneficiary of the revolution.

There is a reversal of the traditionally held image of what formerly were called the "riffraff." Before the revolution these peasants were seen as ignorant, dull, superstitious, dirty, unsanitary, disease ridden, and as having bad personal hygiene habits. Now they are liberated of their oppressions and are becoming wise in judgment, active leading edges in decision making, scientific, pragmatic, oriented to sanitation and health measures, and with improving personal hygiene. The large bulk of China's population is being transformed into the New Man not only in industrial and food production but in health. The key to China's impressive progress in health conduct and public health measures, such as eradication of debilitating diseases, lies in this change and in the peasants' acceptance of their new destiny and role.

Fourth, while the major movement is downward for new techniques, treatments, and preventive health measures, there is an upward flow embodied in the mass line. It contains feedback of effects that need to be taken into account. Local inventions and innovations are also collected and disseminated upwards. Communication flows laterally, and then of course evaluated communication flows downwards to other groups. Systematic attention is paid throughout China to the emulation of model programs and the model New Man.

The mass line emphasizes openness of communication upwards. Furthermore, key linking persons are present who sit in several organizational offices. The same mechanisms operate in coordinating the health workers with local organizations and their management of the clinics and other service facilities, and with supplying old and new types of drugs and herbs, and equipment for testing and diagnosis—that is, all of the new materials necessary for preventive measures and health care. Professional and other health workers, products and materials, and service organizations all operate through these communication links.

Horizontal communication and decision making involving local party, army, and commune brigade leaders are probably achieved by going up to the next echelons above the unit and then down again, although there is reason to believe that cooperation in spirit is present at the same organizational level. The workers and the poor and lower-middle peasants act also as a channel to communicate upwards through these other channels.

Vertical communication among hospital personnel, mobile medical brigades, central clinics, work brigade clinics, peasant doctors, and factory health workers has tremendous potential because of the interchange and movement of individuals up and down by rotation of assignments and for training. While there are divisions of labor according to technical competence, there is an overarching of shared responsibility for providing preventive measures, direct services, training, family planning, or working with local committees on health problems. The latter includes such work as patriotic health committees and committees for the improvement of the ideological consciousness of the people; they also have responsibility for the ideological remolding of health personnel. The most important communication linkages are those that are part of a central hospital, which in turn link in with the research and development groups.

Forces Mobilized for Change

Changing health conduct in the New Man in China is being produced by forces intrinsic to the revolution: its ideology and political stand, its organizational character, and the eager utilization of technical knowledge and modern techniques. Furthermore, the changed concepts and approaches of the people to objective reality—the view of human nature and of the socialist man—reinforce the revolutionary force affecting their own health conduct. In short the procedures and forces in use are embedded in the whole framework of change in other sectors of the new society. The unique characteristics of the change into the New Man is the way in which a total field of forces becomes structured, with reliance on local resources, central planning for setting directions and organizational structures, and a "procedural" emphasis. Health conduct is not treated as different from conduct in work or in education.

The many positive driving forces toward changing health conduct have been discussed in the preceding sections of this paper. In addition there are the information and propaganda campaigns that use all means for communicating the problems and opportunities of medical-health issues, the political-organizational forms, the explicit and implicit cognitive frameworks—all build up to the New Man and his health conduct. The devotion of party, army, production units, and other groups to the health areas is a major force. A common thread and probably the most influential theme running through the propaganda seems to be the contrast between the past and present and the state of living of the poor and middle-lower peasants before the revolution and before the improvements in health conduct, facilities, and services.

Some of the blocks that prevent a falling back in health conduct are intrinsic in the health and medical consumer. Health and medical services and conduct are self-expanding activities. The more consumed, the more provided; the more health needs are seen and behavioral demands made, the more rising expectations take hold.

Identification of the negative driving forces against health conduct was easy to make in prerevolutionary China. Under the present social system there are no discernible negative driving forces against increasing and changing health conduct, although some probably still exist. The blocks against the desired changes are the scarcity of resources and the problem of their allocation. The immensity of the health task would indicate that the central regions, especially the countryside near cities and major urban areas, would make more progress than more remote areas and border regions. There is every reason to believe that the same approach and organizational structures, and the same ability to instill the new cognitive structures, could come with changing the health conduct in these less affected geographical areas.

Epilogue

This brief paper is intended only to provide an analysis. It does not report any data or the reasoning and inference apparatus.

The effect on the reader is untested. The assertions made throughout are not always defendable through evidence and direct observation. As a matter of fact the author had the advantage of reading most of the papers submitted to the conference before finishing this paper. Thus the information and insights of the other papers helped immeasurably.

It would be more modest to state that this paper is a set of hypotheses; such weaseling would deny the convictions of the author and his willingness to take a stand in order to be corrected by others. His basic stand is that we cannot isolate the medical-health system from political factors in China. Politics is not an intrusion into the medical system in China; it is an intrinsic and dominant stand lacing together health conduct and the organizational arrangements in which it occurs.

NOTE

1. Mao Tse-tung, "Talks at the Yenan Forum on Literature and Art, May 1942," in *Selected Readings from the Works of Mao Tse-tung* (Peking: Foreign Languages Press, 1971).

The Role of the Community
and the Patient in Health Care

ఠ

RUTH SIDEL

In his essay *On Practice*, written in 1937, Mao Tse-tung wrote:

> If you want to know the taste of a pear, you must change the pear by
> eating it yourself. If you want to know the structure and properties of
> the atom, you must make physical and chemical experiments to change
> the state of the atom. If you want to know the theory and methods of
> revolution, you must take part in revolution. All genuine knowledge
> originates in direct experience.[1]

This theme of learning by doing runs through essentially all aspects of Chinese life today. A peasant learns the difficulties in determining agricultural priorities by taking part in decision making.
The urban doctor learns about the life of the peasants by moving
to the countryside for a period of time and laboring with them.
The child learns what it is like to be a peasant or a worker by growing vegetables or doing a job on consignment from a factory. And,
according to this theory, the way to teach 800 million people the
principles of health prevention and health care is to involve them
in it.

The mobilization of the masses has been the primary technique
by which the Chinese have accomplished their feats of engineering:
the construction of dikes, canals, bridges, and large-scale irrigation
projects, and the damming of rivers. The mobilization of the
masses has been the primary mechanism in their feats of human
engineering also. Han Suyin has described the process of the education of the masses since 1949 as one that has included the "eradication of the human mind" and

> getting the masses away from the anchored belief that natural calamities
> are "fixed by heaven" and that therefore nothing can be done to

124

remedy one's lot . . . To bridge this gap between scientific modern man and feudal man, the prey of superstition, and to do it within the compass of one generation, is a formidable task.[2]

One of the prime techniques used to accomplish this "formidable task" has been the activating of the "mass." In health care this has meant the broadest involvement of people at every level of society in such campaigns as the Patriotic Health Movement; the training of selected groups of people such as barefoot doctors who are recruited from the population they are to serve; and the exhortation that the individual "fight against his own disease." Individual concern with health reflects the Chinese belief in self-reliance—a virtue as honored today as its converse, mutual help.

This was brought home to us most strikingly while we were observing a kindergarten class for six-year-olds. They were being taught the life story of Norman Bethune, a Canadian thoracic surgeon who provided medical services for Mao Tse-tung's Eighth Route Army in the war against Japan until his death in 1939 from septicemia, secondary to an infection he acquired while performing surgery. Dr. Bethune is a national hero in China, celebrated for his "selflessness," his internationalism, and his self-reliance—all principles that are taught to Chinese children. After the audiovisual presentation, the children were asked what they would do if they came upon a sick person on the street. "I would get water for him," and "I would get medicine for him," were typical replies, all suggesting things the child himself could do for the sick man rather than going to get help from a doctor or other adult.

The Role of the Mass

In 1952 Mao issued his "Four Main Health Principles," widely-quoted in China, one of which is: "Health work should be combined with the mass movement." The Patriotic Health Movement was launched at this time, and Horn states that the Chinese linked the movement to the need to protect the population against the alleged use of germ warfare in Korea by the United States;[3] the Chinese with whom we spoke, however, never mentioned germ warfare. The primary goal of this mass movement in the early fifties, we were told, was the elimination of four pests—mosquitoes, flies, rats, and bedbugs—and the people were mobilized to exterminate them under the guidance of health personnel. The Patriotic Health Movement has been maintained and has been expanded to include the sanitary aspects of food, water, and the environment.

While environmental sanitation is a constant activity, it is attacked with particular intensity around festival days and in preparation for the May 1 and October 1 celebrations. Everyone participates, from retired workers to health activists, and the general population works under the leadership of medical personnel. In Shanghai, Thursday morning is the fixed time for cleaning; all clean their streets and homes. Cadres who work within the government usually do manual labor one day a week, and it often coincides with cleanup day. There is interdistrict inspection, when a group of people from one district can come in and inspect another district and criticize or exchange experiences. We were told by Dr. Hong Ming-gui, vice-director of the Shanghai branch of the Chinese Medical Association, that the criticism most often takes the form of "promoting the strong points of another district, encouraging that district." He also quoted the slogan used around cleanup time: "It's a glorious thing to speak about hygiene and you should be ashamed if you're very dirty." (One assumes this sounds somewhat different in Chinese.) Dr. Hong stressed the importance of the involvement of the masses in breaking with traditional habits and in changing the spirit of the people.

Health workers in a street health center in Hangchow, which serves 7,350 families totaling 28,000 people, reported that they have established three days a month as cleaning days to eliminate pests, and another three days a month as general cleanup days. The entire population has been mobilized into groups, and certain individuals in each group are responsible for wiping out the pests, eliminating the breeding places, disinfecting water, and keeping the neighborhood clean.

The street health center uses more than 100 different herbs to treat chronic diseases, we were told, and residents of this street are mobilized to climb a nearby mountain to plant and gather herbs; the people are also educated as to their use.

"Health propaganda," the Chinese say, plays a crucial role in the participation of the community in health problems. Great attention is paid to educating the populace on the importance of immunizations, the handling of infectious diseases, and the need for "planned birth."

In the twenty-three neighborhood health centers of a district general hospital in Peking, which serves a population of 49,000, we were told of both mass meetings and study groups organized by the health workers in the district to educate the people in hygiene and in the prevention of infectious disease. They are taught to report any infectious disease to the health center immediately. These meetings are conducted on a regular basis, as well as at special times during the year. The health center itself is considered a "mass organization"—the one we visited had been organized by four neighborhood housewives who had been trained as Red Guard doctors, the urban counterpart of the barefoot doctor. The Red Guard doctors are not paid; they do what is called "mass work" and are thought of as volunteers rather than as full-fledged medical personnel. We were told that every district in Peking has been organized in this fashion, although our hosts did state that the one we visited was "better than average."

On the wall of the health center was a list of the responsibilities of the Red Guard doctors. Responsibility No. 3 stated that stress should be put on prevention and on the Patriotic Health Movement—with a general cleaning every week and a thorough cleaning every two weeks—and that emphasis be put on propaganda on how to deal with infectious disease, vaccinations, and combining treatment and prevention.

On the communes the "health workers" receive neither extra pay nor time off from their regular jobs. They do their health work during their lunch periods or at the end of the day. In addition to treating minor illnesses and giving immunizations, these individuals are responsible for disinfecting the water and treating human feces (night soil), which is used as fertilizer. These health workers are trained by, and are under the supervision of, the barefoot doctors.

Leo Orleans and Richard Suttemeier emphasize the importance of mobilizing the masses in dealing with the problem of pollution.[4] They describe people organized in the cities to "remove refuse that had accumulated in residential districts" and, more specifically, "the spring patriotic sanitation movement" of 1970, which was organized by local revolutionary committees to mobilize the people to pick up litter and garbage from residences, farms, and factories, to clean up local waters, to eliminate pests, to collect reuseable wastes, and to advocate public health measures. They also describe the efforts of the Shanghai Municipal Revolutionary Committee in July 1968 to clean up the Huangpu and Suchow Rivers. The authors quote the New China News Agency as stating that

> ... 90,000 persons were mobilized on the industrial and agricultural fronts in Shanghai to form muck-dredging and muck-transporting teams, waging a vehement people's war to dredge muck from the Suchow River. After 100 days of turbulent fighting, more than 403,600 tons of malodorous organic mire had been dug out.[5]

The classic example of the use of mass mobilization in health has, of course, been the campaign against schistosomiasis. According to Horn, this campaign was based on the concept of the "mass line"—"the conviction that the ordinary people possess great strength and wisdom and that when their initiative is given full play they can accomplish miracles."[6] Before the peasants were mobilized to fight against the snails, Horn states, they were thoroughly educated as to the nature of schistosomiasis by means of lectures, films, posters, and radio talks. They were then mobilized twice a year, in March and in August, and, along with voluntary labor from the People's Liberation Army, students, teachers, and office workers, they drained the rivers and ditches, buried the banks of the rivers, and smoothed down the buried dirt. Horn points out that in the fight against schistosomiasis, the concept was not only to recruit the masses to do the work but to mobilize their enthusiasm and initiative so that they would fight against the disease.[7]

This method of fighting the enemy is an adaptation by Mao of the methods used so successfully in Yenan during the war to fire the enthusiasm of the population against the Japanese. Mao has transferred this ideology into a campaign against such "enemies" as illiteracy, disease, famine, and flood. In this case the enemy is schistosomiasis and the technique used to analyze it is the well-known "paper tiger" theory first used by Mao in 1946 to describe the United States–Kuomintang alliance. It states that there is a dual nature to everything—while one's enemies are real and formidable and must be taken seriously, they are at the same time paper tigers that can be defeated by the will of the people. One has to view one's enemies from this dual point of view, Mao teaches, in order to plan correctly one's strategy and one's tactics.

The effort against schistosomiasis is particularly revealing since it mobilized the population in several directions: to move against the snails, to cooperate in case finding and treatment, and to improve environmental sanitation. Yukiang county in Kiangsi Province, for example, had been plagued by schistosomiasis for more than 100 years. According to one report, 1 million m.[2] of the land was infested with snails, and the "average" infection rate among the peasants was 21.4 per cent.[8] After an investigation of the prevalence of the disease, an antischistosomiasis station was set up in the county in 1953. When the campaign started, the personnel of the station began publicizing its purpose, as well as health work in general, using

> . . . broadcasting, wall newspapers, blackboards, exhibits of real and model objects, lantern slide shows and dramatic performances. Related scientific knowledge was also popularized. To help the peasants raise their political consciousness, break their superstitious belief in gods, devils, and fate, and to build up their confidence in conquering the disease, meetings were organized for recalling sufferings in the old society and comparing them with the happiness in the new society. Through these activities, the confidence of the broad masses in the certain triumph of their struggle against schistosomiasis was gradually built up and further strengthened.[9]

Once the population was educated about schistosomiasis, a "people's war" was launched against the snails. From 1955 to 1957, 20,000 peasants in Yukiang county filled up old ditches and old ponds, dug new ditches, and expanded the cultivation area by roughly ninety acres. Special methods had to be used in some areas. For example, three three-feet lotus ponds covering some seven acres had a high density of snails which people had attempted to exterminate by removing the surface soil, by burning aquatic vegetation, and by other methods, but still the snails had not been completely eliminated. Finally the ponds were drained, all the grass and vegetation at the bottom of the ponds was burned, and snail-free mud was then piled on the snail-infested mud and pounded so that the snails were suffocated. Seven square or rectangular fish ponds were then created out of the three former snail-breeding lotus ponds.[10]

After the massive war on schistosomiasis, however, it was still necessary to check for the recurrence of snails, water control, and waste disposal, so that the people had also to be educated in the treatment of human excreta, the provision of safe drinking water, and improved personal hygiene. Production teams under the leadership of health workers are responsible for these public health measures.

Horn reports on the need to educate the population about the importance of regular feces examination. At one commune he was told that the peasants did not always take the necessity of testing seriously and tried to play jokes on the testers by sending in dog or ox dung. The testers met this problem by reminding the peasants of what life was like in the "bitter past" when schistosomiasis was common; cooperation was restored.[11]

Health work in Heilungkiang Province in Manchuria was described in an article in *China's Medicine* in 1968.[12] In order to spread health education in the province, mass meetings were called in sixty cities and counties, leaflets and pamphlets on health were distributed, and students began to engage in health education among the workers and peasants. It was estimated that in two counties 250,000 middle and primary school students were mobilized for health education work. Needless to say the students learned as much as they taught.

The Role of Indigenous Health Personnel

Since the Cultural Revolution it has been common practice in urban neighborhoods and on the communes to recruit health personnel from among the indigenous population. The barefoot doctor in the countryside, the Red Guard doctor in the city, the worker-doctor in the factory, and the health workers in the cities and on the communes are members of the mass recruited to do health work and to communicate what they have learned to their friends and neighbors. In Silvery Lane in Hangchow, a community of 702 families, fifty residents work in the health center in official capacities; in other words, one member of every fourteen families in the lane is directly responsible for health care. The residents in any given neighborhood who are active in health work are responsible for instructing the rest of the community in the need for immunizations, the use of birth control, and the importance of good sanitation.

We were astounded at the high rate of immunizations in a Peking health center that we visited: of the children eligible for measles vaccine, 97.5 per cent were immunized; polio, 100 per cent; DPT, 100 per cent; encephalitis, 94.1 per cent; meningitis,

97 per cent; BCG, for tuberculosis, 98.1 per cent; and smallpox, 80.9 per cent. The rate for smallpox immunization is relatively low because the Chinese do not vaccinate if there are any contraindications. When we inquired about this high rate we were told that the Red Guard doctor in the health station informs the parents when it is time for their child to receive another inoculation. The health center is of course very near their home and therefore very convenient, but if the mother or father is not able to bring the child to the center the Red Guard doctor will go to the home to give the immunization. It became clear that because of the closely knit neighborhood, and the integration of the health center with the neighborhood, few children go unattended.

This is also true in the Hangchow health center we visited, where the personnel keep track of the contraception each family is using by visiting each home once a month. When we asked if the women were reluctant to discuss their methods of contraception we were told that occasionally a newly married woman might be shy but that once the importance of birth control to China is explained she cooperates. The large number of health workers and the commitment to health propaganda combine to make each contact a health education contact.

The Role of the Patient

The third way in which the Chinese people are involved in health is through mobilization of the individual patient. In the psychiatric ward of the Third Peking Hospital we were told that the staff tries to "promote the active factors so that the patient can struggle against his own disease." The patient studies the works of Chairman Mao in order to understand his own illness and to be able to fight against it. The psychiatrists told us that, "Through the patients' studies, the ideology of the patient is much elevated. The patient can then investigate his disease and recognize his own condition in order to prevent relapse." The following description of his illness was given us by a thirty-eight-year-old male patient in the psychiatric ward of the Third Peking Hospital:

My main trouble is suspicion. I think my ceiling is going to fall down; when big character posters are up I think it is criticism of myself; and when somebody is gossiping I think they are talking about me. After I was admitted to this hospital I gradually recognized my illness. As

Chairman Mao says, when we face a problem we have to face it thoroughly, not only from one side. When I am discharged from the hospital, the doctors have said that I should have some problem of investigation in my mind. When I am in touch with people they have suggested that I make conclusions in my mind after investigation not before investigation, in order to see if what I suspect to be true is just subjective thinking or is objectively correct. By studying Chairman Mao, we can treat and cure disease.

The Shanghai Mental Hospital has carried the idea of a patient's disease as his enemy a step further. They have "adopted the system used in the army," and have divided the staff of the hospital into four divisions. The patients on the wards have also been divided into groups, and they now comprise a "collective fighting group instead of a ward." One of the psychiatrists told us, "It is not enough to have the doctors' or nurses' initiative; we need the patients' initiative to work together against the disease." The patients are organized into Mao Tse-tung study groups in order to understand their illness and to be better able to fight it. This view of the patient's relationship with his mental illness is a curious combination of individual responsibility and viewing the illness as an external enemy. This dual attitude perhaps serves to maximize the patient's efforts to fight his illness while leaving him less guilt-ridden if he fails.

Patients are not only expected to participate in their own care—they are also expected to help one another. The Shanghai Mental Hospital has a buddy system whereby the healthier patients who have been in the hospital longer help the newer, sicker patients to adjust to the hospital and to understand their illness.

Horn describes a burn victim whose burns covered 89 per cent of the surface of his body. At one point during treatment the patient's appetite started to diminish and, as days went on, he ate less and less. The dietitian tried to tempt him with delicacies, and chefs in Shanghai restaurants produced special menus to encourage him to eat, but, most important, "his comrades urged him to eat as a political duty, as his contribution to the fight for his life that was being waged with such determination by so many."[13]

In an article entitled, "How We Have Struggled against Unstable Diabetes Mellitus in the Light of Mao Tse-Tung's Thought,"[14] three patients write of their difficulties in dealing with their diabetes over the years, and describe the new approach they took in managing their disease: they studied the "pathophysiology of diabetes," "became familiar with the regulation of insulin dosage," and applied the theory of the paper tiger to their disease, that is, "we despised him and we took him seriously." Thus, the article states, the patients' initiative to fight against their diabetes was mobilized and their disease stabilized.

Summary

In health, as in other aspects of the Chinese brand of socialism, there are no passive participants. One is expected to participate "wholeheartedly" in the public health measures needed by the community, in the organization of medical care in one's community, and in the conduct of all aspects of one's personal life, including one's health. It is a country of mass and individual participation, of mass and individual responsibility. John G. Gurley, an economist, has described China's current view of the role of the people in the following way:

> To gain knowledge, people must be awakened from their half slumber, encouraged to mobilize themselves and to take conscious action to elevate and liberate themselves. When they actively participate in decision-making, when they take an interest in state affairs, when they dare to do new things, when they become good at presenting facts and reasoning things out, when they criticize and test and experiment scientifically, having discarded myths and superstitions, when they are aroused—then the socialist initiative latent in the masses [will] burst out with volcanic force. . . .[15]

In stressing participation and mutual responsibility, the Chinese over the past twenty-two years have accomplished astonishing feats in the field of medicine and public health, and have educated their enormous population to an increased awareness and understanding of preventive medicine and medical care. For the Chinese believe, as Mao teaches, that, "If you want knowledge, you must take part in the practice of changing reality."[16]

NOTES

1. Mao Tse-tung, "On Practice," *Four Essays on Philosophy* (Peking: Foreign Languages Press, 1966): p. 8.

2. Han Suyin, "Reflections on Social Change," *Bulletin of the Atomic Scientists* 22, no. 6 (1966): 80–83

3. Joshua S. Horn, *Away with All Pests . . . An English Surgeon in People's China* (New York: Monthly Review Press, 1969): p. 126.

4. Leo A. Orleans and Richard P. Suttemeier, "The Mao Ethic and Environmental Quality," *Science*, 170 (December 11, 1970): 1173–1176.

5. Ibid.

6. Horn, *Away with All Pests*, p. 96.

7. Ibid., p. 97.

8. "A Great Victory of Mao Tse-tung's Thought in the Battle Against Schistosomiasis," *China's Medicine* 10 (October 1968): 588–602.

9. Ibid., p. 593.

10. Ibid., pp. 598–99.

11. Horn, *Away with All Pests*, p. 99.

12. "Experiences in Health Work and Disease Prevention in Heilungkiang Province in the Past Year," *China's Medicine* 3 (March 1968): 148–53.

13. Horn, *Away with All Pests*, p. 108.

14. Chang Tze-han, Yang Teh-ching, and Tu Jui-fen, "How We Have Struggled Against Unstable Diabetes Mellitus in the Light of Mao Tse-tung's Thought," *China's Medicine* 7 (July 1968): 400–407.

15. John G. Gurley, "Capitalist and Maoist Economic Development," in *America's Asia*, ed. Edward Freedman and Mark Selden (New York: Vintage Books, 1971): p. 336.

16. Mao, *Four Essays on Philosophy*, p. 8.

IV. Health Manpower and Training

Introductory Note

Chu-yuan Cheng, an economist with special interest in science manpower in China, reviewed the demand and supply of health manpower in the People's Republic of China, and Victor W. Sidel, a specialist in social medicine, discussed the general principles governing the role of medical personnel and their training based on his recent visit to the PRC.

Though handicapped by scanty inconsistent data, the best available information suggests that health manpower in the traditional categories—physicians, nurses, midwives, and other health professionals—has increased significantly in the PRC in the last two decades. The gap between the demand for and supply of professional health manpower has been closed considerably, and in 1971 the estimated level of deficiency in most categories was 20 to 25 per cent.

A radically new manpower strategy put into force in 1949 has undergone several modifications, especially since the Cultural Revolution. A novel pattern of manpower utilization and development has now evolved that potentially may meet the long deprived health manpower needs. The main features are: (1) development of a broad spectrum of health workers through the mobilization of community resources; (2) equalization of medical manpower distribution; (3) a new health personnel recruitment policy; (4) reorganization of medical education; and (5) continuing education.

In addition to tapping the manpower resources of traditional medicine, in order to supplement the supply of physicians trained in Western medicine ingenious use has been made of trained lay personnel to take care of local health activities. These include the "barefoot doctor," a subprofessional part-time worker, similar to a *feldsher*, and the "neighborhood (or production brigade) health worker," a kind of community health clerk who supervises and keeps records of health activities of the production brigade or the neighborhood, while serving as liaison with barefoot doctors or health professionals.

For equalization of medical manpower distribution, systematic and intensive deployment of mobile medical teams and rotation or resettling of urban physicians to rural communities (*hsia-fang*) have been the methods of choice. These schemes are intended not only as a way to supplement the supply of much-needed rural health workers rendering curative and preventive services, but as a means to encourage urban physicians to develop a political conscience and a general perspective of the national health services.

Noteworthy is the method employed for recruitment of health personnel based on the community's judgment of the quality of the person, which emphasizes his party loyalty, his performance, and his potential as a responsible member of the community. The method seems to promise the rural communes much-needed health personnel, while gradually erasing from the health care system the image and status of the bourgeois doctor.

As a method of correcting the shortcomings in the large-scale use of barefoot doctors and other indigenous health workers, and of the accelerated training of medical students, continuing education is in extensive use. This is carried out by means of mobile medical teams, rotating health personnel to rural communes, and short refresher courses held in appropriate medical centers.

Health Manpower:
Growth and Distribution

ಞ

CHU-YUAN CHENG

Health manpower—physicians, nurses, midwives, and other medical professionals—is a significant component of the human resources of any society. The ratio of physicians to population has been popularly regarded as an index of the health condition and economic well-being of a society. Ever since the new government assumed power in 1949 great effort has been addressed to improving public health in the People's Republic of China. One of the major goals has been to augment medical professionals to meet the needs of the growing population.

Despite its being a vital component of the overall Chinese development plan since 1953, information and statistics on health manpower are scanty. Not only is there a dearth of data on the various categories of medical personnel, but the aggregate figures are inconsistent and even totally unavailable for many years. A study of Chinese health manpower is thus handicapped on two fronts.

First, official statistics on health manpower have never been clearly defined. The common term, "persons working in public health services," refers to all categories of people working in the public health system regardless of their education and training. In official statistics we can identify the functions of only approximately 20 per cent of the health manpower;[1] there is no indication of the composition of the remaining 80 per cent.

Second, in the PRC, as in Taiwan and Hong Kong, in addition to modern Western medicine there is a system of traditional herbalist medicine. There are more than 500,000 herbalists, who constitute an important element of Chinese medical manpower and exercise significant influence over the rural population. Before 1960 traditional practitioners were excluded from official statistics, but in recent years they have been included. According to Huang K'ai-yun, a member of the Board of Directors of the Chinese Medical Association, "of the more than 1.4 million public health workers in China in 1963, more than 120,000 are senior technicians who have graduated from college; 300,000 from secondary medical schools; and 500,000 are specialists in traditional Chinese medicine."[2] Thus the statistics for various periods before and after 1960 are hardly comparable. The situation became even more complicated when millions of barefoot doctors were incorporated into the medical system in recent years.

In view of data difficulties such as these, estimates of demand and supply of medical manpower in this paper are perforce very tentative. Our purpose is not to arrive at a precise calculation but to trace certain quantitative trends that have great bearing on the recent reforms in medical education and the reallocation of medical manpower in China.

Manpower Requirements for Public Health

Approach and Methodology

The demand for health manpower in a country can be estimated by various approaches. In the past there were attempts to predict demand for physicians and nurses by means of estimates of mortality and morbidity on the grounds that the burden of disease was a basic determinant of a nation's demand for health.[3] This method, based on biological need for health services, is not workable due to the absence of detailed and accurate morbidity and mortality statistics, and to the difficulty in measuring the total health professional time required to combat a given disease.[4]

A simpler method is to use a desired manpower-population ratio to translate "people" into "manpower requirements." In recent years this method has been used in many developed and developing countries—in, for example, the United States, Canada, and Nigeria—to estimate the number of health professionals required by the target year to maintain the manpower-population ratio existing in the base year, or to adopt a standard ratio as a basis for planning.[5]

The obvious advantage of this approach is its simplicity; it has, however, many serious drawbacks. For example, the fundamental manpower problem of a given country may be due more to inappropriate distribution and utilization than to insufficient quantity. Moreover, application of this approach to China immediately confronts a crucial problem: how to select a desirable manpower-population ratio.

The Physician-Population Ratio

While no official manpower-population ratio has been promulgated by the Chinese government, the issue has been mentioned and briefly discussed in one official document that called for the study of the following items to provide a foundation for further planning:[6] (1) the changes of population, including rates of birth and of death; (2) the rate of morbidity for various diseases; (3) current medical organization facilities and the growth of medical personnel; (4) working conditions and living standards of the population; and (5) the number of working days and the norm of work-per-day of physicians.

During the first Five-Year Plan (1953–57) the targets of health manpower set by the government for the final year were extremely low: 0.41 hospital beds per 1,000 population, and roughly one doctor per 10,000 population.[7] The manpower-population ratio adopted by the first plan was apparently circumscribed by limited resources, and was by no means intended to represent a desirable ratio.

While a "desirable" manpower-population ratio for the PRC is hard to determine, empirical data from other developing countries, particularly those from Taiwan, Japan, Hong Kong, and Singapore, may serve as references. According to a recent compilation by the United States Agency for International Development, the manpower-population ratios for ninety-three countries were collected. The data for countries in East Asia and some Latin American countries are particularly relevant to China (Table 1).

The ratios in Taiwan, Hong Kong, Singapore, Brazil, Mexico, and Peru are particularly relevant. The biological need of the populations of the first three countries is basically the same as that of the PRC; the latter three countries have an economic structure similar to that of the PRC. The mean physician-population ratio of these six countries is 1:2,200. Assuming a slightly higher ratio of 1:2,500, the deviation from the general ratio would be insignificant. This ratio would put China in the same position as Brazil and close

Table 1. The Physician-Population Ratio in East Asia and
Selected Latin American Countries, 1966

Country	Population per Physician	
Developed Areas[1]	780	
United States		690
Less Developed Areas[2]	4,000	
East Asia		
Including Japan	2,300	
Excluding Japan	5,200	
Burma		9,300
Cambodia		25,000
Hong Kong		2,800
Indonesia		41,000
Korea, South		2,600
Laos		49,000
Malaysia		6,500
Philippines		1,700
Singapore		2,300
Taiwan		1,500
Thailand		7,300
Vietnam, South		16,600
Latin America	1,800	
Argentina		670
Brazil		2,500
Chile		1,770
Mexico		2,020
Peru		2,150

Source: *Proposed Foreign Aid Program FY 1968*, Summary Presentation to the Congress, Agency for International Development (Washington, D. C.: Government Printing Office, 1967): Table 3. Notes: 1. Including Australia, Canada, Western Europe, Japan, New Zealand, South Africa, and the United States. 2. Including ninety-three countries in the Near East, Africa, East Asia, South Asia, and Latin America.

to the average ratio in East Asia, including Japan. Based on this physician-population ratio, the total demand for physicians in the PRC in 1966 should have been in the neighborhood of 300,000, depending on the population figure one chooses. A 1.5 per cent natural growth rate in the population from 1957 to 1966 would have brought it to about 728 million, with an estimated demand for 290,000 physicians. If one adopts an annual population growth rate of 2 per cent, however, the demand for physicians in 1966 would have been 303,000 for a population of 758.8 million.

Demand for Intermediate-Level Medical Manpower

In the hierarchy of medical manpower, doctors constitute the upper segment which has to be supplemented by a much larger number of auxiliary and supporting personnel on the intermediate and lower levels. In the United States, for each doctor there are two allied professionals and 1.2 auxiliaries, for an overall ratio of 1:3.[8] In Taiwan there has been an acute shortage of nurses—in 1964 there were more than twice as many physicians as qualified nurses. As a result, physicians have to perform inappropriate tasks that would be better delegated to trained nurses, while untrained nurses' aides are assuming nursing responsibilities for which they are unqualified.[9] In the PRC the ratio of high- to intermediate-level medical manpower was set at about 1:2.5. In 1961 there were 100,000 students enrolled in medical and pharmaceutical schools of higher education, while in the same year enrollment in medical and pharmaceutical secondary schools was 235,000.[10] If we apply this ratio of 1:2.35 to 1966, requirements for intermediate medical personnel would range from 680,000 to 712,000 depending on the population figures used.

Requirements for low-level medical personnel are even more difficult to determine. During the first Five-Year Plan period the proportion of doctors, doctors' aides, nurses, and midwives with regular training accounted for roughly 20 per cent of the total medical personnel, which indicated the existence of a rather large supporting force. During the 1959–64 period the growth of these four manpower groups far exceeded that in the first Five-Year Plan period, with the result that they came to represent a larger percentage of the total medical personnel. Assuming that higher- and intermediate-level medical personnel accounted for 30 per cent of the total in 1966, total requirements for low-level medical personnel should have been around 3.3 million. Total demand for health personnel in 1966 may then be estimated (Table 2).

Table 2. Estimated Demand for Health Personnel, 1966

	Calculated at 1.5% Growth Rate of Population	Calculated at 2% Growth Rate of Population
High-level medical personnel	290,000	303,000
Intermediate-level medical personnel	680,000	712,000
Low-level medical personnel	3,230,000	3,380,000
Total requirement	4,200,000	4,395,000

Estimated Manpower Resources

Official Manpower Statistics

The supply of health manpower comes from two sources: those trained before 1949 who are still professionally active, and those graduated after 1949.

Official statistics concerning the overall figures for public health workers have been sporadically reported for various years by the State Statistical Bureau, the Ministry of Health, and the Chinese Medical Association. The available data are summarized in Table 3.

The total number of medical workers shows a continuous upward trend to the year 1958 and a decline after 1961, which may have been caused partly by the financial difficulties of the 1959–61 period and partly by the changing scope of the statistics. Of the total medical manpower reported in the State Statistical Bureau's series, only four are specified (Table 4).

The ratio of the identified to the total medical personnel remains very stable during the years for which these data were reported. They constitute roughly 20 per cent of the total; the remaining 80 per cent is not specified.[11]

Table 3.   Medical Personnel as Reported by Various
Official Sources, 1950–1963

Year	*Total Number*
1950	780,000[1]
1952	1,040,000[1]
1956	1,890,000[2]
1957	1,908,000[1]
1958	2,160,000[1]
1961	1,940,000[3]
1963	1,400,000[4]

Sources: (1) People's Republic of China, State Statistical Bureau, *Ten Great Years* (Peking: Foreign Languages Press, 1960): p. 222; (2) *Jen-min Shou-ts'e 1958* (*People's Handbook 1958*) (Peking: Ta Kung Pao She, 1958): p. 637; (3) "The Success of Public Health Services in China," *ZDraven Front* (Sofia) (October 6, 1962), in *Joint Publications Research Service* 221, no. 19 (May 16, 1963): 105; (4) K'ai-yun Huang, "The Practice of Medicine in New China," *Ajia Keizai Jumpo* (*Asian Economic Report*) (Tokyo) no. 545 (July 1963), in *Joint Publications Research Service* 622, no. 23 (March 11, 1964): 84.

Table 4. Comparison of Identified Medical Personnel with Total Medical Personnel

Years	(1) Total Medical Personnel	(2) Western-type Doctors	(3) Doctor's Assistants	(4) Nurses	(5) Midwives	(6) (2) + (3) + (4) + (5)	(6) ÷ (1) Percent of Identified to the Total
1950	780,000	41,000	53,000	38,000	16,000	148,000	19.0
1952	1,040,000	52,000	67,000	61,000	22,000	202,000	19.4
1957	1,908,000	74,000	136,000	128,000	36,000	374,000	19.6
1958	2,160,000	75,000	131,000	138,000	35,000	379,000	18.1

Source: People's Republic of China, State Statistical Bureau, *Ten Great Years* (Peking: Foreign Languages Press, 1960): p. 222.

The Growth of Higher Medical Manpower

Higher medical manpower refers to physicians, pharmacists, and dentists with college training in Western-type medicine. In 1949 official data listed 41,000 "Western-type doctors" as practicing in China. The bulk of the physicians practicing in 1966 were new graduates trained during the post-1949 period.

Before 1949 China's medical institutes were divided into three categories: university medical schools, independent medical colleges, and medical schools with short courses. At the end of 1949 there were seventeen in the first group, fifteen in the second, and four in the third. During the period 1932–47 there were 80,411 new entrants to these medical institutions, of whom 8,929 graduated. Prior to 1949 most of the medical schools followed a six-year program, although nine years were required in some centers.

A series of reforms and reorganizations have been initiated since 1952, when the medical school course was first reduced to four years; it was increased to five years in 1955; and to six years for some well-established centers in 1960. Medical students in the post-1949 period were required to specialize in particular fields from the very beginning of their studies.

During the Great Leap Forward period in 1958–60, in order to accelerate training, medical colleges were greatly expanded. In 1957 there were only thirty-eight medical colleges, including four of traditional Chinese medicine and two of pharmacology; by the end of 1959 the number had soared to 142, almost four times the 1957 total.[12]

Under the "walking on two legs" policy, many newly-established medical schools offered two- or three-year programs; several leading institutes, however, lengthened their courses to six years. In addition, the China Medical University, founded in Peking in September 1958, offered an eight-year training program stressing basic sciences and basic medical knowledge as well as clinical medicine and scientific research.[13]

In the first decade of the Communist rule, enrollment in the medical colleges sextupled—from 15,200 in the 1949–50 academic year to 103,000 in 1960–61, when medical students accounted for 12–13 per cent of the total college enrollment as compared with 7 per cent in the pre-1949 era.

The training programs have undergone a period of readjustment and consolidation since 1961. Many newly formed institutions that lacked facilities, staffs, and qualified students were closed or merged, reducing the number of medical colleges to ninety-eight by 1963, eighteen of them colleges of traditional Chinese medicine.[14]

The number of medical colleges has been further reduced in recent years as emphasis has been placed on barefoot doctors rather than on doctors with regular training. In 1971 a Japanese government publication listed only sixty-nine higher medical colleges, including twelve of traditional medicine and two of pharmacology. The number had thus been reduced to only half of the 1959 peak.[15]

The vicissitudes of the training programs naturally affect the growth of medical manpower, as is clearly reflected in the fluctuation in the number of graduates between 1949 and 1966 (Table 5).

Table 5. Graduates of Higher Medical Institutions, 1949–1966

Year	Number Graduated	Percent of Total
1949–50	1,391	7.7
1950–51	2,366	12.5
1951–52	2,636	8.2
1952–53	2,948	6.1
1953–54	4,527	9.6
1954–55	6,840	12.4
1955–56	5,403	8.6
1956–57	6,200	11.1
1957–58	5,393	7.5
1958–59	9,000	12.9
1959–60	10,500	7.8
1960–61	19,000	11.7
1961–62	17,000	9.6
1962–63	25,000	12.5
1963–64	23,000	11.5
1964–65	19,000	11.2
1965–66	19,000	11.2
1949–57	32,311	18.0
1958–66	146,893	82.0
1949–66	179,204	100.0

Sources: For 1950–63, Chu-yuan Cheng, *Scientific and Engineering Manpower in Communist China 1949–1963* (Washington, D. C.: National Science Foundation, 1966): pp. 50–51; for 1964–66, Leo A. Orleans, "Communist China's Education, Policies, Problems and Prospects," in Joint Economic Committee, United States Congress, *An Economic Profile of Mainland China*, vol. 2 (Washington, D. C.: Government Printing Office, 1967): p. 55.

From 1966 to 1969 most medical colleges were suspended because of the Cultural Revolution.

During the 1949–66 period some 180,000 students graduated from medical college. If we add the 41,000 doctors professionally active in 1949 to the new graduates, and allow for a 10 per cent attrition, by the end of 1966 there were approximately 200,000 persons who had completed higher medical education.

Before 1965, because of the government's policy of promoting experienced nurses and doctor's assistants to the rank of physician, the actual number of doctors was higher than the total of graduates. A comparison of the official statistics on doctors during the 1950–58 period with the annual increase of medical college graduates shows a discrepancy of 1,689, or about 5 per cent of the total (Table 6).

Table 6. Discrepancies between Implied and Actual Number of Graduates from Medical Colleges, 1950–58

Year	I. Doctors in Practice	II. Annual Increase	III. Graduates from Medical Colleges	Discrepancies between II and III
1950	41,000[1]			
1951	46,500[2]	5,500	1,391	—4,109
1952	52,000[1]	5,500	2,366	—3,134
1953	56,400[3]	4,400	2,636	—1,764
1954	63,000[3]	6,600	2,948	—3,652
1955	70,500[3]	7,500	4,527	—2,973
1956	75,000[4]	4,500	6,840	2,340
1957	74,000[1]	—1,000	5,403	6,403
1958	75,000[1]	1,000	6,200	5,200
1950–58		34,000	32,311	—1,689

Sources: (1) People's Republic of China, State Statistical Bureau, *Ten Great Years* (Peking: Foreign Languages Press, 1960): p. 222; (2) interpolation; (3) *Jen-min Shou-ts'e, 1957* (*People's Handbook 1957*) (Peking: Ta Kung Pao She, 1957): p. 608; (4) *Jen-min Shou-ts'e, 1958* (*People's Handbook 1958*) (Peking: Ta Kung Pao She, 1958): p. 636.

Beginning in 1956 qualifications for the medical degree became more rigid. Not all new graduates were immediately granted the title of "doctor" and they had to serve as interns for a certain period. After 1965 the new principle was that "practical experience and theoretical study supplement one another, and insure for all workers in the medical profession the opportunity to acquire the highest qualification."[16] Following this new approach the government promoted many nurses and technicians to the rank of doctor. In Shanghai, Shenyang, and Hopei, for example, more than 700 nurses were promoted to physicians during 1965.[17]

Assuming that a 10 per cent rate of discrepancy is applied to the post-1958 period, when noncollege graduates were promoted, the total number of doctors in 1966 should have reached 235,000 (75,000 plus 160,000). Subtracting 10 per cent attrition for the entire period, the net total in 1966 would have been around 210,000. According to Orleans, 75 per cent of the medical graduates were specialists in therapeutic medicine, about 10 per cent were pharmacists, and 15 per cent were dentists.[18] The breakdown can thus be estimated as

Physicians	157,500	75%
Pharmacists	21,000	10%
Dentists	31,500	15%
Total	210,000	100%

Intermediate Medical Manpower

Under China's educational system, intermediate medical manpower such as doctor's assistants, nurses, midwives, junior pharmacists, and laboratory technicians were trained in specialized secondary schools. An official report in 1956 listed 176 secondary medical schools throughout the country.[19] The increase in such schools to 200 in 1964 and to 230 in 1965, contrasted with the decrease in the number of higher medical institutions during the same period, signifies the shift of emphasis in priority.

The number of secondary medical school graduates was officially reported as totalling 140,000 before 1949; increasing to 150,000 by 1958; to 250,000 by 1961; to 290,000 by 1962; and to 330,000 by 1964.[20] From these scattered data the increase in secondary medical graduates can be derived as follows:

1949–56	100,000
1957	31,108
1958	18,892
1959–61	100,000
1962	40,000
1963–64	40,000

Although these figures do not complement one another very well they do reveal the general trend: In the 1949–56 period about 15,000 were graduated annually; from 1957 to 1964 annual graduates doubled to 30,000. Assuming a continuation of this trend, by the end of 1966 another 60,000 should have been added, giving a total of 390,000 trained personnel in the 1949–66 period.

The number of people who received comparable training prior to 1949 has been estimated by Orleans at 144,000.[21] A deduction of 10 per cent attrition results in a surviving total of 130,000. Total secondary medical manpower with formal training was to have been around 520,000 by the end of 1966. The categories are estimated in Table 7.

Table 7. Estimate of Secondary-Level Medical Manpower, 1966

		Percent of Total
Doctor's assistants	179,000	34.4[1]
Nurses	193,000	37.2[1]
Midwives	44,000	8.4[1]
Junior pharmacists	52,000	10.0[2]
Laboratory technicians	52,000	10.0[3]
Total	520,000	100.0

Sources: (1) Leo A. Orleans, "Communist China's Education, Policies, Problems and Prospects," in Joint Economic Committee, United States Congress, *An Economic Profile of Mainland China*, vol. 2 (Washington, D. C.: Government Printing Office, 1967): p. 37; (2) assuming the same percentage of higher medical manpower, which is estimated at 10 per cent of the total; (3) residuals.

A Trial Balance Sheet of Demand and Supply

Table 8 summarizes the estimated demand for and supply of medical workers on the higher and intermediate levels in the years 1957, 1966, and 1971. The demands are based on the same medical manpower-population ratio of 1:2,500, and the same ratio between higher and intermediate personnel, 1:2.35. The estimated supplies for 1957 and 1966 are based on official data. Supply for 1971 is derived by adding new graduates between 1967 and 1971 to those previously in practice. During the 1949–55 period, when official statistics were more complete, the enrollment of one year and the total graduates of five consecutive years were almost equal. For example, the sum of graduates of 1949–54 was 13,868, which

Table 8. A Trial Balance Sheet of Demand and Supply for Higher
and Intermediate Medical Manpower in 1957, 1966, and 1971

Category	Demand	Supply	Deficiency
1957[1]			
Higher-level medical personnel	254,000	74,000	180,000
Intermediate medical personnel	597,000	261,000	336,000
1966[2]			
Higher-level medical personnel			
1.5% growth in population	290,000	210,000	80,000
2% growth in population	303,000	210,000	93,000
Intermediate medical personnel			
1.5% growth in population	680,000	520,000	160,000
2% growth in population	712,000	520,000	192,000
1971[3]			
Higher-level medical personnel			
1.5% growth in population	314,000	267,000	47,000
2% growth in population	335,000	267,000	68,000
Intermediate medical personnel			
1.5% growth in population	738,000	620,000	118,000
2% growth in population	787,000	620,000	167,000

Sources: (1) Population in 1957, *T'ung-chi Kung-tso* (*Statistical Work*) no. 11 (June 1957): 25; (2) population for 1966 is calculated on the basis of 1957 official data. At 1.5 per cent growth rate the population was 728 million; at 2 per cent growth rate, 758.8 million; (3) population for 1971, calculated at 1.5 per cent growth rate, was 783 million; at 2 per cent growth rate, 837 million.

comes very close to the 15,200 enrollment in the 1949–50 academic year. From this known relationship, if there were no interruption the total graduates for the 1966–71 period could be estimated at roughly 95,000.[22]

Because of the Cultural Revolution, however, most medical schools were closed between the autumn of 1966 and the summer of 1969. Formal training programs did not resume until 1970. During the 1966–69 period those students admitted in 1961, 1962, and 1963 had already received training varying from two to four years. According to the then new policy of shortening the curriculum from five or six to two or three years these students were probably graduated.[23] Assuming that 19,000 students graduated each year as in the 1964–65 period (Table 5), new graduates for the 1967–71 period would total only around 57,000.

The supply of intermediate medical manpower in the 1962–64 period was about 25,000 a year. Assuming the same rate of growth for the 1966–71 period, approximately 100,000 must be added to the 1966 supply, giving a total of 620,000 in 1971.

The supply of lower-level medical manpower is impossible to estimate because of the lack of statistics and the changing quality of training; a balance sheet of demand and supply has therefore not been constructed.

As shown in Table 8, a physician-population gap existed in each period under study, but it narrowed as time elapsed. Assuming a desired physician-population ratio of 1:2,500, the shortage of physicians declined continuously from 180,000 in 1957 to between 80,000 and 93,000 in 1966, a drop of 50 per cent. By 1971 the shortage was further reduced to between 47,000 and 68,000.

The gap between demand for and supply of intermediate-level personnel also showed continuous closing. The deficiency declined from 336,000 in 1957, to 160,000–192,000 in 1966, and to 118,000–167,000 in 1971. If this trend continues China may soon eliminate the gap between demand and supply in higher- and intermediate-level medical personnel. Should this be the case, why did the government interrupt the trend by introducing the barefoot doctor and the "revolutionary transformation" of medical and public health services in the past few years? The answer to this question cannot be arrived at through quantitative study alone. Inappropriate distribution and utilization may hold the key to the problem.

New Policies and Implications

Partly for the purpose of closing the gap between demand and supply, and partly to correct the uneven distribution of medical manpower in the urban and rural areas, a sweeping reform of Chinese medical and health services has been undertaken since 1965. On June 26, 1965 Chairman Mao Tse-tung issued instructions that "the central gravity of health work be shifted to the countryside."

Ever since the introduction of Western-type medicine to China the facilities and manpower have been concentrated in the large cities, leaving the rural areas, where 80 per cent of the population live, virtually without modern medical care. In the prewar era, 75 per cent of the doctors were located in the main ports of the six coastal provinces.[24] The situation remained unchanged after 1949.

In Kwangtung Province in 1967, two-thirds of the hospital beds, 70–80 per cent of government funds, and 60 per cent of high-level medical personnel were retained in the cities to serve 20 per cent of the province's population. The ratio of doctors to population was 1:600 in Canton, the provincial capital, compared with 1:10,000 in the rural sector.[25] It was due to the extremely uneven distribution of manpower and facilities that in June 1965 Mao voiced severe criticism of public health work in China:

> Public health work is serving only 15 per cent of the population of the nation. The peasants cannot get treatment. They have no doctor and no medicine. The Ministry of Health is not the people's Ministry of Health. It has become a Ministry of Health of the Towns and Mandarins. We would call it the Towns' and Mandarins' Ministry of Health.[26]

Following Mao's directive, several major steps were taken to change the existing medical structures. The first measure involved a wholesale redistribution of medical and public health manpower by means of transferring one-half of the urban hospital staff members to rural areas, setting up "rural health bases," and reinforcing rural medical facilities. Although no nationwide statistics have been published, local newspapers and broadcasts have disclosed a continuous manpower transfer since 1965. In Hopeh Province, for example, the first transfer involved 10,000 medical and health personnel from hospitals above the *hsien* (county) level to form health teams in the countryside.[27] In Heilungkiang Province in Manchuria, by 1968 more than 20,000 urban medical and health workers were serving with circuit medical teams in rural areas.[28]

The second measure was the formation of a rural cooperative medical network. By using the transferred medical personnel as the hard core, a nationwide system has gradually been taking shape. A central hospital has been set up in each *hsien*; health clinics have been established at the commune or village level; each commune production brigade has organized a cooperative medical station; and each production team has a few so-called "red medical rooms" for first aid.

The medical force consists of full-time health workers, barefoot doctors in the production brigades, health personnel on the production teams, and Red Guard medical workers, who are nonprofessionals, in the cities.[29] The barefoot doctors are rural youths in their early twenties who have had at most a primary school education. In the beginning they are given a three-month training course in local hospitals. After working with peasants for a year or more, the talented and most enthusiastic are sent back to urban medical centers for further training. As a typical example, in Lung-hus county in Hopeh Province thirty-seven production brigades in three communes formed a cooperative medical care system that has a force of 105 barefoot doctors whose average age is twenty-four. These "doctors" have in turn helped to train some 1,000 health workers' assistants and acupuncturists.[30] The term "barefoot doctor" is clearly meant to symbolize the orientation of the new basic level of medical work toward the rural poor.

The third measure involved the revision of the system of medical education. Mao was quoted as accusing the current medical training system of being impractical and ineffective. The five- to six-year curriculum was considered too long, and the courses divorced from Chinese reality. Western-type doctors frequently felt contempt for traditional Chinese medicine and its practitioners, even though the latter were indispensable. A dualism of medicine existed and there was no linkage between the two kinds of medicine.

In 1958 the authorities called for the synthesis of Chinese and Western medicine by drafting 2,000 Western-type doctors for a two-year, full-time study of Chinese medicine. More than ten higher institutions of medicine were set up for the study of traditional medicine and, by 1965, 10,000 students had been enrolled. The fundamental idea was that by developing Chinese medicine along with Western medicine the two would eventually merge into a new medical science that would transcend either of them.

Since the Cultural Revolution there has been a renewed emphasis on developing Chinese medicine, and publicity about acupuncture. Acreage sown to medicinal herbs in 1971 was 50 per cent higher than in 1965, and total value of sales rose by 64 per cent.[31]

At the same time a thorough reform in medical education has been underway. Medical schools and their affiliated teaching hospitals have set up branches in the countryside to which more than one-third of the regular teaching staff have been transferred. Most training programs have been cut to three years from the previous five- or six-year courses. The new medical training stresses research on cures for diseases common in rural areas, such as gastrointestinal infections, cataracts, and schistosomiasis. Students are required to learn daily medical and nursing routines—dressing wounds, administering injections, prescribing drugs, and performing acupuncture; very little time is allocated for theoretical studies. When completed, the new reform will require a shift of the students, both physically and mentally, from the "three bigs"—big universities, big cities, and big hospitals—to the "three smalls"—small schools, small clinics, and small towns. The selection of medical students will be based on political attitudes and class origins, in order to change the class composition of medical professionals from bourgeois and intellectual to worker and peasant origins.[32]

While reforms in medical structure and education are still in process, implications for Chinese medical manpower training and distribution have become quite evident.

First, the emergence of millions of barefoot doctors resembles the "backyard blast furnaces" during the Great Leap. Once again the leaders intend to close a gap by a faster and more economical method—the gap now being the lack of professional medical manpower in the rural areas. The traditional system of training intermediate-level medical staffs through the secondary education system is apparently being modified if not totally abandoned.

Second, the attack on the professional mentality of the Western-type physicians, the new curriculum shortening the period of training, and the renewed attention to traditional medicine are designed to destroy the medical dualism that provides an elite corps of doctors too small for China's needs and too individualistic for Chinese Communism.

Third, as the Chinese leaders see it, the problem of medical manpower distribution is at least as significant as the expansion of manpower, if not more so. If new medical graduates continue to be employed in urban hospitals this can only serve to lower the physician-population ratio in the urban sector, but not in the rural sector, which will lead to a wider disparity of medical services between the two. The deployment of one-third of urban medical doctors to the countryside, in addition to the 15 per cent originally serving there, will enable the rural sector to have roughly 48 per cent of Western-type doctors. Based on our estimated supply, this means that 125,000 Western-type doctors were in the rural area in 1971. When distributed among the 75,000 communes and 2,400 *hsiens*, this number would suffice to provide one doctor for each commune and twenty for each *hsien*. With these transferred doctors as a backbone, a rural medical network can now become functioning.

Finally, by setting up clinics in the communes, health stations in the production brigades, and health rooms in the production teams, the Chinese leaders hope to translate the needs for medical care of the vast rural population into mass participation. The rural cooperative medical network, albeit of low quality of service, will become a vehicle to mobilize the entire population to engage in sanitation and public health work; it will also minimize the costs of medical care which in the past the rural poor have not been able to afford. The Chinese experimentation, if successful, may serve as a model for many developing nations where modern medical care is still limited to a small segment of the population.

NOTES

1. People's Republic of China, State Statistical Bureau, *Ten Great Years* (Peking: Foreign Languages Press, 1960): p. 222.

2. Huang K'ai-yun, "The Practice of Medicine in New China," *Ajia Keizai Jumpo (Asian Economic Report)*, Tokyo, no. 545 (July 1963), in *Joint Publications Research Service* 622, no. 23 (March 11, 1964): 84.

3. R. I. Lee and L. W. Jones, *The Fundamentals of Good Medical Care* (Chicago: University of Chicago Press, 1933).

4. Thomas L. Hall, *Health Manpower in Peru* (Baltimore: The Johns Hopkins Press, 1969): pp. 37–38.

5. Report of the Surgeon General's Consultant Group on Medical Education, *Physicians for a Growing America*, Publication No. 709 (Washington, D. C.: Government Printing Office, October 1959): and *Report of the Royal Commission on Health Services*, vol. I (1964) and II (1965) (Ottawa: Queen's Printer).

6. Huang Chi-yin, "The Tabulation of Planning for Cultural, Educational and Public Health Enterprises," *Chi-hua Ching-chi (Planned Economy)*, Peking, no. 2 (1958): 39–44.

7. Ts'ui I-t'ien, *Ti-i-ko Wu-nien-chi-hua-chung ti Wei-sheng Pao-chien Shih-yeh (The Hygienic and Public Health Works in the First Five-Year Plan Period)* (Peking: Chung-hua Chuan-kuo Ko-hsueh Chi-hsu Pu-chi Hsueh-hui, 1956): pp. 2–3.

8. Hall, *Health Manpower in Peru*, p. 63.

9. Timothy D. Baker and Mark Perlman, *Health Manpower in a Developing Economy. Taiwan: A Case Study in Planning* (Baltimore: Johns Hopkins Press, 1967): p. 77.

10. *Kuang-ming Jih-pao* (Peking: October 3, 1961).

11. In 1957 Li Te-chuan, former minister of health, stated that there were 1,890,000 medical workers in 1956, including the following categories: midwives with regular training, 34,000; workers for maternal and child health, 44,000; midwives without modern training, 578,000; and nursing aides, 356,000. These four groups total 1,012,000 (*Jen-min Shou-t'se 1958 [People's Handbook 1958]:* p. 637). Since the total number of medical workers for 1956 and for 1957 differs only

slightly (less than 1 per cent), if we apply the number of Western-type doctors, doctor's assistants, and nurses in 1957 to the 1956 identified groups, then the total personnel in the identified categories would add up to 1,351,000. The remaining 540,000 would be supporting administrative personnel and technicians.

12. Chu-yuan Cheng, *Scientific and Engineering Manpower in Communist China 1949–1963* (Washington, D. C.: National Science Foundation, 1966): pp. 50–51.

13. According to Wilder Penfield, a Canadian physician who visited China in 1962, one-third of the medical colleges provided a six-year curriculum. Penfield reported that only a very few schools had a three-year course. See "Oriental Renaissance in Education and Medicine," *Science*, no. 141 (September 20, 1963): 1155.

14. Huang, *The Practice of Medicine*.

15. Japanese Government, Cabinet Research Office, *Organizations and Who's Who in the People's Republic of China* (in Japanese) (Tokyo: 1971): pp. 343–48.

16. *New China News Agency* (March 3, 1966).

17. Leo Orleans, "Medical Education and Manpower in Communist China," in *Comparative Education Review* (February 1969): 28.

18. Ibid.

19. *Jen-min Shou-t'se 1958* (*People's Handbook 1958*) (Peking: Ta Kung Pao She, 1958): p. 636.

20. *Joint Publications Research Service* 221, no. 19 (May 16, 1963): 105; and *Chung-kuo Hsin-wen* (*China News Service*) (Canton: December 1, 1964).

21. Orleans, "Medical Education and Manpower."

22. According to J. B. Best, an Australian physician who visited China in 1966, "Western-style doctors have increased from 10,000 in 1949 to 300,000 in 1966, and they are being trained at the rate of 25,000 annually." See "Impressions of Chinese Medical Services," in *Eastern Horizon* 6, no. 10 (Hong Kong: October 1967): 34. The figure of 25,000 is for the year 1962–63. Since 1964 the number of graduates has been scaled down to 19,000 due to adjustments made in the training program.

23. According to Victor W. Sidel, who visited China in late 1971, "The most immediate effect of the Cultural Revolution on medical education was to close the medical schools to new classes for three years. Those already in medical school were given accelerated training, graduated almost immediately, and sent to work, usually with faculty members, in the countryside." See "Serve the People: Medical Education in the People's Republic of China," *The New Physician* (May 1972): 288.

24. Sze-ming Sze, former general secretary of the Chinese Medical Association, *China's Health Problems* (New York: China Institute of America, 1942): p. 18.

25. "Canton Forum of Medical Personnel on Tour in Rural Areas," *Union Research Service* 49, no. 22 (December 15, 1967): 289–303.

26. Broadcast of Radio Kunming, Yunnan Province (August 24, 1967).

27. *Kuang-ming Jih-pao* (Peking, August 5, 1965).

28. Broadcast of Radio Harbin, Heilungkiang Province (March 11, 1968).

29. *Kuang-ming Jih-pao* (Peking, January 26, 1971): p. 3.

30. *Jen-min Jih-pao* (Peking, January 10, 1971): 3.

31. *Peking Review* (March 24, 1972): 23.

32. Janet Salaff, "Physician Heal Thyself," *Far Eastern Economic Review* (Hong Kong, October 31, 1968): 291–93.

The Role and Training
of Medical Personnel

VICTOR W. SIDEL

In a brief review of a topic as broad as the role and training of medical personnel in the People's Republic of China, it seems more important to attempt to stress the general principles on which the role of medical workers and their training appear to be based rather than to present detailed job descriptions, statistics, or curricula, some of which are now becoming available in a variety of publications.[1-7]

On the other hand, one month—which was the duration of our visit to China as the guests of the Chinese Medical Association (CMA) in September-October, 1971*—represents an extremely brief period of time in which to observe general principles in a culture totally different from one's own. One must depend on descriptions of duties and curricula, for example, rather than on personal observation. One is also dependent on one's hosts for choice of sites. Although our requests to visit certain types of institutions and to talk with certain types of personnel were almost invariably granted, the institutions we saw and the people with whom we talked were not necessarily typical of the country as a whole or even of the areas we visited. Nonetheless we saw enough different types of institutions and people to make it possible to attempt some generalizations about the role of medical personnel and their training.

- **There is still a relative shortage of resources in,**
but an increasing emphasis on, care in rural areas

Eighty per cent of China's population live in rural areas, a far higher percentage than in the United States where 27 per cent of

---

* In China at about the same time were Drs. E. Grey Dimond, Samuel Rosen, and Paul Dudley White, who together with their wives were independently invited by the Chinese Medical Association; our visits overlapped to some extent.

the people live in areas defined as rural by the Bureau of the Census,[8] or in the Soviet Union where 44 per cent of the population are said to live in rural areas.[9] The rural areas of China prior to 1949 had almost no Western-type medical personnel or facilities; it was estimated by the secretary-general of the CMA in 1943 that 75 per cent of China's doctors of Western medicine, of which he estimated there were only 12,000 to serve a population of some 540 million, were located in the major ports of six coastal provinces.[10] Therefore the only medical personnel to which peasants in the countryside and most of the poor people of the cities had access were doctors of Chinese medicine who used herb medicine, acupuncture, moxibustion, and other traditional techniques. From the time of Liberation in 1949 to the start of the Great Proletarian Cultural Revolution in 1966 there was some improvement in rural availability of health care, but far from enough. One of the issues of the Cultural Revolution was the persisting urban-rural differences, and great efforts have been made since 1966 to rotate medical personnel from the cities into the rural areas and to train indigenous health workers.

A major force in this effort was Mao's directive of June 26, 1965: "In health and medical work, put the stress on the rural areas."

• Most services and training programs are being decentralized

The Chinese are alleged to have been the inventors of bureaucracy—one of the lesser of the many discoveries the world owes to them—and the development of centralization and bureaucracy in the period from Liberation through 1966 was another of the central issues of the Cultural Revolution. In the wake of the Cultural Revolution, medical care services and training facilities for medical personnel have been increasingly decentralized to the city or province and to the urban district or rural commune in which they are located. Each city or province appears to be able to make its own decisions, within certain broad guidelines, about the nature of the training of health personnel and the ways in which they are used. Strangely enough this decentralization is much more similar to certain aspects of medical care organization in the United States— for example, to the way medical auxiliaries have developed through multiple programs such as Medex, physician's assistants, physician's associates, and nurse practitioners, and to the different state laws governing them[11]—than it is to the practice in the Soviet Union where common job definitions and training patterns seem widely prevalent throughout a country covering one-sixth of the earth's land mass.[12,13] Yet despite the decentralization, certain basic principles of the way health care personnel work and the way they are trained seem common to all of the four cities and their environs that we visited.

- **Major efforts are being made to integrate traditional Chinese medicine with Western medicine**

The Chinese use the term *xiyi* (Western medicine) to differentiate the theory and methods used by doctors trained in "scientific" or "modern" medicine—whether trained in China or abroad—from those used by doctors trained in *zhongyi* (Chinese medicine).[14] The reasons for the attempts to integrate Chinese medicine, which Mao has called China's "greatest treasure," into the mainstream of medicine are probably multiple: belief in its efficacy; "cultural nationalism" as in the stress on Chinese painting and Chinese music; the trust that the rural people have had in their traditional doctors, which would often lead them to refuse to accept Western practice even when it was available; and the shortage of other types of personnel. Whatever the reason, the two types of medicine are being increasingly integrated both in practice and in education. Western-type doctors are being trained in the use of techniques such as acupuncture and in the properties of herb medicine, and traditional practitioners are being brought into closer relationships with Western-type institutions and doctors.

- **A broad spectrum of medical care personnel is being developed**

An axiom of current Chinese philosophy is the development and use of every individual up to the highest level of his capacity. This is important not only to achieve the use of human potential in a people-rich, technology-poor society, but to fulfill the ideologic goals of providing opportunities for each person to "serve the public first, self second." One corollary to this philosophy is the development of a broad spectrum of skills, ranging from community members with no special training or skills to superspecialists—but with a difference in attitude, as we shall see, from superspecialists in the United States. In between lie members of the "mass" such as rural health workers and Red Guard doctors; paraprofessionals such as worker doctors, barefoot doctors, and midwives; middle medical workers such as assistant doctors and nurses; and regular doctors.

• **Emphasis is placed on skills rather than on credentials**

Another corollary to the use of each individual up to his fullest capacity is that what a person demonstrates in the way of skills seems considerably more important to his assignment than—as in the United States—the length of his training or experience or the possession of a specific license or credential. The decentralized nature of education and of employment would make nationwide standards for either education or employment very difficult to achieve, even if that were one of the Chinese goals. Since role assignment and promotion are usually done on a local basis, it seems quite possible that these decisions can be made on the basis of direct observation and evaluation of the skills of the person involved.

• **The "mass" is mobilized to participate in their own health care and that of their community**

As described by Ruth Sidel in her paper in this volume, the Chinese make heavy use of essentially untrained community members in health and medical care. This group of what might be called mass workers, volunteers, nonprofessionals, or free-time workers, depending on the context, includes community members who participate in the Great Patriotic Health Movements and who are expected to play a large role in public health measures as well as to participate in their own medical care. We were given the impression that great stress was laid on health education and on a person's being "self-reliant" in relation to his own care and to the care of his neighbors when necessary.

The rural health workers who are trained by the barefoot doctors and who do environmental sanitation and other duties during their lunch breaks and "leisure time" are also examples of this group. A more well-trained worker, who actually falls somewhere between the category of volunteer and paraprofessional, is the Red Guard doctor, who is usually a housewife who lives in the neighborhood and serves in the neighborhood or lane health station. She has had brief formal training—often as little as ten days—and helps provide immunizations, family planning and health education information, and primary care services on a neighborhood basis. She is not paid for her work.

- **Paraprofessionals are widely used**

Although the word paraprofessional has been abused in the United States and has been made to carry whatever positive or negative connotations the user wishes, it would appear to have a real denotative use in describing the barefoot doctor and worker doctor. The words "part-time" would also seem applicable. The barefoot doctor is a peasant who has been given from three to six months' medical training and who spends about half of his time— more during the off-season and less during the planting and harvesting season—providing environmental sanitation, health education, immunizations, first aid, and certain elements of primary care. There are said to be "over a million" barefoot doctors in China.

The training and responsibilities of Liu Yu-sheng, the twenty-six-year-old barefoot doctor of the Double North Production Team (population 509) of the Shuang Chiao (Double Bridge) People's Commune, are typical of the barefoot doctors whom we met. After graduating from junior middle school Liu Yu-sheng worked in a production team. When Chairman Mao issued his June 26th directive Liu was elected by the members of the team to be trained as a barefoot doctor. He was taught for three months in his commune by mobile medical teams of doctors from urban hospitals. Since he began his work as a barefoot doctor he has had opportunities for short leaves of absence for further study. Recently Comrade Liu went to Peking for three months to study traditional Chinese medicine. He focuses on prevention, health education, and the treatment of "common diseases."

Midwives are also trained to provide birth control methods and education and prenatal care, and to perform uncomplicated deliveries on the communes. Their training generally lasts for three to six months. The worker doctor is the analogue in the factories of the barefoot doctor in the communes.

None of these types of workers are paid directly for their medical work but receive regular income—based on work points for the agricultural worker and on wages for the factory worker—with no deduction for the time spent in medical work. The role and training of these personnel, as well as of the closely related Red Guard doctors, are described in detail elsewhere.[15]

- **"Middle medical personnel" were developed
during the period of Soviet influence**

During the period of Soviet influence, from the early 1950s through the early 1960s, the Chinese developed a number of "middle medical schools" following the Soviet pattern. They trained assistant doctors—who seem comparable, so far as I can tell, to the Soviet feldshers—nurses, midwives, and pharmacists. These are clearly full-time, professional medical care personnel. Prior to the Cultural Revolution these personnel required about three years of training; since the Cultural Revolution their training has been reduced experimentally to two years or less.

- **There have been major changes in the recruitment
and training of doctors of "Western" medicine**

Starting from a very inadequate number of doctors, the Chinese after Liberation trained a large number of doctors following Western, and especially Soviet, training patterns. Medical education required about six years after senior middle school, with one school in Peking—the Chinese Medical University which, in about 1962, after a decade's hiatus became the successor to the Peking Union Medical College—having an eight-year program and training researchers and teachers.

This pattern of education was harshly criticized during the Cultural Revolution. The curriculum was said to be "decayed and time-worn" and "copied from capitalist and revisionist countries."

> . . . The curriculum required students to study as long as six or even eight years, but after graduation they were unable to treat independently even the most frequently encountered diseases. Leaving the big hospital, with its laboratories and modern equipment, they found themselves at their wits' end. In the course of six years, three-fourths of the time was spent studying textbooks and reciting abstract theories. . . . The pre-clinical subjects diverged so sharply from their clinical work that the students could find no effective use for the supposedly basic theories which had been drilled into them. Education in the medical colleges over the years was carried out after the fashion of stuffing and fattening Peking ducks. The students memorized the subjects for the examination, and once their ordeals were over, all was well and forgotten.[16]

Since the Cultural Revolution the pattern of medical education has been experimentally reduced to three years or less and the content has been changed. This has been accomplished, we were told, "by eliminating the irrelevant and the redundant, by combining the theoretical with the practical, and by using the 'three-in-one principle' of teachers teach students, students teach teachers, and students teach students." The method of recruitment into medical school was also altered: Candidates are selected by their fellow workers in the communes and factories, and those who have been barefoot doctors and health workers have increased opportunities for medical training.

Chang Sin-yen, for example, is a twenty-two-year-old medical student at the Dr. Sun Yat-sen Medical College in Canton. After graduation from junior middle school in 1966 at the age of seventeen she went to work in a commune. She was trained as a barefoot doctor, and had responsibility for a commune production team of over 100 people. She was chosen by her fellow commune members to enter medical school in 1970. When she graduates she will almost surely return to her commune to practice.

These changes in medical school recruitment and curriculum are described in greater detail elsewhere.[17,18]

• The salary structure is being altered in the wake of the Cultural Revolution

Prior to the Cultural Revolution fairly large salary differentials had developed among medical care personnel. Doctors who were very senior in specialization or academic status often earned four to five times as much as a beginning doctor, and there was a large differential in income between doctors and middle medical workers. Some doctors were even permitted to remain in private practice.[19] As one of the results of the Cultural Revolution all doctors and other medical workers are on salary. It has been decided that the wages at the upper end of the scale will be frozen until wages at the lower end rise to meet them. This is a relatively new policy and its consistent application and effects are not yet clear.

• Professionals and intellectuals are being "reeducated"

One purpose of the Cultural Revolution was to minimize the differences between those who work with their minds and those who work with their hands. As a consequence, all Chinese intellectuals spend some periods of time being "reeducated," usually in "May

7th schools" in the countryside. As another part of this effort, medical workers, including superspecialists, from urban hospitals spend six months to a year, or longer if they wish to take their families with them, in rural areas providing services and training and being themselves educated on the life and problems of the rural Chinese.

One of the most moving stories of an experience in the country-side was told to us by Dr. Chiang Ray-ling, a tall, slim, thirty-seven-year-old internist at the Friendship Hospital in Peking, who spent one year as a member of a mobile medical team in Shensi Province. "After the Cultural Revolution it became clear that conditions in the countryside were more backward than in the city and that the countryside needed more experienced medical care to serve the peasants," Dr. Chiang told us. Her mobile medical team was part of the hospital's effort to put resources into rural medical care and to help urban physicians to become more familiar with the life of the peasants. In the countryside Dr. Chiang lived with the peasants, and ate, worked, and collected herbs with them. She "witnessed how energetic and how revolutionary their ideology is, what a heroic spirit they have." Her "sentiments changed" and she started to look upon them as members of her own family. She told us that before this experience, when she treated a peasant in the outpatient department, she focused only on the disease instead of on the patient—and on how he had managed to come to the hospital and how he lived. Now that she is more familiar with how the peasants live, she considers the relationship between the doctor and the patient, not merely between the patient and his disease.

Although Dr. Chiang practices only internal medicine in Peking, in the countryside she was called upon to treat all kinds of illness; the peasants saw her as a doctor, not as a specialist. Dr. Chiang was in the countryside from May 1970 until July 1971 without once returning to Peking to see her husband and two children, aged eight and two, who were cared for by their grandmother. When we asked why she did not visit, she replied, "There was too much work to do."

From all of those with whom we talked it seems quite clear that these kinds of experiences have given urban medical specialists a new respect for the problems, the work, and the dedication of those who provide primary care, both in the city and in the country.

- **There is a strong emphasis on continuing education**

The Chinese believe that the formal initial period of instruction for all medical workers is much less important than continued on-the-job supervision and training. An example of this in the teaching of the barefoot doctor was given us by Dr. Hsu Chia-yu, deputy chief of internal medicine at the East Is Red Hospital in Shanghai, who was our interpreter while we were in China. Dr. Hsu told us of training barefoot doctors in a county hospital and then returning with them to their communes to provide on-the-job supervision and training. Dr. Hsu described how he lived with a barefoot doctor and his family, sleeping in the same bed and using the same pillow as the barefoot doctor. He told us that this had been quite difficult for him to do because he had been raised in Shanghai and had never shared a pillow with anyone before. Dr. Hsu described how he and the barefoot doctor would talk before going to sleep, both of the patients they had seen during the day and of their hopes and goals for their society.

- **The emphasis is on service rather than on personal reward**

Everywhere we went in China we saw the words *Wei renmin fuwu,* "Serve the People." To the Chinese with whom we spoke this is not at all an empty cliché but the basis for a way of life, and for all human services, including health services. While there was no doubt that health workers gained personal satisfaction from their work, the gratification seemed to come from the opportunity to be of service rather than from the status or financial reward that goes along with it.

In summary, we observed in China a society trying to recruit, train, motivate, and employ medical personnel in ways very different from those used in the West. The methods being used by the Chinese seemed extremely well suited to their special health and medical problems and—even more important—extremely well integrated into the social structures they are attempting to build. Medical personnel are viewed not only in relation to the specific services they perform but as an important part of the society and its overall development. Here, in my view, lie some of the most important lessons that we can learn from the People's Republic of China.

NOTES

1. J. S. Horn, *Away with All Pests . . . An English Surgeon in People's China* (New York: Monthly Review Press, 1969).

2. E. G. Dimond, "Medical Education and Care in People's Republic of China," *Journal of the American Medical Association* 218 (December 6, 1971): 1552–57.

3. R. Sidel and V. W. Sidel, "Human Services in the People's Republic of China," *Social Policy* 2, no. 6 (March–April 1972): 25–34.

4. V. W. Sidel, "The Barefoot Doctors of the People's Republic of China," *New England Journal of Medicine* 286 (June 1972): 1292–99.

5. ———, "Serve the People: Medical Education in the People's Republic of China," *The New Physician* 21 (May 1972): 284–91.

6. ———, "Medical Personnel and Their Training in the People's Republic of China," in J. R. Quinn, ed., *Medicine and Public Health in the People's Republic of China* (Washington, D. C.: Department of Health, Education, and Welfare Publication No. (NIH) 72–67, June 1972): pp. 151–67.

7. ———, "Some Observations on the Organization of Health Services in the People's Republic of China," *International Journal of Health Services* 2 (August 1972): 385–95.

8. U.S. Bureau of the Census, *1970 Census of Population*, PC (VI)–1 (Washington, D. C.: Bureau of the Census, February 1971).

9. *Narodnoe Khoziaistvo SSSR v 1968 Godu* (People's Economy, USSR, 1968) (Moscow: Central Statistical Unit, 1969): p. 7.

10. S. M. Sze, *China's Health Problems* (New York: China Institute of America, 1942): p. 18.

11. J. Hughbanks and D. K. Freeborn, "Review of 22 Training Programs for Physician's Assistants 1969." *HSHMA Health Reports* 86 (1971): 857–62.

12. V. W. Sidel, "Feldshers and 'Feldsherism,'" *New England Journal of Medicine* 278 (1968): 934–40, 981–92.

13. J. E. Muller et al., "The Soviet Health System—Aspects of Relevence for American Medicine," *New England Journal of Medicine* 286 (March 1972): 693–702.

14. R. C. Croizier. *Traditional Medicine in Modern China* (Cambridge: Harvard University Press, 1968): pp. 4–5.

15. Sidel, "The Barefoot Doctors."

16. Revolutionary Committee of the Shanghai First Medical College, "Medical Education Must Be Transformed on the Basis of Mao Tse-tung's Thought," *China's Medicine* no. 3 (March 1968): 159–63.

17. Dimond, "Medical Education."

18. Sidel, "Serve the People."

19. T. F. Fox, "The New China: Some Medical Impressions," *Lancet* 2 (1957): 935–39, 995–99, 1053–57.

V. Disease Control, Nutrition, and Preventive Care

Introductory Note

Four papers are included in this chapter, which is concerned with various aspects of disease control, nutrition, and preventive care in the People's Republic of China. Robert Worth, an epidemiologist who had lived in China and worked in Hong Kong and Macao, discusses the general strategy of the PRC in combating its rampant infectious diseases on a nationwide scale. Tien-hsi Cheng, a parasitologist, describes the achievements made in, and the various methods used for, the control of parasitic and other diseases. W. K. Ng and G. R. Wadsworth, both nutritionists, discuss food, food habits, and malnutrition. A. Minkowski, a French pediatrician who has visited China twice in recent years, gives an account of developments in maternal and child health care.

Though still lacking in precise disease data and evaluative information on the effectiveness of various control measures, the available evidence suggests a remarkable reduction in widespread disease and malnutrition, once regarded fatalistically as always being part of China. The reported achievements include, among others, the control of syphilis and other venereal diseases, cholera, plague, smallpox, kala-azar, malaria, trachoma, schistosomiasis, filariasis, hookworm, and, to a lesser extent, leprosy and tuberculosis.

In all disease control programs an orderly sequence of events appeared to be taking place, starting with treatment of the affected; long-term social engineering to minimize social risks; technical decisions on diagnostic methods; decisions on methods of identification of high-risk segments of the population; field trials of experimental control techniques; assessment and validation of the results of the experiments; dissemination of knowledge and techniques through conferences and training programs; and, finally, extension to other areas, nationwide, with maintenance of maximum local autonomy in implementation. The control programs apparently represent a unique mixture of epidemiological judgment and innovative sociopolitical action for translating biomedical knowledge into practical application, and making maximum use of available human, material, and sociocultural resources.

With the increased production and improved distribution of food, the peasants' nutritional condition has apparently improved to a great extent, although precise information on the actual situation is still unavailable. Disease conditions due to nutritional deficiency appear to have greatly decreased, but again much more information will have to be obtained to gain a clearer understanding of the nature and extent of the decline.

As a priority program in health, maternal and child health care has made significant progress, as witnessed, for example, in the reduction of infant mortality rates and the incidence of prematurity. Extensive preventive services are available, often carried out by nonprofessional health workers, at all stages of care of mother and child from prenatal to birth and, later, up to school age. Information is still unavailable, however, as to the comprehensiveness of the coverage and the quality of the services. One recurrent observation reported by many people points to the determination of the government and the willingness of the people to improve their own health by effectively carrying out preventive programs such as vaccinations and attendance at prenatal checkups.

New China's Accomplishments
in the Control of Diseases

ROBERT M. WORTH*

When I was growing up in a small town up the river from Shanghai, several vivid images about diseases were imprinted in my memory:

—When I was about seven years old my mother told me that during the summer of 1924, when I was born, there had been six other babies born in our immediate neighborhood of whom only one had survived with me to reach his seventh birthday.

—I was not allowed to go swimming in the canals or lakes because of the danger of schistosomiasis.

—I was not allowed to eat or drink anything unless an elaborate boiling, cooking, or peeling ritual had first been followed.

—I recall how hard my missionary-doctor grandfather worked, along with the other doctors and nurses, to give intravenous fluids to cholera victims brought to the hospitals during an epidemic; I also remember wondering why there was not at least an equivalent effort to fix the village wells.

It was these early childhood images of "old China" that led me into preventive medicine, and have continued to sustain my interest in the public health accomplishments of "new China."

Health Strategy

When I was in my first few months as a student at an American school of public health I was taught that the priority list for the control of diseases should be something like this:

1. Political priorities—to gain public support:

  (a) Concentrate resources first on the control of those diseases that cause a great rate of morbidity or premature mor-

* The author wishes to express his gratitude to Mr. Koji Ariyoshi of Honolulu, Dr. Joshua Horn of London, and Dr. Ma Hai-teh of Peking for their kindness in reading and criticizing a draft of this paper. Any errors remaining in the text are the sole responsibility of the author.

tality *and that you know how to control easily or quickly in that society*—rapid results will be clearly visible to the people and will result in gratitude, increased public co-operation, and continued political support.

(b) Then move into control programs that take longer to accomplish and/or require a large measure of public cooperation and/or changes in ways of living.

2. Technical priorities—to reduce the incidence of new cases to as near zero as possible:

(a) Where a specific vector can be identified and is suscepti-ble to control, a direct environmental attack on it will usually give maximum, long-term, benefit-cost ratios, particularly in places with a high population density.

(b) Where vector control is not available, if feasible, immu-nize to produce long-lasting artificial immunity; if not, short-lasting immunization or mass chemoprophylaxis may be alternative approaches.

(c) Where neither vector control nor immunization is feasi-ble, try to minimize transmission by early case-finding and treatment—mass treatment is a variant of this approach.

(d) As a supplemental approach to any of the above, or as a long-term alternative, attention should be focused on education to change behavior in order to promote avoidance of exposure and/or improvement in non-specific resistance through improved nutritional status of those who are exposed or potentially exposed.

When the leaders of the present regime took over China in 1949 they were faced with about 500 million people with a very high prevalence of many diseases, and malnutrition was rampant. The situation had been aggravated by the recent war and by the abject poverty in which a majority of the peasant population had lived for generations. Resources of trained manpower were very limited, and medical services did not reach the rural population. It is in-structive to see how the Chinese went about the tremendous tasks that faced them and how their priorities and strategies compare with those that I was taught.

Rifkin and Kaplinsky have characterized health systems along three different axes:

1. Health program—preventive versus curative emphasis;
2. Delivery system—labor intensive versus capital intensive;
3. Target population—rural versus urban (also masses versus elite).[1]

It is their contention that the Chinese health system is characterized by more emphasis on prevention, by being more labor intensive, and by being more focused on the rural masses than is the case in virtually every other developing country. Let us test this analysis by looking both at the official pronouncements of the government and by examining the actual character of the health system of China with regard to a major aspect of its responsibility— the control of diseases in the population.

The first National Health Conference was convened in Peking in August 1950 and received the following directive from Mao Tsetung: "Unite all medical workers, young and old, of the traditional school and the Western school, and organize a solid, united front to strive for the people's health work."[2] Ma Hai-teh writes that,

On this political and ideologic basis a series of four principles were set down for all health work:
1. Health work should be directed towards serving the masses—the workers, peasants, and soldiers;
2. Chief emphasis should be placed on preventive work, with prophylaxis and treatment combined;
3. Close unity between traditional Chinese doctors and modern trained doctors;
4. Health and hygiene work should be integrated with mass movements.[3]

Early Campaigns Against Specific Major Diseases (1949–60)

The first political priority listed at the beginning of this paper was quickly followed by the Ministry of Health, which in 1950 began to organize medical teams to design and execute six specialized, disease-specific campaigns. A massive smallpox immunization campaign was started, and by 1953 about 307 million people had been vaccinated, thus virtually eliminating smallpox, an ancient, highly prevalent, and highly visible disease in old China.[4] Disease-specific campaigns were also started against kala-azar, schistosomiasis, hookworm, malaria, and filariasis.[5-9] Syphilis was another disease that was singled out for special attention in the early 1950s, and the skillful use of politics in that successful campaign is illustrative of the special Chinese style and strategy in public health practice. I will therefore outline that campaign as an illustration.

The most obvious foci of syphilis in China were:

1. The urban prostitute, largely a by-product of poverty, of war, and of the depressed feudal status of women;

2. Certain national minority groups (serologic surveys 10–48 per cent positive)[10] whose cultural and economic patterns had been different from the majority, the Han people.

The initial emphasis was on urban prostitution, and by the end of 1950 all brothels had been closed and the prostitutes had been treated for venereal disease. As many as 96 per cent of some groups were found to have at least one type of venereal disease. In addition to medical treatment they were given basic education and social and vocational rehabilitation.[11] Ma Hai-teh has given us a very revealing account of how the antisyphilis campaign was extended during the following ten years to bring about full control in the general population.[12]

First, the eradication of the social and economic causes of prostitution came about through "social engineering," analogous to the long-term benefits ascribed in my priority list to environmental sanitation engineering. The peasants were relieved of debts, usury, exorbitant taxes, and land rents—all of which used to force them to sell their daughters into prostitution. The development of agriculture and industry, both with a labor-intensive style, opened up jobs for all, including women. Women were given equal rights with men in political, economic, and cultural life.

Second, it was decided that instead of trying to do serologic screening for case-finding in the whole population, a high-risk group could be screened out of the general rural population by a ten-item questionnaire that had yielded a 5 per cent confirmed case rate in a previous test situation in Hopei Province. The cooperation of the people was sought through telling them, "Syphilis is a legacy of the old society. . . . It is no fault of your own that you are afflicted. . . . Care is sure and free. . . . Comrades, we cannot take syphilis with us into socialism."[13]

A large-scale rural field trial was done in an entire county in Kiangsi Province in 1958, using not only existing health personnel but every existing social and political organization. Almost 3,000 activists, largely nonmedical, were given an intensive seven-day training program involving a pilot field trial of 3,000 people. Over 80 per cent of the trainees passed a qualifying test at the end of training and then carried out a two-month campaign to distribute and discuss the questionnaires with the entire population of the county, to register and examine those screened, and to treat those found to have venereal disease. Out of a population of 318,000 in the county, the questionnaire identified over 49,000 people who were then examined as VD suspects. Not only were diagnosed cases of VD treated, but cases of filariasis, malaria, hookworm, ringworm, and leprosy were also diagnosed and treated. The seropositive rate in the county was found to be 3.8 per cent.

This large-scale field trial was evaluated through a random sample of 2,000 people drawn from each of the fifteen communes that had been processed by the mass methods. This sample was given an examination and a Kahn test by personnel at the Research Institute of Dermatology and Venerealogy. The evaluation showed that the mass campaign personnel had correctly identified 90.2 per cent of the VD patients in the sample, and had made a correct diagnosis in 89.8 per cent of the VD cases discovered in the sample by the research institute personnel.

This demonstration project in Kiangsi served as the focus of a Ministry of Health national, on-the-street conference in 1958 to which personnel from all regions of China came to observe and discuss the techniques used. The approach was then taken back for nationwide application, with important variations for special groups; in high-prevalence national minority areas, total population surveys were used; in cities the screening techniques were focused on special age groups, premarital and prenatal examinations, and entrance examinations for the army and for certain schools.

An essential ingredient of this mass campaign was an intensive health education campaign by means of pamphlets, lectures, posters, plays, radio, wall newspapers, and small-group discussions. The messages were:

1. The role of the old society in fostering VD;
2. The role of the new society in eliminating it;
3. The need for active participation and self-reliance; and
4. How to prevent the transmission of VD.

As Dr. Ma put it:

When they learned how the disease was contracted, and what to do to treat it or prevent it, and applied this knowledge through their political consciousness, they were enabled to defend themselves. They became or could become "immune." This "immunity" through knowledge had the advantage of being acquired by all at no material cost and with little effort or pain. This . . . mass "immunity" . . . can be as efficient as medically induced immunity, . . . and was instrumental in ridding the county of venereal disease.[14]

Here we have a very good illustration of what is meant by the "mass line," and a clear indication that health education and "social engineering" are regarded in China as being of *primary* importance in the control of disease.

A similar combination of political ideology, "mass line," and technical competence has led to remarkable and well-documented programs in other specific campaigns against kala-azar, hookworm, schistosomiasis, malaria, and filariasis, which are discussed by T. H. Cheng in another chapter in this volume.

The Patriotic Health Movement (1952—Onwards)

Another very revealing illustration of the new Chinese style arose from the attack on environmental sanitation problems in the early 1950s. There is ample documentation of the deplorable state of urban and rural environmental sanitation in old China; the resulting diseases would place this problem high on any priority list. The lack of satisfactory, long-term, artificial immunization for many infectious and parasitic diseases transmitted by the fecal-oral route leaves no alternative but engineering and behavioral approaches to control. Yet how was this to be done with a huge population in which most of the people did not believe in the germ theory of disease causation? Here again China has shown innovation and vigor in attacking the problem, with apparent success.

Public education about environmental sanitation received a massive, skillfully managed, emotional boost in the spring of 1952 with widely publicized claims of United States attempts at bacteriologic warfare in North Korea and northeastern China. There was wide distribution of movies of captured American pilots confessing to participation in bacteriologic warfare, as well as reminders of well-publicized attempts at bacteriologic warfare with plague by the

Japanese Army in north China during World War II. "This bar-
barous act aroused deep indignation in the Chinese people everywhere," and resulted in "aid to the government in anti-epidemic
and health work,"[15] with "unconditional support of all classes of
the population."[16] The public attention, anger, and anxiety thus
aroused were organized into a Patriotic Health Movement focused
on specific tasks to be carried out by every person in his home and
at his place of work. There were two main tasks:

1. A massive onslaught against flies, mosquitoes, rats, fleas, lice,
bedbugs, and stray dogs;

2. A tremendous improvement in water supplies and fecal disposal systems, emphasizing self-reliance and labor-intensive methods, with appropriate technical supervision.

The overt message was that if the United States dropped plague-
infected fleas, cholera-infected matter, or other infective material
into your neighborhood, could they be disposed of quickly enough
to prevent the spread of an epidemic? The covert message was, perhaps, that if the Japanese Army and the United States Air Force
believed in the germ theory sufficiently to have tried to use it, and
if the Chinese government felt that this was a clear and present
threat, then maybe it was true. Visitors to cities in China since that
time have consistently expressed their amazement at the lack of
flies and at the general cleanliness of the streets. Continuing efforts
have been made to push this campaign in rural areas, with mention
of training large numbers of volunteer rural health workers for
these tasks and of teaching them first-aid skills.[17] Joshua Horn has
reported that one of the six specific responsibilities of the mobile
medical teams dispatched from urban hospitals to rural areas in
increasing numbers since the middle 1960s was to assist the Patriotic
Health Movement activists in their tasks of eliminating pests and
improving village sanitation.[18]

I was in Hong Kong during the time of severe agricultural problems in China in the early 1960s when there was a temporary influx
of southern Kwantung Province village people into Macao and
Hong Kong. During 1961–62 I had the opportunity to examine
eighty children, aged five to seven years, within forty-eight hours
after they arrived in Macao from neighboring Kwantung villages.
Although these children could in no way be construed as a representative sample of others in their villages, the results of examinations of their feces and blood gave us some clue as to the disease

control status of their villages at that time of maximum economic stress. Although the children's feces showed 98 per cent with helminth ova (largely ascaris and trichuris), we found no schistosome ova, and only 10 per cent had hookworm ova, which were apparently very light infestations since they were hard to find even with a concentration technique; none of the children was anemic as judged by microhematocrit.

These data suggested that the problem of fecal contamination of the soil in these particular villages had not been completely solved by 1961. While hookworm and malaria were both present, this small sample showed no evidence of a severe incidence of either of these diseases, which had formerly created major health problems in that region. The fact that 90 per cent of the children had vaccination scars and that none had smallpox scars was an indication that the smallpox campaign had reached effectively into these villages. One may therefore infer that by 1961 the specific disease campaigns and the Patriotic Health Movement had had some impact on the health of small villages very far removed from the seat of government in Peking.[19]

Emphasis on Industrial Health

The early admonition by Mao Tse-tung to care for the health of the workers and the peasants was followed in a systematic way. Studies of the health of miners in the early 1950s revealed a serious problem with hookworm, whose larvae thrived in contaminated mining shafts. This issue was solved by education and by provision of proper facilities for the miners.[20] Silicosis was one mining hazard that was attacked very early and vigorously through dust control, frequent examinations, supplemental diet, and extra rest in sanitoria when appropriate.[21,22] By 1964, five specialized "secondary medical schools" had been set up in mining and industrial regions to train several levels of health workers specializing in occupational health.[23] Each major industrial plant or mine has its own primary health-care unit responsible for safety, first aid, and ambulatory care.

Programs Related to Local Health Services (1958—Onwards)

The development of a widespread system of local health services had its first great rural impetus when the formation of the communes in 1958 provided the necessary administrative structure to maintain them. There are many disease control and preventive activities that function better as adjuncts of a local organization than as specialized campaigns, as was emphasized by those trying to control malaria in China by various combinations of chemotherapy and antimosquito measures.[24]

Another way in which curative services support preventive efforts is through the building of confidence. One member of an urban mobile medical team who went to Hunan in 1965 wrote about "propaganda through treatment." The people were willing to believe his preventive advice *only* after the team had first demonstrated that it could cure. He observed that the most common diseases seen were trachoma, dysentery, ascaris, tuberculosis, bronchitis, and asthma.[25]

An early emphasis in the development of local health services was the provision of modern midwifery and well-child care, including immunization of infants and children with smallpox vaccine, diphtheria-pertussis-tetanus vaccine, typhoid-paratyphoid vaccine, and BCG. In some high-risk urban situations the "Hong Kong-style" BCG vaccination of newborn infants had reached a 90 per cent coverage by 1964, and had been followed by a sharp drop in the incidence of acute miliary tuberculosis and tuberculous meningitis.[26] As polio vaccine became available it was added to the routine list of childhood immunizations; large-scale urban campaigns began in 1963.[27] At the 1959 National Conference on Communicable Diseases, measles was identified as a high priority item, and measles vaccine was added to the routine immunization list as it became available.[28,29] A controlled trial in various districts in Peking showed that preventive services for children were more acceptable and more effective when combined with curative services given in a local clinic or at home, with each assistant physician serving about 500–600 children. Their responsibility also extended to health guidance in local nurseries and kindergartens.[30]

In many countries, including the United States, tuberculosis mortality rates have been shown to fall gradually with improved living conditions, and rapidly with the widespread use of effective case-finding techniques and carefully managed chemotherapy. Tuberculosis was a very severe problem in old China, particularly in the cities, where crowded housing conditions and poor nutrition set the stage for annual mortality rates ranging from 200 to 500:100,000 population.[31-33] Mass chest X-ray screening was being done in Shanghai by 1958,[34] and a very careful prospective study was done in Peking from 1953 to 1960 to identify the optimum management of various kinds of tuberculosis patients on ambulatory chemotherapy. It was found that the duration and continuity of chemotherapy were the crucial variables, *not* the amount of physical activity, age, sex of the patient, or the extent of the lesion.[35]

It is instructive to read that in 1963 the tuberculosis mortality rate in Peking was 1.6 per cent of what it had been in 1949.[36] Unfortunately, I have not been able to find in English any tuberculosis mortality data expressed as actual rates, nor have I found comparative statements of trends in locations other than Peking.

Summary and Speculation

It seems to me there is ample evidence that the Ministry of Health and other authorities in Peking have done a most commendable and imaginative job of sharply reducing the incidence and prevalence of the most troublesome diseases that oppressed the people of China before 1949. They have done so by a unique mixture of sound epidemiologic judgment and innovative social-political action. They have demonstrated that they have both the will and the ability to translate biomedical scientific knowledge into a form for practical application that results in improvement in the health status of the people. One of the most remarkable aspects of this accomplishment is that although it started from a very small economic and professional base, it has gone so far in only two decades in such a massive population. I think the evidence supports the analysis of Rifkin and Kaplinsky,[37] who point out the preventive, labor-intensive, and rural emphasis of the Chinese health system. I believe there are many lessons to be learned from China by those responsible for health planning in other countries.

If the Chinese people have been able to accomplish this great task it may not be impossible for them, using similar approaches, to also accomplish the task of bringing their population growth quickly under control. But that is the topic of another chapter in this volume.

In closing I would like to speculate on the possible impact of the Cultural Revolution on the health system of China. It seems likely to me that some of the short-term effects are and will be:

1. A rapid acceleration of the process started in the 1950s of

improving the local health services, both preventive and curative, available in rural areas.

2. A temporary slowing of the rate of growth of urban health services by moving more health workers to rural areas and, as a by-product of recent changes in higher education, by slowing the rate of production of more highly skilled health workers.

It seems to me that the crucial *long-range* question with regard to the Cultural Revolution is whether the Chinese will be able to maintain a close fit between the real needs of their health system and the actual health manpower they produce. Many nations have come to face the reality that while producing the highly skilled practitioners, researchers, and teachers needed in a health system, they have also produced an elite group that becomes increasingly maladapted to the needs of the society it serves. The Cultural Revolution was one answer to this problem. But this answer bears within itself the seeds of another problem—the failure of production of the small number of very highly skilled people needed by the health system. It will be very interesting to see if the Chinese can solve that problem without again producing a maladapted elite.

NOTES

1. S. Rifkin and R. Kaplinsky, "Health Strategy and Development Planning: Lessons from the People's Republic of China" (University of Sussex: Science Research Policy Unit, December 1971).

2. Mao Tse-tung, *Chinese Medical Journal* 82 (1963): frontispiece.

3. Ma Hai-teh, "With Mao Tse-tung's Thought as a Compass for Action in the Control of Venereal Diseases in China," *China's Medicine* 1 (1966): 52–68.

4. Kung N. C., "New China's Achievements in Health Work," *Chinese Medical Journal* 71 (1953): 87–92.

5. Chung H. L., "A Resume of Kala-azar Work in China," *Chinese Medical Journal* 71 (1953): 421–64.

6. Chinese Medical Delegation to the U.S.S.R. Academy of Medical Sciences, Tashkent, September 1954, "Some Aspects of Research in the Prevention and Treatment of Schistosomiasis Japonica in New China," *Chinese Medical Journal* 73 (1955): 100–106.

7. Wang C. Y., "Studies on Ancylostomiasis in New China," *Chinese Medical Journal* 78 (1959): 257–66.

8. Ho C., "Studies on Malaria in New China," *Chinese Medical Journal* 84 (1965): 491–97.

9. Li H. H., "Studies on Filariasis in New China," *Chinese Medical Journal* 78 (1959): 148–60.

10. Ma, "With Mao Tse-tung's Thought as a Compass."

11. Hu C. K. et al., "The Control of Venereal Diseases in New China," *Chinese Medical Journal* 71 (1953): 248–58.

12. Ma, "With Mao Tse-tung's Thought as a Compass."

13. Ibid.

14. Ibid.

15. Fu L. C., "Achievements of the Association in the Past Ten Years," *Chinese Medical Journal* 79 (1959): 208–18.

16. International Scientific Commission for the Investigation of the Facts Concerning Bacterial Warfare in Korea and China, "Hygiene in New China," *Chinese Medical Journal* 70 (1952): 390–91.

17. News and Notes, *Chinese Medical Journal* 83 (1964): 481.

18. Joshua S. Horn, *Away with All Pests . . . An English Surgeon in People's China* (New York: Monthly Review Press, 1969): pp. 129–46.

19. R. M. Worth, "Health Trends in China Since the 'Great Leap Forward,' " *American Journal of Hygiene* 78 (1963): 349–57.

20. Wang, "Studies on Ancylostomiasis."

21. News and Notes, p. 132.

22. Wang S. H., Hu F. C., and Lu C. H., "Roentgenologic Observations on 412 Cases of Anthracosilicosis in Coal Miners," *Chinese Medical Journal* 83 (1964): 551–57.

23. News and Notes, p. 270.

24. Ho, "Studies on Malaria."

25. Huang C. S., "Our Medical Team in the Countryside," *Chinese Medical Journal* 84 (1965): 800–803.

26. Chu F. T., "Progress of Pediatric Work in China in the Past Eight Years," *Chinese Medical Journal* 83 (1964): 795–802.

27. News and Notes, p. 480.

28. Ibid.

29. Hsueh C. P. et al., "An Experimental Study of the Organization of Urban Child Health Services," *Chinese Medical Journal* 84 (1965): 563–70.

30. Ibid.

31. C. F. Bume, "The Tuberculosis Problem in China," *Chinese Medical Journal* 47 (1933): 124–37.

32. Chen C. C., "The Rural Public Health Experiment in Tinghsien, China," *Chinese Medical Journal* 50 (1936): 1125–27.

33. F. Oldt, "Tuberculosis in Kwangtung," *Chinese Medical Journal* 47 (1933): 110–27.

34. News and Notes, p. 317.

35. Li S. S. and Hsiao, C. C., "Factors Affecting the Results of Ambulatory Chemotherapy in Pulmonary Tuberculosis," *Chinese Medical Journal* 83 (1964): 201–208.

36. News and Notes, p. 480.

37. Rifkin and Kaplinsky, "Health Strategy."

Disease Control and Prevention

ψ

TIEN-HSI CHENG

As one born and brought up in "Old China," I remember vividly
my visits to villages and to cities during my youth. The beautiful
and serene landscape was marred by evidence of apathy towards
public hygiene in general and unsanitary latrine habits in particular. The focus of my memory then shifts to outbreaks of cholera and
bubonic plague and to widespread infections by schistosomes and
other parasites. The experience of witnessing the horror of death
en masse left an indelible mark on me over these years. As far as I
can remember, hospitals were few and far between and were located
mostly in the cities. Their services were available primarily to the
relatively well-to-do. The peasants and workers who constituted
the vast majority of the population were left to the mercy of un-
licensed, self-appointed healers. Western-trained doctors formed
an elite of their own, accessible only to a selected segment of society.

Against this background, control and prevention of diseases in a
country of some 800 million people is indeed an undertaking of
tremendous magnitude. Instead of being overwhelmed by difficulties, however, the present regime has demonstrated its determination to conquer them. By establishing new priorities in health
care, planners in Peking have shown imagination and a grasp of
realities. And by placing emphasis on rural areas instead of on cities
and towns, and on workers, peasants, and soldiers instead of on
intellectuals and other urbanites, they have chosen the long-op-
pressed majority over the traditionally privileged small minority.

To meet the demands of the new policy, the quality of trained
doctors necessarily has to suffer in order to achieve quantity, at
least during the initial period. Mao Tse-tung is a believer in mass
power and a denouncer of elitism. The masses, now the privileged
class, are willing, able, and ready to answer the call of health cam-

185

paigns that have transformed China from a land of sick people to a nation of vigor and cleanliness.

In the last two decades numerous innovations and changes have been instituted in China for disease control and prevention. Included in this report are highlights of some major programs dealing with parasitic diseases, cancer, and mental disorders.

Parasitic Diseases

Organization

Control of parasitic diseases is directed by the Institute of Parasitic Diseases which was established under the Academy of Medical Sciences shortly after the People's Republic of China came to power in 1949. Preventive and therapeutic programs were focused as rapidly as possible on *Schistosomiasis japonica*, malaria, filariasis, ancylostomiasis, and leishmaniasis.

The same cardinal principles govern all projects for control of diseases in China, and measures for the suppression of schistosomiasis are applicable, at least in part, to the other four major parasitic diseases. Hence this paper will review the highlights of antischistosomiasis activities to illustrate the *modus operandi* of the nationwide campaign for eliminating those parasites that for centuries have caused untold sorrow to millions of Chinese.

The antiparasitic disease campaign was organized on a vast scale in the early years of the present regime. For the antischistosomiasis program alone, by 1958 a total of 197 prevention and treatment stations had been established in endemic areas, manned by more than 1,200 medical teams and 17,000 specialized personnel.[1] Technical organizations and manpower grew in quality as well as in quantity until mid-1966, when control of schistosomiasis and other parasitic diseases, and indeed most areas of scientific pursuit, was temporarily disrupted by the outbreak of the Cultural Revolution. As of 1968 approximately 330 research workers with authorship standing—better trained scientists as differentiated from hundreds of semitechnical assistants—were engaged in schistosomiasis studies in more than fifty research institutions and hospitals.

Prevention

The major emphasis of the antischistosomiasis program gradually shifted from treatment and cure toward active prevention, as did programs for the control of other parasitic diseases. Preventive measures are concerned primarily with destruction of the eggs produced by various parasites and extermination of intermediate hosts or vectors.

Destruction of eggs. Studies have shown that ammonia is toxic to schistosome and hookworm eggs and that its potency increases with its concentration. Storage of human feces mixed with urine, widely practiced in all farm districts, destroys schistosome eggs in three to seven days depending upon seasonal temperatures.[2] Before being used as fertilizer, human and animal excrement is stored for fifteen to thirty days, during which time the viability of schistosome and hookworm eggs is destroyed. Storage facilities vary from large, tightly sealed earthenware containers to cement-walled pits divided into compartments separating waste matter of different ages.[3]

Where human waste is in urgent demand to meet fertilizer needs, such procedures as boiling the excrement or treating it with urea, ammonium bicarbonate, and calcium cyanamide have been adopted. Manure preparation by boiling is credited also with reduction of housefly populations.

For ancylostomiasis control, mixing urea, wettable BHC, calcium cyanamide, quicklime, and Dipterex with feces serves to kill hookworm eggs.[4]

In Chinese experience, the utilization of the heat of fermentation generated in manure composts to achieve ovicide is a highly practical method for control of schistosomes as well as ascaris and flies.[5]

Extermination of intermediate hosts or vectors. The use of chemicals in the form of sprays, dust, and fumigants for exterminating the *Oncomelania hupensis* snail, mosquitoes, and sandflies constitutes an important phase of China's program for parasitic disease control, although manual labor plays a dominant role. Insecticides such as DDT and BHC as well as those of plant origin are manufactured in state-owned factories and commune shops.

For the control of schistosomiasis, various snail-extermination practices are employed; one of the most effective is to bury them. A widely adopted practice before installing new irrigation systems is to fill in old snail-infested waterways, ponds, and wells, thereby suffocating the intermediate host; this minimizes the hazard of spreading the disease to newly irrigated areas. In practice Chinese peasants first remove 10 to 15 cm. of soil from infested ditch walls and dump it in the bottom of the ditch. The waterway is then filled to ground level with dry dirt. Of the twenty-four districts and municipalities declared free of schistosomiasis by 1964, twenty-one are located in hilly regions where the practice of burying snails is the principal measure of control.[6] Other snail extermination practices have varied from cleaning irrigation ditches and applying molluscicides to scalding, burning, and even hand-picking the snails. The nation's massive manpower has been further utilized to reclaim thousands of acres of marshlands for crop production, thus rendering the environment unfit for the snails to survive. Such efforts also have contributed to the nationwide destruction of mosquitoes.

Environmental sanitation. Prior to 1949 farmers and their families often lived under the same roof as their cattle, hogs, and other domestic animals; in old Chinese village communities it was quite common for dilapidated animal shelters and manure pits to be scattered all over the land. Such traditional living conditions aided the spread of diseases. Public latrines and shelters with collective animal feeding facilities have now been built; at the same time strict management of human and animal wastes and of water sources has been instituted.[7] Vigorous enforcement of these measures, together with draining swamps, filling-in stagnant ponds and puddles, and removing wild vegetation have been responsible for a sharp decline in schistosomiasis infection centers. Such environmental sanitation projects have also led to the virtual elimination or subsidence of malaria, filariasis, kala-azar, taeniasis, and cysticercosis.[8]

Personal protection. For protection against infection by schistosome cercariae, people are warned against unnecessary contact with infected waters. Farmers are advised to wear double-puttees sprinkled with powder made from the fruit of *Thea (Camellia) oleosa*. A water emulsion of 15 per cent dibutyl phthalate applied to the skin of experimental animals gives good protection for four hours.[9] Oil extracted from the seeds of the weeping cypresses, *Cupressus funebris*, also has been found to yield encouraging results. Tests on the efficacy of other protective agents are in progress. In addition, stockings and gloves made of cloth or plastic effectively protect wearers against infection.[10] Because of the inconvenience involved, however, especially in farming activities, the use of stockings and gloves has not been widely adopted. Personal protection is believed to be a relatively weak phase of the otherwise intensive antischistosomiasis campaign.

Treatment

Combined use of Chinese and Western medicines. Treatment of *Schistosomiasis japonica* infection is based on the combined use of traditional Chinese and Western remedies involving both internal medicine and surgery. Current therapy involves various prescriptions of herbs and animal and mineral products, three-day intravenous injections of tartar emetic, and oral administration of a nitrofuran compound, *N*-isopropyl-(5-nitro-2-furyl)-acrylamide. Splenectomy is performed whenever necessary. Acupuncture and moxibustion are used for treatment of hepatomegaly and ascites and for prevention of antimony toxication. Moxibustion, little known in Western countries, consists of burning on the skin a moxa made of the dried leaves of *ai, Artemisia argyi (compositae).*[11] This species of perennial herb has been found to contain cineol (eucalyptol), α-thujon, sesquiterpen alcohol, adenine, choline, amylase, and vitamins A, B, C, and D.[12,13]

Artemisia apiacea, Dichroa febrifuga, and *Vitex negundo* are among the plants from which effective antimalarial medicines are derived. Acupuncture is used in treating malaria. Hetrazan and carbarson have been found to yield good therapeutic results against filariasis. Injections of sodium stibogluconate have significantly reduced the incidence of kala-azar. Principal remedies for ancylostomiasis include tetrachloroethylene and 1-bromo-2-naphthol.[14]

Coordination of treatment with production activities. Treatment of patients is administered with a minimum of interference with regular farm activities. In the case of schistosomiasis, able-bodied peasants are treated in February and March before spring plowing is in full swing; treatment of women and other villagers who do not have full-time farming assignments is deferred until April or May; schoolchildren and other farm workers are treated during the late summer lull before harvest time; those who work during the day are given treatment at night. Measures such as these have reduced loss of productive labor to a minimum, which to a large extent accounts for ths sustained popular interest among China's peasantry in combating schistosomiasis and other parasitic diseases.

Summary of Achievements in Disease Control

In a vast antischistosomiasis drive, by 1961 more than 5 million Chinese had been treated, and as of 1964, or earlier, half the nation's 7 million victims of the disease had been cured.[15] Thus significant progress has been achieved in comparison with pre-1949 days when the number of sufferers was estimated to exceed 10 million. Before the advent of the Cultural Revolution a number of well-known centers of the infection such as Ch'ingpu County in Kiangsu Province, Yüchiang County in Kiangsi, and Jiashan County in Chekiang had fully recovered from the ravages of the schistosome parasite. During the three years beginning in mid-1966, however, schistosomiasis research and control programs were interrupted, and the disease raged again in some localities where it had earlier been brought under control.[16] Although the antischistosomiasis program was reactivated in the spring of 1970 the disease remains a major cause of concern to Chinese authorities.

The number of malaria victims in China before 1949 was estimated to be 30 million a year.[17] If this figure is taken as 100 per cent, the incidence of malaria dropped to 19.4 per cent in 1955, to 10.3 per cent in 1956, and to 2.6 per cent in the first eight months of 1958.[18] It was the professed aim of the Chinese to basically free the country of malaria by 1960, and they appear to have come close to achieving that goal—in a report dated December 1969 malaria was listed among the diseases that had been brought under control.[19]

The geographical distribution of filariasis covers fourteen provinces and affects 20 to 30 million people. By 1958 more than 700,000 filariasis patients had been treated and the disease had been virtually eliminated in twenty-two counties and cities in Hunan and in four coastal provinces—Fukien, Chekiang, Kiangsu, and Shantung. Good groundwork for filariasis control had been laid with the help of the Patriotic Health Movement which was credited with extermination of mosquitoes and improvement of environmental sanitation in many localities. In one year, 1957–58, 13 million kg. of mosquitoes reportedly were destroyed.[20]

According to an estimate made shortly after 1949, 600,000 people residing in provinces north of the Yangtze River were infected by kala-azar. Efficient administration of preventive and therapeutic measures had reduced the number to about 3,000 by 1958.[21]

Ancylostomiasis is endemic in almost all parts of China with the rare exception of some cold, dry regions—of 100 million people infected, 22 million had been treated by September 1958.[22]

It is not clear whether the Chinese have yet succeeded in completely wiping out most of the major parasitic diseases as they confidently predicted they would more than a decade ago. With the probable exception of schistosomiasis, however, none of these diseases poses a serious threat at present or in the foreseeable future. Progress in the disease control programs has brought with it such rewards as an increase in productive manpower, the extension of irrigation facilities, and the reclamation of wastelands for crop production. It has created a new healthy environment in the countryside through improvements in sanitation and through mass extermination of mosquitoes, flies, sandflies, rats, and stray dogs. And in large measure it has been responsible for bringing about a revolutionized medical care delivery system in both rural and urban China.

Delivery of Medical Care in Rural Areas

In compliance with Mao Tse-tung's decree of June 26, 1965, that health care and medical services should be emphasized in the countryside, hospitals and/or clinics have been established in counties, communes, and production brigades (Figure 1). While county and commune hospitals are equipped with relatively modern facilities and manned by more experienced personnel, clinics and health stations at less sophisticated levels are often improvised in vacant buildings and manned by medical workers of varied training and skill. When the need arises, makeshift wards are set up in living quarters evacuated by peasants, and doors are used as beds.[23]

Aside from physicians and health workers with various levels of training and experience, a group of healers known as barefoot doctors have become increasingly active in the rural areas since the Cultural Revolution. These are part-time medical workers with rudimentary skills, who work alongside the peasants and answer calls for medical care. They are trained to treat common and endemic diseases such as schistosomiasis, malaria, measles, pneumonia, and influenza. They are adequately experienced in administering both Chinese and Western drugs, in applying acupuncture, in providing first aid, and in delivering babies. Their primary contributions, however, include enforcement of disease control measures, such as disinfection of drinking water, construction of sanitary latrines, careful management of night soil, and maintenance of a clean environment. These projects, which are largely responsible for the amazing transformation of China's countryside,

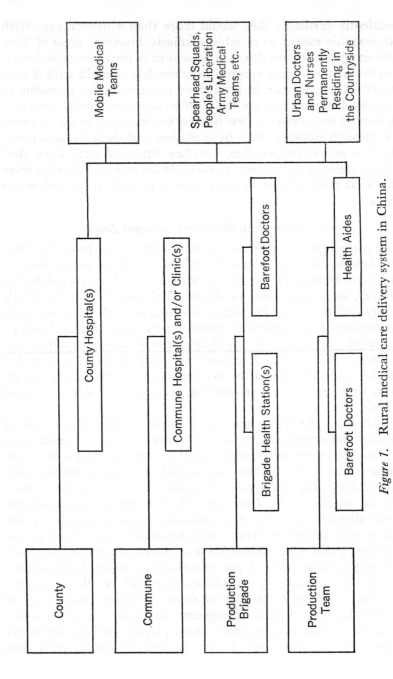

Figure 1. Rural medical care delivery system in China.

are carried out with the help of health aides trained by more experienced barefoot doctors to work in production teams.

The great majority of barefoot doctors are the children of peasants. Most are in their early twenties and have had only primary or junior middle school education before receiving paramedical training, which consists of a short course or an apprenticeship of two to four months at a commune hospital, often under the auspices of a mobile medical team. With a view to enhancing the quality of their services a limited number of barefoot doctors of outstanding achievements are selected for advanced studies in medical colleges. Upon graduation they return to their original communes to practice and to train younger barefoot doctors and health aides. From time to time an exchange is arranged between barefoot doctors and physicians at commune hospitals, a procedure designed to improve the former's professional competence and to reinforce the latter's interest in serving the less privileged peasants.

It is not unusual for a barefoot doctor to handle as many as 1,500 sick calls a year, frequently under the most trying circumstances. When advanced professional service or modern facilities are required, the patient is dispatched by the barefoot doctor to the county or commune hospital. Thus he serves as a valuable link between the hospital and the masses. In the Chiangchen People's Commune southeast of Shanghai, for example, in 1969 a population of 28,000 was served by forty-two barefoot doctors, two in each of twenty-one production brigades. Their activities were coordinated with those of the commune central hospital, which was manned by thirty-seven professional and semiprofessional medical workers.[24]

The annual income of a barefoot doctor corresponds to that of a poor or lower-middle-class peasant, and ranges from U.S. $85 to $130, including remuneration for both his farming and medical services. The latter, paid by the production brigade in which he serves, amounts to approximately two-thirds of his income. Fees collected for delivering babies, making injections, etc., are turned over to the brigade treasury. Thus the net expense of having a barefoot doctor available is equivalent to three cents per peasant per year.[25]

Today barefoot doctors provide the bulk of basic medical care in the rural districts. The number of these peasant medical workers increased from 500,000 in 1969 to over 1 million in 1970, and it is still growing.[26] They are in fact gradually taking command of the nation's rural health service. However unsophisticated their backgrounds may be by Western standards, they receive the warm support of a huge segment of the population and constitute an ingenious health care delivery organization that reaches the grassroots level of Chinese society.

To further facilitate delivery of medical care and to supplement the barefoot doctors' services, mobile medical teams have been organized by physicians and nurses in urban hospitals and medical institutes. Most hospitals have committed one-third of their professional manpower to tours of duty among the masses, offering services to peasants and their families at home, on farms, and in schools. Since the emergence of the Cultural Revolution 400,000 doctors and nurses have participated in this project.[27] Each mobile team may consist of fifteen to twenty members, divided into groups of four or five, who eat, live, study, and work with poor and lower-middle-class peasants. Besides treating parasitic diseases, especially schistosomiasis, and various ailments common to the countryside, the mobile teams conduct training courses and sponsor clinical sessions for the benefit of local barefoot doctors and health workers.[28]

In addition to mobile medical teams, other medical groups volunteer to serve in isolated regions. The "Spearhead Squad," for example, organized by young medical workers of the Shanghai First Medical College, has settled permanently in Taiyong, a mountainous district of Kweichow Province.[29] Having resolved to dedicate their lives to the service of minority nationals residing in the district, the young medics live in very primitive conditions; lacking electricity and any modern communications system they are virtually cut off from the outside world; and their lives are constantly threatened by venomous snakes and wild animals. Harsh as the living conditions are, clinical facilities are no less primitive. In attending the sick in the outlying villages the squad members have to tax their ingenuity in constructing substitutes for whatever equipment they lack: for want of an operating table, planks are used; for lack of electricity, a flashlight provides illumination for surgery. Their devotion to the program of disease control and prevention in rural areas is shared by other teams of medical workers, such as those in the People's Liberation Army.[30] All work toward a common objective—that of protecting the health of the peasants, workers, and soldiers who form the overwhelming majority of China's population. According to a recent report, in 1971, 330,000 urban medical workers were settled permanently in the countryside.[31] The combined efforts of various groups and organizations already have exerted a notably favorable impact on the health of the people in the vast countryside.

Delivery of Medical Care in Urban Areas

City dwellers are of course also subject to infection by parasitic diseases although to a lesser extent. Difficulties arising from a shortage of hospital beds and the heavy demand for outpatient services used to be commonplace in urban areas, a condition that became a cause for serious concern. A revolutionary urban medical care system was initiated early in 1965 in the city of Tientsin, an industrial center with a population of over 3 million. Reportedly the system has worked well in terms of improvements in quality and efficiency of medical service, deployment of technical manpower, and alleviation of overcrowded conditions in the hospitals. There is evidence that in the last several years the new system has in essence been put into practice in other cities.

Under this system the urban core of Tientsin is divided into a number of districts, each responsible for providing medical care to its residents and for promoting disease control programs within its limits. These tasks are executed by health organizations of various categories—comprehensive hospitals, health institutes, factory health protection stations, street Red Cross stations, and group health stations.[32] These district organizations are so closely coordinated in their activities that they form a network through which medical care is channeled to every segment of the populace (Figure 2).

In Tientsin there are seventeen comprehensive hospitals, each serving as a nucleus of the district health network. Affiliated with, and under the guidance of, the hospitals are fifty-eight health institutes and over 1,000 factory health protection stations that constitute the "basic health care category" responsible for supplying primary medical service and treating common ailments and occupational diseases. As a rule, employees of large factories are taken care of by factory health protection stations; those of small factories and shops, as well as residents of streets and lanes, are served by health institutes in cooperation with street Red Cross and group health stations.[33] Under the auspices of the health institutes, in 1965 over 300 factory worker doctors, the equivalent of barefoot

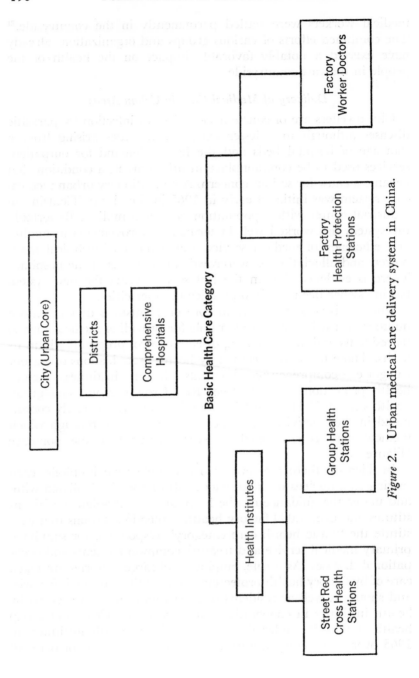

Figure 2.   Urban medical care delivery system in China.

doctors on farms, were trained to treat minor diseases and injuries.

Besides taking care of patients, the comprehensive hospitals stand ready to provide professional guidance and technical support to all categories in the health system. When the need arises it has become established practice for a hospital to send medical personnel to factories, health institutes, and stations in any part of the district in which it is located. Hospital specialists make daily rounds, perform surgery, and give scheduled lectures in affiliated health organizations at lower levels. To fulfill their respective assignments, whenever feasible different categories in the city's health structure share available manpower and facilities.

Because of this on-the-spot delivery of medical care to workers in factories and shops, and to residents in their homes or in street Red Cross or group health stations, the pressure on both outpatient and inpatient services in the city's hospitals has been alleviated significantly. Overcrowding in hospitals has been further relieved by the expansion of house-call services to include registration of sick children, payment of fees, delivery of drugs, and performance of simple clinical tests.

Administration of inpatient service has undergone profound changes in recent years, notably in the integration of medicine and nursing. The rigid professional division between doctors and nurses, which for years has hampered inpatient services, has been abolished. The two groups are prospering under a new-found unity based on equal voice and democratic exchange of ideas in professional matters.[34] According to recent reports, doctors are encouraged to assist nurses in washing patients and making beds, while nurses are expected to have competence in the diagnosis and treatment of common diseases.[35,36]

Evaluation of the merits of the new medical care system based on one year's experience shows that the demand for outpatient services in hospitals in Tientsin dropped by 25 to 35.9 per cent. By late 1965 Tientsin was in a position to contribute one-third of its hospital personnel to serve in rural and urban areas throughout Hopeh Province. Absenteeism in factories has been reduced by 37.3 per cent, and medical expenses by 24.3 per cent.[37] As a result of innovations, Chinese authorities claim that patients receive better and more efficient care. It is said that in Tientsin No. 2 Hospital the rate of child mortality caused by toxic dysentery was reduced from 8–9 per cent in 1964 to zero in 1965, and by epidemic Type B encephalitis from 25 to 8.26 per cent in the same period.

Of particular importance to the Chinese government is the fact that well-trained physicians and nurses who were once self-centered, aloof, and indifferent to the working class have been introduced to the world outside of their hospital wards and clinics. They have had an opportunity to observe life in factories and homes, to measure the stamina of working-class people striving to achieve production goals, and to appreciate the enormous strength demonstrated by ordinary people in all lines of pursuit. Such experiences have inspired sympathy, humility, and selfless devotion, resulting in the elimination of elitism in the medical profession.

Cancer

Owing to the urgent sanitary and health problems posed by infectious and parasitic diseases, cancer treatment and research was not given attention in China's health program until 1958. Initial measures taken included mass surveys, public education, and organization of research on a national scale. The First All-China Tumor Conference was convened in 1959, and guidelines were drafted for the nation's cancer program.[38] Since then, specialized hospitals and clinics have been set up in Peking, Tientsin, Taiyuan, Shanghai, Nanchang, Canton, and other cities. In rural districts medical services are available to peasants through commune clinics. Short courses for physicians, lasting from six months to a year, are offered regularly in a number of hospitals and clinics.

To meet the demands of the new program, factories in China have been producing practically all the surgical instruments needed.[39] Modern diagnostic and therapeutic practices involving radium, X-rays, isotopes, ultrasonic waves, and cytochemical techniques have been adopted in varying degrees.[40,41] In many instances medical centers reportedly have been provided with 1 to 2 g., and possibly more, of radium tubes and needles—a far cry from the old days when there were fewer than 2 g. of radium in the whole country.[42]

Prior to 1959 China had to import most of the anticancer drugs it needed. More recently, Chinese pharmaceutical laboratories have succeeded in duplicating a variety of imported anticancer drugs as well as hormonal products. As of 1965 more than 1,000 chemicals had been synthesized and tested by Chinese scientists; of these, from twenty to thirty were found to have antitumor properties.[43] Among the more noteworthy is N-formylsarcolysine, which was synthesized by the Institute of Pharmacology in Peking. Clinical observations indicate that large inoperable seminoma tumors have been shrunk and rendered operable by administration of this drug.[44] Also, according to a clinical report by researchers at the Peking Union Hospital,* 6-mercaptopurine used in combination with surgery has given promising results in the treatment of choriocarcinoma and chorioadenoma destruens.[45]

Surveys of cancer incidence conducted since 1958 in large and medium-sized cities have been extended to rural and mountainous districts.[46] Data gathered from twenty-six provinces and cities show that among some 4 million persons examined almost 2,000 had some form of cancer.[47] For the first time in China's history these surveys provided valuable information on the status of cervical, esophageal, and nasopharyngeal carcinomas in different parts of the country.

In the last decade or so cancer research in China has covered a surprisingly wide area—from tissue culture, histopathology, cytogenetics, etiology, and mechanisms of tumor development, to surgical techniques, radiation therapy, chemotherapy, virology, and immunology. Efforts have been made to link basic research with clinical and applied treatments and to correlate morphological observations of tumor cells with their biological activities. Serious attempts have been made to explore the mechanism of tumor development. Some of this work was reported at the Eighth International Cancer Congress held in Moscow in July 1962.[48]

Progress in cancer research since 1960 was reviewed at the Second All-China Tumor Conference held in 1965 under the auspices of the Chinese Medical Association.[49] This ten-day conference was attended by 198 delegates from twenty-seven provinces and cities throughout the country. Of the more than 900 papers submitted, 158 were presented, among them the work of scientists from Sinkiang, Tibet, and Yunnan. Despite inadequacies in certain areas of the studies, as revealed in group discussions, Chinese scientists had achieved excellence in some clinical and basic phases of cancer control during a brief period of five or six years.

---

* Recently renamed Capital Hospital.

In certain areas China has reached or even surpassed international levels. For example, an analysis of five-year data shows that China has achieved a 70 per cent cure of cervical cancer in Stages I-IV, as compared to 66 per cent for the United States and 57 per cent for Great Britain.[50] The mortality rate due to choriocarcinoma has dropped from approximately 90 per cent to less than 47 per cent as a result of combined treatment with 6-mercaptopurine and surgery.[51] Moreover, an accuracy of 98 per cent has been achieved in early diagnosis of cancer of the uterine cervix by the methylene blue-triphenyltetrazolium chloride test-tube smear method.[52]

China's cancer program is directed toward research and treatment of six major carcinomas—cervical, esophageal, nasopharyngeal, mammary, hepatic, and pulmonary. In basic research, continued emphasis is placed on the biochemical and biophysical aspects with special reference to the mechanism of carcinogenesis. Further investigations in tumor cytogenetics, tissue culture, virology, and immunology complete the list of priorities for the near future. Clinical studies will center on so-called "comprehensive therapy" involving combined application of antitumor drugs, radiation, and surgery.

Reports indicate that traditional Chinese medicine plays an active role in cancer treatment; certain unspecified native drugs have been found to alleviate cancer symptoms and prolong the lives of patients.[53]

In spite of great progress and painstaking effort by all concerned, cancer work in China is on the whole a good distance behind world standards in quantity if not in quality. Even with the steady increase in technical personnel, and improvements in equipment and facilities, the needs of China's huge and expanding population can hardly be met adequately in the foreseeable future. Furthermore, many gaps remain to be filled with respect to both the training and experience of the younger generation of Chinese scientists.

Mental Diseases

The New Program and Its Objectives

The program for treatment and prevention of mental diseases in China has been revamped since September 1965. Emphasis is placed on integration of services in hospital wards, outpatient clinics, and patients' homes. Thus the responsibility of mental hospitals continues after the release of patients, and the patients' relatives play a significant role in minimizing the chances of relapse.

The major objective of the new mental disease control program is to rectify the mistakes of previous years, which included lack of coordination between inpatient and outpatient services, concentration on treatment at the expense of prevention, preoccupation with physiological aspects of mental diseases while neglecting environmental factors affecting the patients, excessive reliance on the use of medications, and insufficient efforts to encourage the patients' cooperation.[54]

Much stress is now placed on active participation by the mentally ill instead of passive reliance on doctors and specialists. Patients are encouraged to learn the nature of their illnesses through personal contacts and group discussions, to develop initiative and self-reliance, and to establish constructive relationships with doctors and nurses. They are encouraged whenever possible to participate actively in daily chores and in social, recreational, and even therapeutic activities.

The present trend in Chinese mental hospitals is to shun the use of electric and insulin shock treatments, chlorpromazine in large doses, and restraints such as solitary confinement and straitjackets.[55] New treatments for the mentally ill allow a combination of Western and traditional practices, involving, among other things, acupuncture, herbal applications, and small doses of chlorpromazine.[56] Invariably medical treatment is accompanied by ideological discussion therapy based on Mao Tse-tung thought, conducted either individually or in groups.

Posthospitalization Care

Care of a patient does not end with his release from the hospital. Instead, members of the hospital staff assume full responsibility for providing guidance to prevent relapse, especially in schizophrenic cases. Before leaving the hospital and during "discussion therapy" sessions the patient is fully advised of the nature of his illness and instructed to observe the rules guarding against recurrence. In his final meeting with the hospital staff he is required to report on highlights of his experience during hospitalization and to recount the instructions for posthospitalization care. Finally, members of the patient's family are invited to participate in the discussion sessions, during which details of their role in connection with the continued health of the patient are elucidated. Within half a month of the date of his release the doctor in charge or the head nurse makes a house call to check on the patient's progress, his living conditions, and follow-up medication; to provide whatever guidance is required; and to impress upon members of the family and the neighborhod Red Cross station the importance of their contribution toward the patient's lasting recovery, with particular reference to his living and working environments.[57]

On the basis of experience, professional and livelihood problems constitute major causes of relapse. Accordingly, in post-hospitalization visits attention is focused on ways and means to relieve the former patient of pressures traceable to these problems. As part of the operational routine a hospital representative calls on the patient's employer to advise him of the circumstances and to suggest occupational adjustments consistent with the patient's state of health. Likewise, domestic difficulties are resolved or alleviated by appeals for sympathy and understanding on the part of those concerned. Thus, under the revolutionized system, the hospital is as much committed to posthospitalization rehabilitation as it is to inpatient service. Since the former is achieved at home, duration of hospitalization has been considerably shortened, and this has relieved the shortage of hospital beds and reduced the expenses incurred by patients.[58]

As far as we know, China is making good progress in the control of mental disease. In the mental hospital at Chenchow prefecture in Hunan Province, for example, the rate of recovery of the mentally ill during 1970–71 came close to 80 per cent. Improvement in different degrees was noted in almost 99 per cent of the patients, some of whom had been deranged for more than twenty years.[59]

Cost of Medical Care

Medical care and medicine are provided to Chinese peasants either free of charge or at a nominal cost. In some communes patients pay whatever they can afford; in others, villagers contribute a few days' labor a year to the commune medical fund and pay a registration fee equivalent to 2 U.S. cents when admitted for treatment. In Ch'ingpu County, Kiangsu Province, in 1956 the cost of treating schistosomiasis patients was $3.00 per person; this was reduced by one-half the following year. In 1971 peasants in the Chengtzushan production team in a tiny village in Yunnan

Province spent an average of 5 cents on medical care and medicine.[60] In some brigades a fee of $1.50 is charged for delivering a baby, and 2 cents for administering an injection. On the whole, medical expenses do not constitute a financial burden for low-income peasants.

Pharmaceutical Industry

In recent years China's pharmaceutical industry has undergone rapid expansion. The nation is now self-sufficient in all major drugs for disease treatment and prevention, and some medicines have been exported. As of March 1972 the prices of sulfa drugs, many kinds of antibiotics and hormones, antipyretics, antituberculous drugs, vitamins, and medicines for endemic diseases were reduced to one-fifth of what they were in the early days of the People's Republic, when chemicals needed for pharmaceutical production had to be imported.[61, 62]

Conclusions

Plans for disease control and prevention are based on the realization that agriculture will remain the lifeline of China's destiny for a long time to come, and that improvements in public health are a prerequisite to a prosperous agricultural economy. Consequently, the emphasis on health and medical care has shifted from urban to rural areas. Adopting the same strategy in disease control and prevention as in food production, China has resorted constantly to the use of "human sea" tactics in waging health movements and agricultural campaigns. In the antischistosomiasis movement this is illustrated by the massive manpower employed to fill in snail-infested waterways and to build new ones, and in the reclamation of marshlands for snail extermination; the labor-intensive approach in agriculture is manifest in the conversion of rocky mountains into terraced rice fields. As a result, China is succeeding in providing food for its almost 800 million people, and has made remarkable progress toward the elimination of certain devastating diseases and the effective control of others.

Appeals for mass participation, however, made either in the name of patriotism, as in the Patriotic Health Movement, or in the name of war preparation, will ultimately lose the momentum that has been maintained so far by intensive indoctrination based on Mao Tse-tung thought. It follows therefore that China is struggling against time to close the gap between population growth on the one hand, and increase in food supply and advancement in health care on the other. Reports by Western observers indicate that as of March 1972 China was making headway in its enormous birth control efforts.[63] Chinese authorities are confident that with the guidance of the four cardinal principles—following "mass line," stressing service to workers, peasants, and soldiers, integrating Chinese and Western medicine, and placing emphasis on disease prevention—in due time she will be able to provide adequate medical care to everyone in need, just as she has succeeded in feeding the entire population.

On a long-term basis China will continue to improve both the quality and quantity of paramedical personnel as well as the training of specialists for medical research and practice. That investigations on a sophisticated level have been in progress, probably less intensively than in pre-Cultural Revolution days, is attested by a recent report that reveals successful determination of the structure of crystalline pig insulin at a resolution of 2.5 A.[64] The work began in the summer of 1967 at the height of the Cultural Revolution and is a follow-up on the chemical synthesis of bovine insulin accomplished by Chinese scientists in 1965.

At the present time China is too engrossed in making available to villages and communes the much needed medical personnel, equipment, and drugs to afford to devote serious attention to basic research. For the time being, at least, Chinese scientists will have to rely more heavily on their colleagues abroad for information on new developments in basic medical studies. Knowing the nature of the Chinese people and considering Mao Tse-tung's strong advocacy of independence and self-sufficiency, I believe that theoretical studies of disease control and prevention will gradually assume equal importance with applied aspects.

NOTES

1. Ch'ien Hsin-chung, "Summing Up of Mass Technical Experiences with a View to Expediting Eradication of the Five Major Parasitic Diseases," *Chinese Medical Journal* 77 (1958): 521–32.

2. Mao S. P. and Huang M. S., "Schistosomiasis Control and Its Theoretical Basis," *Kexue Tongbao (Scientia)* 11 (1964): 963–72. (In Chinese.)

3. Joshua S. Horn, *Away with All Pests . . . An English Surgeon in People's China* (New York: Monthly Review Press, 1969). (Translated into Chinese by N. N. Kung.)

4. Feng L. C., Mao S. P., and Liu E. H., "Research on Parasitic Diseases in New China," *Chinese Medical Journal* 80 (1960): 1–20.

5. Ibid.

6. Mao and Huang, "Schistosomiasis Control."

7. Editorial, "The First County to Wipe Out Schistosomiasis," *China Reconstructs* 17, no. 7 (1968): 12–16.

8. Feng, Mao, and Liu, "Research on Parasitic Diseases."

9. Mao and Huang, "Schistosomiasis Control."

10. Ibid.

11. Liu Shen-ngo et al., *Record of Medicinal Plants in Northeast China* (Peking: Science Press, 1959): p. 198. (In Chinese.)

12. Ibid.

13. Institute of Pharmacology, Chinese Academy of Medical Sciences; Chungshan Botanical Garden, Nanking Academia Sinica; Department of Pharmacology, Peking Medical College; Tientsin Pharmaceutical Co.; Peking College of Chinese Medicine; and Peking Pharmaceutical Co., *Chung Yo Chih* (*Record of Chinese Medicines*, 4 vols. (Peking: People's Health Press, 1961). (In Chinese.)

14. Ch'ien, "Summing Up of Mass Technical Experiences."

15. Mao and Huang, "Schistosomiasis Control."

16. Tien-hsi Cheng, "Schistosomiasis in Mainland China. A Review of Research and Control Programs since 1949," *American Journal of Tropical Medicine and Hygiene* 20 no. 1 (1971): 26–53.

17. Ch'ien, "Summing Up of Mass Technical Experiences."

18. Ibid.

19. Anna Louise Strong, "These Twenty Years," *Letter from China* no. 69 (December 30, 1969): 1.

20. Ch'ien, "Summing Up of Mass Technical Experiences."

21. Ibid.

22. Ibid.

23. Culture, Education, Health and Antischistosomiasis Section of Revolutionary Committee of Yukiang (Yüchiang) County and Yukiang Antischistosomiasis Station, "A Great Victory of Mao Tse-tung's Thought in the Battle Against Schistosomiasis: The 10 Years Since the Eradication of Schistosomiasis in Yukiang County in 1958," *China's Medicine* 10 (1968): 588–602.

24. Editorial, "The 'Barefoot Doctors'," *China Reconstructs* 18, no. 3 (1969): 34–38.

25. Editorial, "The Orientation of the Revolution in Medical Education as Seen in the Growth of 'Barefoot Doctors,' Report of an Investigation from Shanghai," *China's Medicine* 10 (1968): 574–81.

26. J. Bonner, "Medicine and Public Health," *China Science Notes* 3, no. 1 (1972): 6.

27. Ibid.

28. Revolutionary Committee of the Shanghai Institute for the Prevention and Treatment of Eye Diseases, "Resolutely Implement Chairman Mao's Great Call, 'In Medical and Health Work, Put the Stress on the Rural Areas'," *China's Medicine* no. 12 (1968): 744–45.

29. Section of Politics and Education under the Revolutionary Committee of Shanghai First Medical College, "The 'Spearhead' Squad, Young Medical

Workers Nurtured by Mao Tse-tung's Thought," *China's Medicine* no. 12 (1968): 724–34.

30. Medical Team for Supporting Agriculture of a P.L.A. Hospital, Kirin, "Let Chairman Mao's Brilliant Thought Light Up Our Villages," *China's Medicine* no. 12 (1968): 735–43.

31. Bonner, "Medicine and Public Health."

32. Chang Chao-ming, "Develop Revolutionary Medical Service to Achieve Unity of Production and Disease Control," *Chung Hua I Hsueh Tsa Chih* (*National Medical Journal of China*) 52 (1966): 140–45. (In Chinese.)

33. Ibid.

34. Internal Medicine Branch of the First Subsidiary Hospital, Chinese Communist Peking Medical College, "The Rationale for Instituting Revolutionized Ward Service, a Political Innovation," *Chung Hua Nei K'o Tsa Chih* (*Chinese Journal of Internal Medicine*) 14 (1966): 299–303.

35. Ibid.

36. Anna Louise Strong, "The Revolution in Education," *Letter from China* no. 61–62 (November 20, 1968): 4.

37. Chang, "Develop Revolutionary Medical Service."

38. Editorial, "China's New Achievements in Tumor Control and Prevention," *Kuang-ming Jih-pao* (March 14, 1965). (In Chinese.)

39. Wu Hoan-hsing, "Conditions for Cancer Work Yesterday and Today," *China Reconstructs* 12, no. 2 (1963): 27–29.

40. Ibid.

41. Li Ping, "The Second All-China Tumor Conference," *Kexue Tongbao* (*Scientia*) 4 (1965): 373–74. (In Chinese.)

42. Wu, "Conditions for Cancer Work."

43. Li, "The Second All-China Tumor Conference."

44. Wu Hoan-hsing et al., "A Preliminary Clinical Report on the Efficacy of N-formylsarcolysine in the Treatment of Some Malignant Diseases," in *Cancer Research* (Shanghai: Scientific and Technical Publishers, 1962): pp. 84–105.

45. Soong H. C., Wu P. C., and Ho T. H., "The Treatment of Choriocarcinoma and Chorioadenoma Destruens with 6-Mercaptopurine and Surgery—A Clinical Report of 67 Cases," in *Cancer Research* (Shanghai: Scientific and Technical Publishers, 1962): pp. 441–63.

46. Editorial, "China's New Achievements in Tumor Control."

47. Li, "The Second All-China Tumor Conference."

48. Editorial, "Scientists from Various Countries Discuss the Cause and Cure of Cancer at the International Cancer Congress," *Jen-min Jih-pao* (*The People's Daily*) (August 1, 1962). (In Chinese.)

49. Li, "The Second All-China Tumor Conference.'

50. Ibid.

51. Soong, Wu, and Ho, "The Treatment of Choriocarcinoma."

52. Koo J. R., Huang Z. M., and Teng W. M., "A Study on the Cyto-Chemistry of Cancer of the Uterine Cervix, II. Methylene Blue-Triphenyltetrazolium Chloride Test Tube Smear Method in the Early Diagnosis of Cancer of the Uterine Cervix—A Preliminary Analysis of 5,969 Cases," in *Cancer Research* (Shanghai: Scientific and Technical Publishers, 1962): pp. 314–24.

53. Li, "The Second All-China Tumor Conference."

54. Mental Disease Institute of the First Subsidiary Hospital, Peking Medical College, "Follow the Guidance of Mao Tse-tung Thought, Break Through Old Regulations and Outmoded Doctrines, and Render Better Service to Patients," *Chung Hua I Hsueh Tsa Chi* (*National Medical Journal of China*) 52 (1966): 203–208. (In Chinese.)

55. Editorial, "New Treatment for the Insane," *China Pictorial*, no. 11 (1971): 13.

56. Mental Disease Institute, "Follow the Guidance of Mao Tse-tung Thought."

57. Ibid.

58. Ibid.

59. Editorial, "New Treatment for the Insane."

60. Editorial, "Everybody Works for Good Health," *China Reconstructs* 22, no. 11 (1971): 20–22.

61. "Our Pharmaceutical Industry Has Expanded Drastically," *Ta Kung Pao* (Hong Kong) (February 26, 1972). (In Chinese.)

62. Editorial, "Big Advances in Pharmaceutical Industry, *Peking Review* no. 11 (March 17, 1972): 22.

63. J. Unger, "Chinese Make Headway with Birth Control, *The Christian Science Monitor* (March 14, 1972).

64. Editorial, "Determining Insulin Crystal Structure—Another Step Forward in Protein Research," *China Reconstructs* 21, no. 1 (1972): 38–40.

Nutrition

ਵ਼

W. K. NG AND G. R. WADSWORTH*

The preparation of a paper on the subject of nutrition in the People's Republic of China today is presumptuous, as neither writer has recent first-hand knowledge of that country, and very little information is available outside of China about the current state of the population's nutritional status. Furthermore, there is the inherent difficulty of disentangling nutritional factors from the number of others that interact to determine standards of health in any community. Finally, a meaningful review of food supplies and nutritional status in China is especially difficult because of its vast size and marked regional differences.

Characteristics of the Chinese People

Because of China's geographical features, dense populations have built up along the coast and the alluvial plains at the mouths of the great rivers that flow from the mountains eastwards into the China Sea. Some areas are among the most densely populated in the world.

Throughout recorded history the Chinese have suffered greatly from periods of pestilence, famine, and internal warfare. In spite of these disasters, with their heavy tolls on human lives—the Taiping Rebellion of 1854–82 directly and indirectly took 20 million lives, and another 23 million died in the floods and famines of 1846, 1849, and 1877—the population has steadily increased and the conglomerations have become more dense and widespread.

These conditions stimulated migration to other lands, where the Chinese have been settling for a great many years—in 1882, for example, over 100,000 Chinese migrated to Malaya and Singapore. The adventurous nature of the Chinese has thus been important in

---

* Dr. Wadsworth did not attend the conference.

motivating them to emigrate on a large scale. Many of those who braved the unknown outside world were men of great energy, with business acumen and an ability to thrive and live frugally under various climatic conditions. These characteristics developed as a result of the necessity to survive, and were rewarded by outstanding success.

By contrast, immigration to China has been extremely limited. Thus while Chinese ideas and food habits have been widely disemminated, foods consumed in other parts of the world, with few exceptions such as maize, chili, and tomatoes, have not entered into the Chinese diet. Some modifications in the diet of overseas Chinese have been made by a sort of "hybridization" of local and Chinese dishes. There is reason to believe, however, that the customs and food habits in Chinese communities overseas reflect closely those of the homeland.

The Chinese People's Republic was proclaimed in Peking on October 1, 1949. Of significance for the nutrition of the population are the policies set by the government since then. Particularly important was the 1965 decree whereby support was provided for agriculture, instead of subordinating it to industry—a policy that has resulted in an increased production of food. Also of relevance is the emphasis on preventive health services, especially in the rural areas where the food is produced and where three-quarters of the people reside—500 million of them in villages.

Agriculture

Chinese agriculture is typified by the intensive farming of small areas. The average size of a farm is about 2.5 acres: cultivable land is on the average less than half an acre per head. Most of the usable land is tilled, and terracing and planting is often carried to the tops of hills. Few open areas are available for woodlands, orchards, or livestock grazing. Emphasis is on raising cereals for human, not animal, consumption. This pattern of farming must therefore lead to diets that contain little animal protein. The danger of protein deficiency is not quite so great as would appear, however, because use is made of all possible edible parts of animals and fish.

Due to geographic features and the vastness of the country, transportation of food is limited. Thus a crop failure may be disastrous to a particular area because of the difficulty of getting food to it from elsewhere. The long distances that food must travel necessitate special methods of preservation, such as milling rice and other cereals. Undermilled rice soon becomes rancid because of the presence in the grain of fat; hence highly-milled rice has become the accepted form. Many sauces and other products of household food technology have become essential items in the Chinese diet, arising from the need to preserve some foods. At the same time, because of bacterial fermentation the processes used in preservation lead to the synthesis of some vitamins.

While productivity of the farmers was always restricted because of the small size of the holdings and the lack of adequate communications, this situation has been overcome since the establishment in 1958 of "people's communes." All farmers contribute to the central organization, which is responsible for managing the farms, constructing highways and irrigation systems, supplying electricity, and providing other amenities needed for the efficient production and distribution of food.

For the purpose of describing agricultural production, China can be divided into three regions.

North China

This region lies for the most part north of latitude 33°, and the climate differs considerably from the rest of the country. North China includes almost all of the Yellow River valley where the worst floods and famines have occurred. Light rainfall and often very severe, cold winters make farming in this region particularly hazardous. Wheat, sorghum, and millet are the main crops. In Manchuria and along the northern border, wheat is planted in the spring to provide the single annual crop. In some parts, however, wheat can also be sown in the winter, thus producing two crops a year. Barley, oats, peas, soybeans, peanuts, maize, and sesame are also grown, as well as a variety of vegetables, including sweet potatoes, Irish potatoes, carrots, onions, cabbages, and stringbeans. Fruits include melons, pears, persimmons, apricots, and peaches.

As considerable use is made of draft animals there is comparatively little manual labor; modern farming machinery is employed in Manchuria. Because of the severe winters, higher levels of physical activity are presumably limited to other seasons of the year. Thus although food supplies are perhaps not abundant they may be sufficient to meet the energy requirements of the population.

Central China

This region lies between latitude 26° and 33°. It includes almost all of the Yangtze basin, the Hwai valley, and the Chengtu plain. The plain covers an area of 3,600 square miles and is watered by a highly-developed irrigation system dating from the third century B.C., which makes it one of the most productive agricultural areas of China.

While rice is the most important crop, wheat, tea, and vegetables are also produced. The climate does not fluctuate greatly throughout most of the year, although the summers are hot and humid, with regular rainfall. In some parts of the region two annual crops of wheat and rice can be produced.

South China

The mountainous southern region is below latitude 26° 30'. The large deltas of the two main rivers are among the most fertile areas in the world and usually sustain three crops a year.

The tropical and subtropical climate encourages the growth of a great variety of foods. Rice is the most important cereal, but tung seeds, bamboo, sugarcane, and many kinds of vegetables are common. Along the south coast, citrus fruit is abundant. Other areas produce peaches, pears, apricots, persimmons, walnuts, and chestnuts.

There is much wildlife in China and many birds, but preoccupation with intensive farming probably precludes much exploitation of this source of food. Cattle are raised to a small extent; the main farm livestock are pigs, sheep, and goats. The population of domestic animals is increasing (Table 1).

Freshwater and saltwater fish are important items in the diet of many Chinese. Before 1950 there were few modern facilities for

Table 1. Development of Animal Husbandry in China 1949–59

	1949	1959
Large animals	50,776	85,360
Pigs	57,752	180,000

Source: People's Republic of China, Bureau of Statistics, *Communique on Results on Execution of 1955 National Economic Plan* (Nung-yeh-Kie-heueh Tung Hsin: January 31, 1959.)

handling fish on a large scale, and fishing fleets were not mechanized. The situation is improving. The catch from the sea rose from 448,000 tons in 1949 to over 2 million tons in 1956.

The massive administrative reorganization since 1949, the development of administrative policies in recent years, and the occasional untoward effects of natural hazards have all influenced food production, but there has been an overall upward trend (Table 2). The greatest rates of increase were in the years 1952, 1955, and 1958, partly due to favorable weather conditions. In 1952, however, reforms were completed that led to a redistribution of the land among the farmers. There was also a progressive increase in the number of farming families who joined cooperatives, so that by 1956 over 90 per cent were so involved. The people's communes were instituted in 1958. Apparently there were food shortages in 1959 and 1962, but in recent years the situation has improved.

Food Consumption

Snow has stated that in about 1958 some students in a school in Changsha showed evidence of protein deficiency.[1] At that time, however, surveys in 586 communes showed that the average intake of food per capita was 2,265 calories in August, and as many as 4,000 calories during the busy harvest season. Snow states that in recent years he has seen no starving people in China.

Observations on ten types and amounts of foods available for consumption by Chinese in China, Singapore, and elsewhere suggest the possibility of a deficiency in riboflavin in China. Ariboflavinosis was in fact known to occur.[2-4]

The Chinese diet is largely vegetarian[5]—80 per cent of the total food intake is in the form of cereals, and over 90 per cent of the protein is of vegetable origin. The nutritional value of the diet is enhanced by the frequent inclusion of leaf greens and bean sprouts. Soybean curd and other special products are also of high nutritional value.

A number of traditional beliefs and customs may affect the nutrition of the Chinese. Special attention is given to women after childbirth, which is probably beneficial to lactation and hence to the nutrition of the infant. Use is made at this time of a preparation of ginger and vinegar which, among other nutrients, is rich in iron. During pregnancy, women by tradition often avoid ingestion of foods classified as "raw," "cold," "sour," and "irritant";[6] unfor-

Table 2. Output of Principal Farm Crops 1949–58

(Units in 100 million *katis*; 1 *kati* = 605 g.)

Years	Total Food Grain	Rice	% Increase	Wheat	% Increase	Miscellaneous Food Crops	% Increase	Potato	% Increase
1949	2,162	973		276		716		197	
1950	2,494	1,102	13.3	290	5.1	854	19.3	197	Nil
1951	2,701	1,211	9.9	345	19.0	865	1.3	280	42.1
1952	3,088	1,369	13.0	362	4.9	1,030	19.1	327	16.8
1953	3,138	1,425	4.1	366	1.1	1,014	1.6	333	1.8
1954	3,209	1,417	0.7	467	27.6	985	2.9	340	2.1
1955	3,496	1,560	10.1	459	1.7	1,099	11.6	378	11.2
1956	3,650	1,649	5.7	496	8.1	1,068	2.8	437	15.6
1957	3,700	1,736	5.3	473	4.6	1,053	1.4	438	0.2
1958	5,000	2,274	31.0	579	22.4	1,239	17.7	908	107.3

Source: People's Republic of China, State Statistical Bureau, "Ten Great Years," *Jen Min Jih Pao* (January 23, 1960).

tunately, such foods, for example, fruits, are valuable sources of vitamin C and folate. Owing to this abstinence, together with seasonal variation in supplies of fruits and vegetables, pregnant women in some areas may reach deficiency levels of vitamin C and probably of folate also.[7] Folate deficiency in pregnancy, even if of short duration, may be a cause of abnormal development after conception, and may also be a cause of placental insufficiency and dysmaturity.[8] That dysmature, or "small for dates," births occur in China is suggested by records of "malnutrition" among causes of prenatal death.[9] Folate deficiency is particularly liable during pregnancy and may lead to the development of anemia in the mother and her offspring.[10,11] Y. S. Ch'en et al. observed megaloblastic anemia in infants in Shanghai,[12] and the condition may not be uncommon.[13] The importance of lack of vitamin C in pregnancy is not known, although it has been suggested that it may lead to premature rupture of the membranes.

The Use of Night Soil in Agriculture

The danger of hookworm infestation in China, due to the use of human excreta (night soil) as manure, requires discussion here because of its importance in food production.

The shortage of available cultivable land requires intensive fertilization, and the use of night soil has allowed the production of food essential for the survival of the Chinese nation. The custom dates back to antiquity, and specific reference is made to it in agricultural rites formulated over 3,000 years ago. It was said that:

> They shall collect it into vessels, where it will ferment for six days; and after that it shall be used dilute with ten parts of water. For rice it should be spread during growth, not before, as often as it is needed, but not more often, for it is not the earth which must be nourished, but the plant. . . . By acting thus with wisdom and economy little of it will be expended, abundant harvest will be obtained, and the people will be happy. In the northern provinces, which have no harvest during the winter, the surplus manure is to be mixed with earth, and bricks made of it which are to be transported to the southern provinces.

Exploitation of natural products and resources, as in the hunting-gathering stage of man's history and in primitive agriculture, leads eventually to progressive diminution of food supplies as populations increase. Only with the return to the soil of materials removed from it is productivity maintained. It has been noted that areas of increased fertility surround the cities due to the use of human feces as fertilizer. Dramatic changes in food production in Europe after the seventeenth century were to an appreciable extent the result of regularly spreading manure on the fields. Thus the use of night soil in China was deemed an economic necessity. Stoll and his colleagues calculated that, with a population of 400 million people in 1926, 43 billion pounds of excreta were produced a year,[14] of which two-thirds, or 28 million pounds, may have been saved and used as fertilizer; this would provide about 180 million pounds of nitrogen, 57 million pounds of phosphoric acid, and 68 million pounds of potash—a very suitable proportionate mixture of essential plant nutrients which, if used locally, might not involve any capital expenditure.

The following conclusions can be made: First, the use of night soil is so entrenched in Chinese agricultural practice that perhaps little change is to be expected. Second, the production of food to sustain the population in the past, and perhaps to an increasing extent in the future, has and will depend on the use of night soil. Thus any danger to health because of this practice must be nullified by appropriate modifications to the natural material or to the manner in which it is used. At the same time, production and the use of chemical fertilizer is increasing in China.[15]

Malnutrition and Dietary Deficiency Diseases

The mean weight of Chinese children in China in the past, compared with that of Chinese children in Hong Kong recently, suggests that their intake of food was not optimal for growth. More recent figures from China indicate, however, that children in China are now bigger.[16] That the small size of the children in older studies was not genetically determined is indicated by the large size of many Chinese children presently residing in Singapore and Hong Kong.[17]

It is difficult to measure improvement in specific nutritional diseases. Those previously known to be common, such as rickets, osteomalacia, beriberi, and pellagra, are certainly not generally manifest. Rickets was described over 1,000 years ago and may still occur. Hsueh et al., for example, found that in one community in Peking over 12 per cent of a group of children under the age of two years had rickets, although only a small proportion were in an active stage of the disease.[18] In that area, prophylactic doses of Vitamin D were prescribed for children under one year of age, so the incidence of rickets may be declining. There also seems to have been much osteomalacia among women in recent years.[19]

Iron deficiency anemia, with or without ancylostomiasis, may still be common today, and megaloblastic anemia, probably of dietary origin, occurs especially in the northwest.[20]

Beriberi is a constant hazard to people when their diet consists mainly of rice. The disease has been known in China from the earliest times. Chen Chuang Kie in the eighth century described the ill effects of eating highly milled rice: "It softens one's body, bends and paralyzes dogs' and cats' legs, limits the activities of horses."[21] Chen Sze Liang at about the same time noted an effect on the heart of a prolonged diet of highly milled rice.[22] References in the ancient literature to "wet paralysis" may have been to beriberi, although the cases described might also have been ancylostomiasis or hypoproteinemia edema.

In some places, notably Hong Kong, there has been an appreciable fall in the incidence of beriberi; the drop has occurred spontaneously and there is no certainty as to why. One opinion is that in the past greater use was made of rice that had undergone some degree of spoilage, thus decreasing its content of thiamine. A similar decline in cases of the disease, although less marked, has been observed in Singapore; it has probably occurred in China also.

The foregoing general observations clearly need to be supplemented by data on the nutritional status of the Chinese people. Unfortunately, specific information is lacking and one must rely on rather general and unquantified observations and impressions. Chief among these are the repetitive reports from returning visitors who have known China for decades that the frequently observed malnutrition and starvation of the old days are absent. One hears that the Chinese people "appear to be well fed." More specific information on such improvements is not available.

Conclusion

In the absence of detailed information about actual food intake and nutritional status, assessment of the nutritional problems of China must be speculative.

The present review indicates that in this vast country a great range of products is available. The state of the Chinese farmers and the nature of the traditional Chinese diet suggest that when circumstances permit, poor nutrition should not be a general health problem. The present situation has been described by Whyte:

> The general situation seems to be best summarized by accounts of refugees and visitors who have said that everyone in China has food but no one has enough.[23]

NOTES

1. Edgar Snow, *Red China Today* (New York: Random House, 1971).
2. Hou H. D., "Riboflavin Deficiency Among Chinese: 1. Ocular Manifestations," *Chinese Medical Journal* 58 (1940): 616.
3. ———, "Riboflavin Deficiency Among Chinese: 1. Cheilosia and Seborrheal Dermatitis," *Chinese Medical Journal* 59 (1941): 314.
4. Hou H. D. and Dju M. Y., "Liveriary Excretion of Riboflavin," *Chinese Medical Journal* 62 (1944): 140.
5. Wu H., *Introduction to Nutrition* (Shanghai: Commercial Press, 1946). Quoted by Huang K'o-wei and Hang Chen-piao, *Chinese Medical Journal* 80 (1960): 455.
6. Lu Yi-ch'in, Hu Hwei-lien, and Chou Yen-ch'wan, "Plasma Vitamin C Levels of Chinese Pregnant Women," *Chinese Medical Journal* 75 (1957): 127.
7. Ibid.
8. B. M. Hibbard and E. D. Hibbard, *British Medical Journal* 44 (1968): 452.
9. Yen Ching-ch'ing and Liu Ch'ung-hsuen, "Death Rates in the City District of Peking," *Chinese Medical Journal* 78 (1959): 27.
10. I. Chariarin, *The Megaloblastic Anaemias* (Oxford: Blackwell's, 1969).
11. M. K. Strelling et al., "Megaloblastic Anemia and Whole Blood Folate Levels in Premature Infants," *Lancet* i (1966): 898.
12. Ch'en Y. S. et al., *Chinese Medical Journal* 67 (1949): 519.
13. Sung Shao-chang and Yang Chung-li, "Advances of Clinical Hematology in China in Recent Ten Years," *Chinese Medical Journal* 80 (1960): 46.
14. W. W. Cort, J. B. Grant, and N. R. Stoll, *Researches on Hookworm in China*, American Journal of Hygiene Monograph Series No. 7 (Baltimore: Johns Hopkins Press, October 1926): p. 257.
15. Snow, *Red China Today*.
16. Chao Lin, "Anthropometric Measurements of Shanghai Students and Preschool Children in 1954," *Chinese Medical Journal* 75 (1957): 1018.
17. Chang K. S. F. et al., *Far East Medical Journal* 1 (1965): 101.
18. Hsüeh C. P. et al., "An Experimental Study on the Organization of Urban Child Health Services," *Chinese Medical Journal* 84 (September 1965): 563–70.
19. Lim Kahti, "Obstetrics and Gynecology in the Past Ten Years," *Chinese Medical Journal* 79 (1959): 375.
20. Sung and Yang, "Advances of Clinical Hematology."
21. Chen Chuang Kie, "Pen T'sao Shih I" (Eighth century).
22. Chen Sze Liang, "Shih Hsing Pen T'sao" (Nang Tang).
23. Robert Orr Whyte, *Rural Nutrition in China* (New York: Oxford University Press, 1972).

Care of the Mother and Child

℣

ALEXANDER MINKOWSKI

The following notes, based upon personal observation and discussions during visits to China in 1965 and 1968, are not intended as a comprehensive presentation of maternal and child health in China but as a compilation of material in certain selected areas of the care of mothers and children. One general observation is important—while the living conditions could be described only as barely acceptable to a Westerner, health status seemed reasonably good.

Data on Natality and Mortality

Specific data on the usual indices of maternal and child health were not available, but some measure of the situation may be obtained from data covering the newborn for 1957 and 1964 supplied by the First Maternity Institute of Shanghai (Table 1). The statistics shown in the table were prepared with a punched-card system not generally available elsewhere in China.

There were usually 5,000 deliveries a year in this hospital, with approximately 800 cases of dystocia and about 250 caesarean sections. There were some 1,000 gynecological operations a year. The service had 160 beds, eighty-five cots for newborns, fifteen cots for prematures, and six incubators, the latter of modern design manufactured in Shanghai. The hospital staff consisted of thirty doctors, 150 nurses or diploma midwives, and 135 administrative workers and cleaners. There were three qualified pediatricians responsible for the care of newborn babies.

It is not known whether the much smaller total number of births in 1964 was due to an actual decrease of births in the hospital, or whether the data cover a shorter period of time. In any event the decline in overall mortality, over 60 per cent, is impressive; the 1964 rates are not very different from those to be expected in a large hospital in metropolitan France. Particularly to be noted is that in the seven-year interval there was substantial improvement

Table 1. Neonatal Deaths and Mortality Rate of Newborns—
1957 and 1964
(First Maternity Institute of Shanghai)

Birth Weight (in grams)	1957			1964		
	Total Live-Born Infants	Number of Deaths of Live-Born Infants	Neonatal Mortality Rate %	Total Live-Born Infants	Number of Deaths of Live-Born Infants	Neonatal Mortality Rate %
Total	5,392	105	1.95	2,794	21	0.75
Total 2,500 or less	338	60	17.75	183	13	7.10
501–1,000	8	8	100.00	1	1	100.00
1,001–1,500	26	17	65.38	6	4	66.67
1,501–2,000	60	16	26.67	27	4	14.80
2,001–2,500	244	19	7.79	149	4	2.68
Total 2,501 or more	5,052	43	0.85	2,611	8	0.31
2,501–3,000	1,373	13	0.95	843	4	0.47
3,001–3,500	2,451	22	0.90	1,268	2	0.16
3,501–4,000	1,077	8	0.74	440	2	0.45
4,001–4,500	141	0	0	55	0	0
4,501–5,000	10	0	0	5	0	0
5,001 or more	0	0	—	0	0	—
Unknown	2	2	100.00	0	0	—

in the weight groups over 1,500 g. where better obstetrical and newborn care may be more readily manifest.

The author was told that a similar improvement had been seen in Peking, where an overall mortality rate of 17:1,000 in 1957 had fallen to 12.4:1,000 in 1963. Furthermore, the Peking rates may have been conventional neonatal mortality rates covering the first twenty-eight days of life, rather than, as seems to be the case in the Shanghai figures, death rates based only on the period before discharge from the hospital.

The three leading causes of death in the neonatal period, verified at autopsy, were in the following order: perinatal asphyxia, intracranial hemorrhage, and hyaline membrane disease—the same causes as one observes throughout the world. Autopsies were done on 95 per cent of those who died.

Much of the seven-year improvement in the First Maternity Institute of Shanghai seemed to be related not only to the size of the staff and the facilities available but to the fact that adequately *trained* staff were available for competent care at night and on Sundays as well as on weekdays. Comparatively one has the impression that in situations where there may be one attendant in France there are five to ten in China. Furthermore, whereas in the public hospitals in France the staff is perpetually changing, in China the staff seems to be far more stable and permanent.

Staff of the institutes cited many measures as being influential in reducing mortality—better nursing care, isolation of individual infants, breast feeding, continual nasal gavage for small, weak infants, continuous observation of underweight infants in "humidicribs"—totally enclosed transparent containers with constant temperature and humidity—and the use of the Apgar system for scoring the status of all newborn infants. Respiratory obstruction was treated with laryngoscopy, a method used rather reluctantly in France, and by the use of respirators. In general one can say that these measures were comparable to those used in good obstetric and newborn centers in the Western world.

The information given in the table also permits some observations on the incidence of prematurity. In China it would appear that the frequency of premature birth varies between 4 and 5 per cent, in comparison with most other countries where it is between 8 and 12 per cent. While the Chinese figure could not be verified, its authenticity is supported by the small number of premature babies seen in the ten obstetrical hospitals visited by the author.

A related factor is that most of these premature babies are in the higher weight groups, of presumably longer gestation, with a better prognosis. In 1957, 72 per cent of infants under 2,500 g. weighed over 2,000 g.; this figure had gone up to 81 per cent by 1964. On the other hand it may be further calculated from the data that the mean birth rate in 1957 was 3,175 g. and that in 1964 it had fallen slightly—to 3,127 g.

A decline was also noted in the proportion of infants under 1,500 g.—those at highest risk. While the death rate in this group did not improve in contrast to the other weight groups, there was an actual saving in babies because, in 1957, 10 per cent of infants under

2,500 g. —0.6 per cent of all infants—weighed under 1,500 g., while in 1964 these figures had dropped to 3.8 per cent and 0.2 per cent respectively.

The author attributes the low incidence of prematurity and the low percentage of very small fetuses to the quite extraordinary measures taken to supervise Chinese women during pregnancy that he observed everywhere.

Prenatal Care

The remarkable attention given to women during pregnancy is said to be the same throughout the country. The women receive check-ups in the factories, in the country areas, and in the communes. This method of supervision could set an example to any Western country.

The initial visit to the midwife takes place during the first month of pregnancy. In factories the pregnancy is noticed immediately because every woman has a menstruation card; as soon as a few days' delay is observed by the health worker responsible for keeping the cards, biological tests for pregnancy are performed.

While this system might be criticized because of its obligatory character and because it is perhaps a little coercive, it is very representative of the way the Chinese regard medicine: *to have responsible health workers everywhere* educate the public concerning health and *take prophylactic measures at the slightest alert.*

For pregnant women working in a factory or in a country area there is a complete scale of progressive measures for resting. She works for seven hours a day after the twenty-eighth week; in the country, pregnant women are not allowed to work in the rice paddies. There is a midwife in every people's commune who is able to take blood pressure and to supervise normal deliveries; any rise above 120/80 in arterial pressure, which is checked every month, is regarded with suspicion. This makes what the Chinese say believable: That there is almost a complete elimination of toxemia of pregnancy and a very considerable reduction in the incidence of prematurity.

Following delivery, all women have fifty-six days' rest on full pay. Breast feeding is almost universal. Back in the factory the mother places the baby in a nursery and is relieved from work to feed it every few hours. In the rural areas the babies are looked after in a day care center or by the grandmother. The mothers come in from work in the fields to feed their babies.

Prophylaxis against uterine cancer includes urinalysis and systematic vaginal examination of all female workers every year.

Birth control measures for family planning do not seem to be coercive. In factories and in communes educational conferences are held, but the real instruction is given following delivery of a child. The measures are decided *individually, in each case*, depending on the number of children, housing conditions, psychological condition of the couple, etc. In some cases of extreme necessity, sterilization of the man or woman, or even abortion, is considered, but the consent of *both husband and wife* for any such measure is obligatory.

Specific Measures for Childhood Diseases

Information on childhood diseases was obtained from visits to pediatric hospitals in Peking, the Pediatric Hospital of the Second Faculty of Medicine of Shanghai, the municipal hospital of Wuhan, and from conversation with Professor Chu Fu Tang, vice-president of the Academy of Medical Sciences. Dr. Chu, who received his training in Great Britain, is very knowledgeable about modern pediatrics.

Measles Vaccine. Since 1960 the Chinese have concentrated on attenuated live virus vaccine, giving it in association with human globulin. Six million children had been vaccinated by 1963, and estimates of the effects suggest that there has been a considerable drop in morbidity among those receiving the vaccine.

Live Oral Poliomyelitis Vaccine. From 1960 to 1963, 40 million children between the ages of two and seven, or roughly half of the total population in that age group, received the vaccine in liquid form. More recently, preparations of the vaccine incorporated in candy have been used in some of the more remote rural areas. Ten million children had received this vaccine by 1963. Success of this effort is attested by the report that there was a 92 per cent reduction in the incidence of poliomyelitis in Shanghai between 1959 and 1963. Similar reductions are reported in the provinces of Kwangtung and Yunnan, as well as in large cities such as Peking and Shanghai. There are no longer summer or autumn peaks of poliomyelitis in epidemic form. This change and the general decrease in the incidence of poliomyelitis is, however, attributed to earlier vaccination campaigns using killed (Salk) vaccine.

Tuberculosis. A combined program using BCG vaccination and general prophylactic measures has been going on for some time. Treatment of severe tuberculosis, that is, miliary tuberculosis and tuberculosis meningitis, led to a reduction in fatality rates from 100 per cent in 1949, to 18 per cent in 1959, to 1.6 per cent in 1968.

Kala-azar. In 1949 there were 650,000 cases of this disease, the majority of victims being children; the mortality rate was 5 per cent. It is now reported that through the use of insecticides and antimony preparations, and the extermination of stray dogs, the disease has been almost completely eliminated.

Other Diseases. Although data were not available, we were told that the problem of infant diarrhea, particularly the role of pathogenic colon bacilli and viruses, is being studied intensively. One has the impression that virology is one of the best developed branches of research in China.

Other aspects of pediatric care worth noting, and the hospitals in which the work is concentrated, are: neonatal and childhood surgery (Pediatric Hospital of the Second Faculty of Medicine of Shanghai); cardiac surgery (Fu Wai Hospital in Peking); accident surgery (Hsin Hua Hospital in Shanghai); management of burns (Kuang Tse Hospital in Shanghai); and fluid and electrolyte therapy, with specific reference to the management of severe dysentery, (municipal hospital in Peking).

General Plan of Health Services for Children

In larger cities the major elements for health supervision of children under seven years of age include:

1. Supervision of newborn babies, including three visits to the home by a qualified worker to supervise the care of the infant;

2. Special intensive follow-up in the homes of premature babies born in the hospital, with supervision and advice by specially trained child health workers.

3. Regular visits to child health stations for prophylactic measures against the principal infectious diseases;

4. Supervision of all creches and kindergartens;

5. Education of the whole population in child health care.

Special attention should be drawn to the last point since one observes generally that the level of knowledge about health procedures is remarkably high, even among those living in primitive dwellings. Similarly, health knowledge is taught to teachers so that they can do a better job of supervising the health of the school children. The system may appear to be coercive but it seems to bear fruit.

To illustrate the experimental approach toward finding the best way to provide child health services it is pertinent to summarize a comparative study carried out in 1963 in two districts of Peking, both of which were in a sector with 15,000 inhabitants, 3,700 of whom were under the age of seven years.

In District A in the southern part of the city each medical assistant was responsible for 500 to 600 children. His duties included: (1) organizing services and clinics for supervision of noninfectious diseases; (2) conducting periodic examinations to help prevent rickets and malnutrition; (3) engaging in practical supervision of newborn babies; (4) supervising the crèches and kindergartens in his area; (5) keeping track of infectious diseases; and (6) giving a course of instruction in health education.

In District B in the northern part of the city each medical assistant was responsible for 800 to 1,000 children. Thus he had almost twice as many children but fewer resources. While there were no clinics for regular health examinations, more emphasis was put on the care of newborn babies and on infectious diseases.

It was found that the incidence of rickets in District B was nearly twice that in District A. This was attributed to longer intervals between examinations of the children and advice to the parents, with a consequent delay in the administration of Vitamin D. District B also had a greater number of cases of infectious diseases, notably measles, whooping cough, poliomyelitis, infectious hepatitis, scarlet fever, and dysentery.

This and similar studies were used by the Ministry of Health to guide it in deploying health personnel and helping to achieve the goal of care of equal quality for all segments of the population. This goal of equality appeared frequently in all aspects of the health services and seemed to be a very central theme of the organization. In contrast, in many Western countries wide differences in the availability of services exist without causing great concern.

Child Rearing and Education

There are 200 million children in China, and those seen on the streets radiate cheerfulness and vitality. Much of their play is organized in groups, with one child carrying a small red flag acting as supervisor. They march to school in groups. On Sundays they generally go to the park where they play under the watchful eyes of their parents. They dress in bright colors of pleasant design. In fact the sight of children in China is perhaps the only bright note in an otherwise severe and puritanical country.

As a matter of principle, the state takes charge of children while the families are at work during the day, and it sometimes takes charge of them even more extensively. Teachers appear to be plentiful, of high quality, with great enthusiasm for their work. Although the system would appear not to lend itself to individualization, there seems to be a strong effort to preserve the individual personality of the child.

Up to the Age of Two Years

In the day care centers in the factories and in the communes there is always a qualified children's nurse in attendance. She not only looks after the physical needs of the children but plays with them from the time they are only a few months old. The supervisors are constantly finding ways to keep the children busy, whether they are in nursery school or at a more advanced grade.

From Two to Seven Years: Kindergarten

Observations in many kindergartens in urban and rural areas revealed the typical picture of children kept occupied with artistic activities—acting, dancing, and singing—as well as with ordinary games. A prototypal institution, the "Kindergarten of Good Health" in Wuhan, is for the children of "cadre" members, that is, community political leaders. In a sense this special grouping is surprising because in other sectors the Chinese government seems to practice a scrupulous equality, mixing all classes of society together. At this kindergarten the children wear colorful clothes representing the national costumes of the main provinces of China, as well as the national costume of Vietnam. With advanced technique, considering their age, the children perform very gracefully the ballets of the provinces of their particular dress. During our visit the little North Vietnamese girls, between four and six years of age, mimed with a pointing fist, a gesture indicating "the American imperialist aggressor." Little boys of only three years were practicing the handling of wooden guns—a somewhat disturbing motif. Although all adolescents are taught that they should fraternize with the people of all nations of the world, including specifically the American people, war themes constantly appear in their instructive games, in singing, in acting, in ballet, and in art classes. While this emphasis is perhaps reflective of the situation in which China finds itself, a pediatrician cannot help but be disturbed over this emphasis in early childhood education.

From Seven to Fifteen Years

After school, usually from 4:30 to 6:00 P.M., these children go to the "houses of pioneers" a number of times a week. These are really art and technical schools where children may be seen playing electronic games with apparatuses of their own construction, designing instruments with transistors, building small-scale airplanes and boats, playing music of a very high standard, including orchestral works, learning acting, ballet, and singing, and making art objects. In these pioneer houses in the cities and in the rural areas one finds an extraordinary degree of interest, cheerfulness, enthusiasm, and technical ability.

Organization of Health Services

The People's "1st of July" Commune

This commune in the environs of Shanghai has 2,700 families, with a total population of 12,500, cultivating an area of 12,500 hectares. The members of the commune are grouped in nine production brigades and seventy-seven production teams. Cotton, wheat, rice, and cabbage are grown, and mushrooms are a special crop. They also raise cattle and pigs—the pigsty being a model facility, better kept than many dwellings.

In 1964 the commune produced 8,159 kg. of cereals, 855 kg. of raw cotton, 130,000 1. of milk from fifty-six cows, and raised 10,300 pigs. Each peasant has an annual income of approximately 340 yüan, and each family has a small plot of land on which to grow vegetables. No rent is charged for this land nor is there a charge for water.

The health care centers are simple but adequate and are designed so as to minimize the movement of patients. (That this goal is generally considered important was also illustrated in Shanghai and Wuhan where most of the commercial traffic is by means of heavily loaded carts, very often pulled by hand by old women. In the heart of the city of Wuhan, sick people are often carried on stretchers on bicycles, merely covered by a blanket, while a nurse rides alongside keeping check on the patient's condition.) In the commune health service facility there is a maternity ward, a surgery adequate for appendectomies, and an X-ray installation. The hospital equipment is very simple and reminds one of the medical equipment used by an army field unit. There are qualified staff, particularly midwives.

The Lungorchan Commune

This commune is near Peking and is dedicated to the friendship between China and Rumania. It is made up of 5,110 families totaling 42,000 people and covers an area of roughly 60–65 km.², about 6,000 hectares. There are five production brigades and 148 production teams, with five health stations or polyclinics—one for each brigade. The medical and nursing staff in the commune total ninety persons. While the health care organization is roughly similar to that of the "1st of July" Commune, there is greater emphasis on acupuncture and traditional medicine. For example, if towards the end of a pregnancy the baby is in an unusual position, instead of performing external maneuvers, a plant called moxa is burned on the feet of the woman for nine consecutive days. The fetus is said to assume the normal position in 90 per cent of the cases, presumably because of reflex action. This level of effectiveness was reported to us by well-trained physicians.

State Textile Factory No. 19 in Shanghai

This factory, with 2,100 cotton-weaving machines and 68,000 bobbins, employs 4,800 people of whom 80 per cent are women, most of whom have young children. Sixty per cent of the women live in the immediate neighborhood of the factory. The nursery can take care of 400 children and the mothers come there regularly to feed their babies. If a woman does not have help at home she can leave her child in the nursery for twenty-four hours whenever it is more convenient for her to do so. The working day is eight hours for each shift and the factory is in operation for twenty-four hours. After the seventh month of pregnancy a woman's workday is reduced to seven hours, but further modification is readily arranged at the slightest hint of complications. She makes a compulsory visit to the factory clinic each month during pregnancy and blood pressure determinations are made routinely. In addition to the regular fifty-six-day postpartum rest, a woman may be given an extra period of up to seventy days if, for example, she has had dystocia or has given birth to twins.

The polyclinic and nursery in this factory appeared badly managed and were rather dirty. The staff consists of twenty-three people—three "fully-trained doctors," and twenty nurses, medical assistants with three years' training, and traditional doctors. As in many other places, the medical and nursing staff spend part of every day studying the works of Mao Tse-tung.

Working conditions in this factory were not as good as might have been expected. A number of the pregnant women were working in a noisy room and were continuously being shaken by vibrations. The danger of this to the embryo was pointed out to the managing staff who apparently took note of the comments.

About 1,200 workers in this factory attend night school or technical school; 35 per cent of the supervisors are recruited from among the ranks of ordinary factory workers.

There was one interesting sidelight in this factory: Many of the workers were Mohammedans who had their own cafeteria which provided their ritual food.

The Wu Han Steel Works in Central China

This is one of the most important steel works in China, employing 36,000 workers. It represents one of the high points of Chinese nationalism for it was from this installation that in 1960 all Soviet technicians were withdrawn on short notice before the Chinese had quite learned how to operate it.

In this factory protection of workers against pneumoconiosis was rather elementary; even visitors found themselves in an atmosphere of iron dust. No cases of pneumoconiosis were said to have occurred, but precautions seemed to be inadequate. The medical staff admitted that they had difficulty in organizing proper methods of protection. Only 10 per cent of the employees are women, and they leave the factory when they become pregnant.

The health service employs 800 people, which seems a very large number for the tasks to be performed; 500 are doctors, nurses, and laboratory technicians. There is a 400-bed hospital, a 200-bed sanitorium for patients with tuberculosis and occupational diseases, and satellite services consisting of five polyclinics and seven sanitary stations; at both of the latter, services are available all night.

Hospital Facilities

The Municipal Children's Hospital in Peking

This is one of five children's hospitals in Peking. Established in 1955 it has 600 of the 2,000 children's beds available in Peking. Although the hospital was clean, it seemed less well kept than others visited. There are facilities for research on infectious diseases as well as for patient care. The hospital has an excellent surgical service that is particularly concerned with the newborn; it has a highly sophisticated procedure for megacolon. In this hospital, as in all of the centers visited, acupuncture is used widely in treatment. Electroencephalographic studies are also done.

The hospital also has a highly developed technique for rehydrating patients on an outpatient basis; they receive intravenous therapy and then go home. A Western observer might consider that many of these cases could be handled by oral fluid therapy, but the Chinese believe that using intravenous fluid requires less follow-up, is more efficient, and is safer.

An interesting aspect of this hospital is its emphasis on teaching the young child to speak by repeatedly reproducing in front of him the gesture corresponding to the verb.

Fu Wan Hospital in Peking

This hospital is well known to heart and lung surgeons because of its highly sophisticated open-heart surgery. In one year its surgeons performed 500 operations under hypothermia; 400 of these patients had extracorporeal circulation. The observers saw a large number of children who had recently undergone open-heart surgery; all appeared to be in good condition and cheerful. The children appear to be relatively free of emotional problems, apparently because they are accustomed to being away from their parents for periods of time, beginning with their nursery and kindergarten experiences, and because there are many attendants who keep them fully occupied.

Hospital No. 2 of the Wuhan Faculty of Medicine

This is a teaching center where faculty increased from 135 in 1949 to 749 in 1965, while the number of students rose from 480 to

2,665. In 1965, 554 doctors were graduating each year. The hospital has a center that specializes in traditional medicine, particularly for the treatment of renal stones. X-ray evidence was produced of dozens of patients who have been cured by medicinal plants. Similar results were reported on patients with ascaris infection. The newborn nursery was remarkably clean: it is disinfected once a week with phenol-lysol, and once a month with formaldehyde; ultraviolet light is used every day. A neonatal mortality rate of 0.88 per cent was reported, which is somewhat higher than the rate reported in Table 1. The incidence of prematurity was 5 per cent, with an overall mortality rate of 15 per cent.

One special focus of this hospital is the localization of organs, the fetus, and tumors by an ultrasonic-ray apparatus made locally.

Hospital No. 2 Sia Huan in Shanghai

This hospital, built in 1958, is affiliated with the Second Faculty of Medicine and is situated in an industrial section. In many ways it was one of the most interesting hospitals visited. Especially to be noted are:

1. All pediatric specialties are represented;

2. There are four operating rooms, and the surgery is really remarkable. They have developed to a high degree the treatment of intussusception by insufflation of air;

3. Modern laboratory techniques are used, including ultramicro methods in biochemistry. There is an excellent cytogeneticist on the staff;

4. The staff includes 230 physicians, 260 nurses, and 100 technicians for a total of 600 beds, 250 of them for children. The hospital is especially designed for teaching, and accepts students in the last three years of the medical school. Some 400 students at the hospital concentrate on a special subject, such as pediatrics. There is also a school for nurses. The newborn service appeared to be particularly well run.

Health Manpower

By 1965 there were eighty-five faculties of medicine producing what were called "complete" or fully qualified doctors. At seventy-three faculties the course was five years in duration and at eleven it was six years. At Peking Medical College it was eight years, the first three spent in a premedical course outside the faculty and the final five in clinical medicine within it.* All medical faculties are attached to universities but come under the control of both the Ministry of Higher Education and the Ministry of Health.

In order to meet the country's needs, a large number of institutions have been set up to produce "medical auxiliaries" after a three-year training period; the extent of their ability to treat patients is carefully defined. Every graduate of such a program has the possibility ultimately of completing the entire medical course. Technicians also take a three-year course at a medical technology school. An active program of postgraduate training for doctors in practice is more highly developed than in many Western countries.

Because of the enormity of the health care problems to be solved and the early policy decision that equal care would be provided to the whole population, there has been great expansion of the health manpower program under which a health worker is trained in three or four months. There is at least one part-time health worker in every production team and one medical auxiliary who works part time with every production brigade. Every commune has at least one medical station with four or five medical auxiliaries. There is a hospital in every large commune, and a larger hospital with fully qualified doctors in each district. At the time of this visit there were approximately 150,000 fully trained physicians and 1.7 million health workers in China. It was impossible to find accurate data on the number of medical auxiliaries or traditional doctors.

A striking feature of medical practice in China is that a majority of the physicians practicing in the cities are obliged to spend time working in rural areas, participating not only in medical care but in other aspects of rural life. Recently, for example, the president of the Academy of Medical Sciences undertook such an assignment as part of a general program of interchange between city people and rural workers. There seems to be general acceptance of this principle. One important result is that rural health services are being developed to a higher standard than would otherwise be possible.

Research

There is considerable emphasis on research, and most workers are fully qualified doctors. Those who are most interested and able

---

* This program apparently has been changed in the last few years.

are assigned according to individual skills and to the needs of the particular research institutes. The Academy of Medical Sciences has fourteen such institutes employing 2,000 research workers and 4,000 technicians and administrative workers. A number of biologists were seen working alone in the laboratory of the Academy of Sciences. A strange phenomen was that, despite the emphasis on care of the newborn, and the record rates in the field of neonatology, it was only in the hospital of the Second Faculty of Medicine in Shanghai that any real experts in this field were found.

General Conclusions

Emphasis on the care of mother and child appears to be a basic policy of the Chinese health service. Given the limitations of personnel and facilities, there appears to be concentration on valid priorities for preventive care. As far as one can tell the results are quite good.

VI. Population Planning

Introductory Note

Pi-chao Chen, a political scientist, discusses population planning and its effects on the demographic transition in the People's Republic of China. In his view, China seems to have the distinction of being the first nation in history to have effected a significant fertility transition through an organized promotional program. China's population policy has evolved in stages over the last two decades in response to the changing political climate and social and economic circumstances, ranging from pronatal on the one hand to antinatal on the other, and including implicit and explicit political coercion such as the advocation of delayed marriage. One again sees in it the display of pragmatism and the surprising flexibility of the Chinese policy makers.

Since 1968, when the direct manifestations of the Cultural Revolution subsided, the action program for family planning seems to have been in full swing—zero population growth was proclaimed as its long-term goal. No data are available to measure the rate of population growth objectively, however, or to assess the effectiveness of the various programs, or of the contraceptive methods employed. The accumulated evidence suggests that there has been a considerable decrease in the number of children per family, and that urban-rural differences in the number of children per family still exist.

Several factors are considered to be operating to explain the reported fertility decline: changes in intrafamily relationships, the liberation of women, collectivization of agriculture, improvement in the literacy rate, improved health and lowered infant mortality, and easy access to birth control measures. The extent to which the Chinese government has been able to reach its citizens to rearrange their daily lives, to change and replace their old values and norms with the new socialist, or Mao Tse'tung, thought, and to manipulate reward and punishment to induce compliance and deter defiance seems to have played a decisive role in the effective execution of the population program.

235

Population Planning:
Policy Evolution and Action Programs

ॐ

PI-CHAO CHEN

Since 1949, when Chairman Mao Tse-tung categorically refuted any suggestion that China had population problems, China's attitude toward the question of population has undergone several dramatic changes. Currently there is every indication that the government is doing and will do everything it can to bring about further fertility reduction, with zero growth rate as its long-run goal. Drawing upon available information this paper purports to: (1) reconstruct the evolution of China's population policy since 1949; (2) describe the Chinese birth control action program; and (3) appraise the prospects of demographic transition.

Policy Evolution

The history of China's evolving population policy may be viewed as a sequence of decisions made at different stages:

1. 1949–53—Initial confidence and no official antinatal policy;
2. 1954–56—Shift to antinatal position and initiation of some pilot projects;
3. 1956—Decision to launch a national birth control action program;
4. 1958—Decision to suspend the action program;
5. 1962—Decision to reactivate the action program;
6. 1968—Decision to intensify the action program.

In each of the stages a different set of factors operated on the policy makers and shaped their choice.

In September 1947, on the eve of the Communist conquest, Chairman Mao spurned Dean Acheson's diagnosis that China had population problems, and confidently held that, if indeed they did exist, under the leadership of the Communist Party, China would solve them within a very short period of time.[1] In the years immedi-

236

ately following Liberation the official position, if articulated, was pronatal.[2] During this period there was no systematic and reliable information about China's economic and demographic reality; a nationwide census to determine the size and dynamics of the population was not taken until mid-1953. This lack of information undoubtedly sustained the policy makers' optimistic outlook.

Initial optimism notwithstanding, the Ministry of Health had quite early initiated a series of vital-rate sample surveys in selected areas that revealed a significant rate of natural growth.[3] The information derived from the surveys must have caused considerable disquiet among certain high-level policy makers, and must have generated a climate of opinion favoring an antinatal policy, for it was revealed that as early as August 1953 the then Government Affairs Council had ratified the Ministry of Health's revised "Regulations on Contraception and Induced Abortion" and instructed the ministry to facilitate the practice of birth control.[4] Subsequently, in July 1954, the Ministry of Health drew up another set of "Measures Concerning Contraception."[5] None of these steps were reported at the time, however, and there is no evidence that a birth control program was introduced.

In mid-1953 the government undertook a census, in conjunction with which a large scale sample survey of vital statistics was also conducted. The census revealed a population of 583.3 million as of June 30, 1953, and the sample survey, a birth rate of 37:1,000, a death rate of 17, and hence a natural growth rate of 20.[6] If these figures are accurate, in the early 1950s China's population was growing by more than 12 million a year[7] (Table 1).

Although the official reaction to the census and the survey results was one of jubilation and confidence, the feedback seems to have alarmed some high-level policy makers and strengthened the opinion favoring immediate adoption of a national population planning policy. This was evidenced by a speech made by Shao Li-tze, a deputy to the recently elected National People's Congress and a member of the Government Affairs Council, at the first session of the First National People's Congress in August 1954, in which he advocated adoption of an antinatal policy.[8] More significantly, in December 1954 Liu Shao-ch'i called a conference to discuss the problems of birth limitation, following which the Second Office of the Government Affairs Council appointed a small group to study and submit recommendations on ways and means of promoting

Table 1.   The Population of the People's Republic of China,
by Province 1953, 1958, and 1964

	Population (in Thousands)				Rate of Growth (Percent)	
			1 July 1964			
	1 July 1953[a]	1 January 1958[b]	As Reported[c]	Projected[d]	1953– 1958	1958– 1964[e]
Southern Region						
Kiangsu[f]	47,137	52,130	57,000	60,290	2.26	1.38
Anhwei	30,663	33,560	35,000	38,234	2.03	0.65
Chekiang	22,866	25,280	31,000	29,224	2.26	3.19
Fukien	13,143	14,650	17,000	17,137	2.44	2.32
Hupeh	27,790	30,790	32,000	35,704	2.30	0.59
Hunan	33,227	36,220	38,010	41,025	1.94	0.74
Kiangsi	16,773	18,610	22,000	21,624	2.34	2.61
Kwangtung	36,740	37,960	40,000	39,794	0.73	0.81
Kwangsi	17,591	19,390	24,000	22,318	2.19	3.34
Szechwan	65,685	72,160	70,000	82,656	2.11	−0.47
Kweichow	15,037	16,890	17,000	19,977	2.62	0.10
Yunnan	17,473	19,100	23,000	21,721	2.00	2.90
Northern Region						
Hopeh[g]	43,348	48,730	54,000	57,705	2.63	1.59
Shansi	14,314	15,960	18,000	18,677	2.45	1.87
Liaoning	20,566	24,090	28,000	30,273	3.58	2.34
Kirin	11,290	12,550	17,000	14,622	2.38	4.78
Heilungkiang	11,897	14,860	21,000	20,489	5.07	5.47
Shensi	15,881	18,130	21,000	21,952	2.99	2.29
Shantung	48,877	54,030	57,000	62,447	2.25	0.83
Honan	44,215	48,670	50,000	55,909	2.16	0.42
Western Region						
Inner Mongolia	7,338	9,200	13,000	12,754	5.15	5.46
Kansu and Ninghsia	12,928	14,610	15,000	17,433	2.76	0.41
Tsinghai	1,676	2,050	2,000	2,742	4.58	−0.38
Sinkiang	4,874	5,646	8,000	6,964	3.30	5.53
Tibet	1,274	1,270	1,320	1,264	0.07	0.60
Total	582,603	646,530	711,330[h]	752,935[i]	2.34	1.48

Sources: Robert Michael Field, "A Note on the Population of Communist China," *China Quarterly* no. 38 (April–June 1969): 162; a) John S. Aird, "Population Growth and Distribution in Mainland China," in Joint Economic Committee of the United States Congress, *An Economic Profile of Mainland China*, vol. 2 (Washington, 1967): p. 370. The figures from the 1953 census, which are adjusted to the boundaries of 1957, are taken from *Chung-Hua jen-min kung-ho-kuo ti-t'chi* (*Atlas of the People's Republic of China*) (Peking, 1957); b) People's Republic of China, State Statistical Bureau, *Ten Great Years* (Peking, 1960): p. 11; c) these figures, collected from provincial newspapers, regional broadcasts, and New China News Agency releases, are listed under 1 January 1964, on the assumption that they are the results of the 1964 registration; d) projected from the data for 1953 and 1958 on the assumption that growth rates remained constant; e) derived from the 1958 and 1964 data as reported; f) the figures include the population of Shanghai; g) the figures include the population of Peking and Tientsin; h) derived as the sum of the data reported for individual provinces; i) derived as the sum of the data projected for the individual provinces.

birth limitation.[9] In spite of this, almost two more years elapsed before the government formally promulgated an antinatal policy, although during the interval it had been quietly promoting birth limitation among cadres and had initiated some pilot projects.[10]

There is reason to believe that the delay in launching a birth control action program was due to internal disagreement concerning the urgency and feasibility of such a program. In the course of the first Five-Year Plan period (1953–57), as more information about China's socioeconomic and demographic environment became available, and as the implications of rapid population growth became increasingly clear, antinatal opinion within the decision-making council gained further credence. As a result, in mid-1956 a major decision was adopted to launch a nationwide campaign to promote birth limitation.[11]

In June 1956 Madame Li Teh-chuan, then the minister of health, announced the government's intention of initiating an education and publicity campaign to promote birth limitation and to expand birth control facilities and guidance clinics.[12] In September, in a major speech before the Eighth Party Congress, Premier Chou En-lai announced the government's approval of birth limitation,[13] which to all intents and purposes amounted to official adoption of an antinatal policy.

Following these announcements a mass campaign began to evolve that gathered increasing momentum with the passage of time. Mass organizations such as the youth leagues, the women's federations, the trade unions, and the Red Cross were mobilized to popularize the idea of birth limitation and the various methods of contraception. Pamphlets, films, and slides were released in large quantity; planned childbirth exhibitions made their appearance, first in major urban centers, then in lesser cities and towns, and finally in rural villages; and neighborhood meetings and small group study sessions were held in which the benefits of planned childbearing were explained and methods of contraception diffused.

In April 1957 the National Committee on Technical Guidance was established under the Chinese Medical Association, and soon thereafter technical guidance committees were set up at lower administrative levels throughout the country. Guidance clinics were introduced, birth control cadres trained and deployed, and a manufacturing and supply network of contraceptives was expanded and strengthened.

In February 1957 Chairman Mao, in his "On the Correct Handling of Internal Contradictions among the People," spoke in favor of birth limitation:

> Steps must therefore be taken to keep our population for a long time at a stable level, say, of 600 million. A wide campaign of explanation and proper help must be undertaken to achieve this aim.[14]

On March 5 the authoritative *Jen-min Jih-pao* editorialized on behalf of limitation,[15] and in that same month scores of delegates to the National People's Consultative Conference pledged their support for planned childbearing;[16] as late as June 1958 there was still an indication that the program was being vigorously implemented and expanded.[17] All these activities were given detailed coverage and wide publicity in the national and local press.

Toward the end of the summer, however, the action program was abruptly albeit quietly terminated, and exhibitions, small-group meetings, and other such activities were suspended; beginning in August the press ceased to carry any progress reports on the campaign. It should be noted that the abrupt suspension of the program coincided with the initiation of the Great Leap Forward and the people's commune movement.

No sooner did the press cease to report on the work of the birth control program than it started to print voluminous reports on the fantastic accomplishments on the economic front; throughout the remainder of 1958 the papers were full of statistics registering the Great Leap Forward in various sectors. At the same time there appeared in the press frequent complaints of a severe labor shortage and suggestions as to its solution—whereas previously the problem had been one of unemployment and underemployment, it was now one of a severe labor shortage.

In this euphoric atmosphere the birth limitation program was suspended, and between 1959 and 1961 the government neither promoted nor discouraged the practice of birth control.

In the aftermath of the Great Leap the government reappraised the wisdom of its earlier decision and decided to revive the program. As a first step it reactivated the now largely defunct planned childbearing guidance committees at various administrative levels.[18] The spring of 1962 witnessed the launching of a press campaign involving virtually all national newspapers urging delayed marriage for the single and birth limitation for the married. Reflective of the high priority status of the campaign was the fact that many newspapers set up a "planned childbirth column." The advantages of delayed marriage and planned childbearing, as well as the disadvantages of early marriage and failure to practice birth limitation, were cited repeatedly. While the arguments were more or less similar to those of the 1956–58 campaign, the new drive placed decided emphasis on delayed marriages.

Concurrently, planned childbearing exhibitions began to reappear. The manufacture of contraceptives, largely halted for three years, was resumed and expanded; distribution networks for contraceptives and technical guidance clinics were reactivated and expanded; and more counseling and guidance cadres were trained. Meanwhile the search for more reliable and less expensive contraceptives was intensified, resulting in the mass manufacturing of IUDs in 1963–64; another result of the search was the successful synthesis of birth control pills, which since 1968 have been mass produced. Another research accomplishment was the perfection and improvement of induced abortion by vacuum (suction) methods.

The year 1963 saw the campaign take on new vigor and intensity with the government resorting to all the resources at its disposal to encourage delayed marriage and birth limitation. The approach was multifaceted, combining education and persuasion on the one hand and administrative measures that rewarded the compliant and punished the defiant on the other. For unknown reasons the publicity campaign via the mass media was terminated in mid-1963.

At the height of the Cultural Revolution in 1966 and 1967 the birth limitation program was disrupted to some extent due to the almost total breakdown of the nation's administrative apparatus.[19] Since order was restored in 1968 the program has resumed its operation and has gained further momentum with the passage of time.

In short, the evolution of Chinese population policy has been a process through which the policy makers finally learned the correct response to a new situation for which orthodox Marxism-Leninism had ill-prepared them.

The Birth Control Action Program

An organized birth control action program has to tackle two related tasks:

1. To inform the public of the possibility of family planning, and to make information and the various means of birth control easily accessible and widely available;

2. To inculcate the small family idea of, say, no more than two children per family, depending upon the long-term goal of the population planning policy.

Success in the first task is in itself a great accomplishment, and will go a long way toward reducing fertility and the rate of natural increase. But if the long-term goal is zero population growth, the organized program will have to address itself squarely to the second task as long as the ideal number of children the average married couple want is above two. China has set for itself the goal of reducing the natural increase rate to 2 per cent in "the near future" and to below 1 per cent by the year 2000.[20] While we do not know for sure the ideal number of children desired by the average Chinese married couple, we do have scattered evidence that it is well over two.

The Chinese government therefore really has no alternative but to carry out the two tasks. This section purports to dwell on two aspects of the action program: the government contraceptive service system and the education campaign. Inasmuch as there already exist quite a few studies of the Chinese birth control action program[21] we propose to concentrate on more recent developments, with emphasis on the post-1965 public health reform and the recent breakthrough in the research and manufacture of contraceptives.

Innovative Approach to Public Health

Prior to 1949 China had a small number of trained medical personnel, few hospitals, and no nationwide public health service. Both modern doctors and hospitals were concentrated in urban centers and treaty ports, and their services were unavailable to the majority of the Chinese people.

Determined to improve medical care rapidly, but having limited resources, since Liberation in 1949 the government has opted for the "walking on two legs" approach, that is, combining maximum utilization of existing medical manpower, modern and traditional doctors, with a labor-intensive mass movement approach to public health such as the "Patriotic Hygienic Campaign."[22] Concurrently it took steps to rapidly expand the training of more medical personnel. As a result of these measures the last two decades have witnessed a tremendous increase in China's medical manpower. One estimate is that as of 1968 there were 115,000 Western-style doctors with at least five years training after middle school, not including doctors in the People's Liberation Army (PLA), for which figures are not available. In addition there were an estimated 500,000 doctors practicing traditional medicine and acupuncture.[23]

In spite of this tremendous increase, the aggregate medical manpower of all types as of the late 1960s remained grossly inadequate for a population of over 700 million. Assuming the above figures are not far off the mark, the ratio of doctors to population was less than 1:1,000. Even if the PLA doctors were included, the ratio could not possibly be significantly higher. Furthermore, there was apparently an uneven distribution of medical personnel, with a high but unknown proportion concentrated in the cities.[24] This meant that in spite of the progress since 1949, medical care in the late 1960s remained largely unavailable to the majority of the rural population, which comprised about 80 per cent of the total population.

Against this background it becomes easy to understand why Chairman Mao issued his now famous June 26, 1965 directive calling for a mass migration of medical personnel to the rural villages: "In medicine and public health put the stress on the rural areas . . . Urban hospitals should retain some doctors who graduated only one or two years ago and who are not very experienced. All the others should go to the countryside." Since then, urban medical hospitals have dispatched one-third of their personnel to villages as mobile medical teams on a rotation basis, the usual period of service lasting one year or so. Since the outbreak of the Cultural Revolution this program has been intensified and has resulted in a mass migration of doctors from urban and county hospitals to the countryside; some have even taken up more or less permanent residence there (Table 2).

As the table indicates, Peking alone has organized 6,000 medical and health personnel into 430 medical teams that have traveled as far as Szechuan, Yunnan, and Inner Mongolia. In addition to general mobile units, there are teams that specialize in eye, ear, nose, and throat disorders, dental care, and birth control. They were as-

Table 2. Number of Doctors Rotated to the Countryside:
Selected Areas

Kiangsi	11,000
Kwangtung	5,000
Hunan	5,000
Heilungkiang	8,400
Kweichow	4,000
Kansu	1,400
Inner Mongolia	1,000
Hopei	2,000
Peking	6,000

Sources: Figures other than those for Peking are all from "The Mao-Liu Controversy Over Rural Public Health," *Current Scene* 7, no. 12 (June 15, 1969): 17; the figure for Peking apparently refers to 1970 and is from Edgar Snow, "Population Care and Control," *New Republic* (May 1, 1971): 22.

signed six tasks, of which two are of great importance to the work on birth control: to train auxiliary medical personnel (feldsher-type field workers) and barefoot doctors; and to bring birth control information and services to the countryside.[25]

The provisional plan calls for the mobile medical teams to train four or five doctors for each health clinic in a commune, one or two barefoot doctors for each production brigade, and one or two midwives and one or two health workers, not divorced from production, for each production team.[26] The training program is expected to be carried out within three to five years after being initiated. The curriculum, in addition to disseminating information about fundamental and general medical care, includes imparting knowledge about the various methods of contraception. The provisional plan also calls for the barefoot doctors to have at least three periods of full-time retraining, lasting from four to six months, at yearly intervals.

Barring unforeseeable developments this program promises to create an army of paramedical personnel over the next few years. With the deployment of this army China will overcome one of its greatest obstacles to introducing birth control to the countryside. Whatever the political or humanitarian rationale for such an approach to public health, it will fulfill one of the organizational prerequisites to any serious attempt to provide birth control services in the vast number of rural villages.

Breakthrough in Research on and
Manufacturing of Contraceptives

The Intrauterine Device. The search for an IUD began in the late 1950s, and by the mid-1960s it had emerged as the most popular contraceptive device in China, surpassing even the condom.[27] The type of IUD developed earlier dropped out easily, especially among rural women doing heavy manual labor in the fields. To remedy this an improved plastic IUD called "flowers" was devised which does not fall out easily.[28] Summarizing some twenty articles published in Chinese medical journals in the early 1960s, Leo Orleans concludes that

> almost all the reporting doctors agreed that the IUD is a simple and effective birth control device, is most suited to the requirements of rural women, is "most welcome by these women," and that an intense campaign to popularize IUDs in rural areas should be accompanied by more attention to the quality and size.[29]

The Pill. Research on oral birth control pills began in 1957. By 1964 an oral pill was successfully synthesized but proved to be unsatisfactory. A completely satisfactory twenty-two-day pill was developed in 1967; the improved pill is "free of side effects" and is "100 per cent effective if taken daily." According to Edgar Snow, China is now manufacturing the pill "in the billions, in the largest chain of labs of this nature in the world."[30] Han Suyin has also reported on the widespread use of the pill.[31] Medical organizations, mobile medical teams, barefoot doctors, PLA medical teams, factories, and shops all participate in distributing the pill either free of charge or for a nominal cost. Evidence seems to indicate that it is available to women factory workers free of charge,[32] while in the countryside it is either distributed free or at a small cost.[33] As of 1970 the demand for the pill exceeded current production. Given time, this imbalance should be overcome.

Induced Abortion by Vacuum Method. In the early 1960s the Chinese medical profession improved upon induced abortion by the vacuum method, which apparently originated in Eastern Europe. Quite a few ingenious and simple procedures and methods are in wide use today.[34] Trained nurses as well as doctors perform the operation using acupuncture for anesthesia if the patient so chooses. Abortions are performed free of charge, on demand of the mother alone;

if she is a working woman she is entitled to two weeks leave with full pay.[35]

The Education Campaign

The education campaign is directed toward achieving two goals: (1) To persuade young people to accept and practice delayed marriage; and (2) to induce married couples to accept and practice the ideal of two children per family.

Article 4 of the Marriage Law promulgated in 1950 provides that "a marriage may be contracted only after the man has reached twenty years and the woman eighteen years of age." In 1956 Shao Li-tze proposed that the legal age of marriage be raised to twenty-three for men and twenty for women,[36] but this proposal was not taken up by the government. In March 1963[37] the government quietly handed down a recommendation on the optimal age of marriage: it ranged from twenty-five to thirty for men and from twenty-two to twenty-eight for women. In making the recommendation the government made a careful distinction between the "legal age" and the "optimal age." "Marriage is more appropriate for men between twenty-five and thirty, and for women between twenty-two and twenty-eight, for only at this age has a person's physical development completely matured, a certain degree of knowledge and skill be grasped, and economic life is reliant, and the capability for an independent life is achieved."[38] Furthermore, the young should devote their entire energy and time to study and to the socialist construction of the fatherland, and should not allow themselves to be diverted into "talking love" and marriage.

The fact that the government sees fit not to raise the legal age does not mean that it has confined its promotion efforts to recommendations and persuasion. Whenever feasible it has not hesitated to back up its persuasion with subtle or outright sanctions against those who have the audacity to decline the recommendation. Administrative sanctions available to the government include punitive job assignments, separating defiant married couples upon graduation, and discriminatory promotion policies. Needless to say, such sanctions or threats are applicable only to high school and college students and graduates, employees in the urban-industrial sector, civil servants, and cadres in general.

While the government is in a position to apply sanctions or threats in order to force its advice on certain segments of the young married population, it cannot and has not attempted to exert the same pressure on the rural population,[39] where discriminatory job assignments and promotions are not applicable except for those aspiring to or occupying cadre positions. The compliance rate is thus more likely to be higher among educated urban youth than among rural youth. Scattered evidence seems to confirm this.

If delayed marriage became widespread, by reducing the theoretical number of children a woman may bear before reaching forty-five, it would make a significant contribution to fertility reduction.[40] But since this pattern cannot be forced upon the rural youth, who constitute the majority of the young population, its impact on the overall fertility rate is likely to be limited.

Due to the limitations of a policy of enforcing delayed marriage, the main thrust of the education campaign has been centered on inculcating the concept of the small family norm. While we do not know the ideal family size preferred by the population of China it seems safe to say that it is well above the replacement rate. The data collected from women refugees in Hong Kong and Macao by Robert Worth and Janet Salaff tend to confirm this statement.[41]

Since the early 1960s the government has carried out an intensive education campaign to promote the idea of small families. Two of the most oft-repeated slogans are: "Two children are just right, three too many, and four a mistake"; "Extol one, praise two, criticize three, and avoid four." In this campaign the government has not only mobilized the mass media, but "transmission belts" such as trade unions, small groups, women's federations, the educational system, and public health networks. Ad hoc birth control propaganda teams have been dispatched to the countryside, and planned parenthood exhibitions are sponsored periodically. In addition the government has utilized posters, slide and film presentations, and face-to-face persuasion.

As in its efforts to promote delayed marriage the government has not confined its efforts to publicity and persuasion. It has shown no hesitation about exerting pressure or resorting to administrative measures when feasible. These include denial of ration coupons for clothing for a third baby, as was done in certain areas in the mid-1960s, and group criticism of those bearing or wanting to bear many children.[42] There have been unconfirmed reports that for those employed in the urban-industrial sector, the first two children are delivered free of charge, but not the third.

Closely paralleling the persistence of the traditional large family idea is the traditional preference for male offspring. Chinese leaders, including Chairman Mao, have repeatedly singled out this sex bias as one of the greatest obstacles to the efforts to spread birth control practices in the countryside.[43] If this complaint is based on statistical information, then, given its long-term goal, the government obviously has no alternative but to combat this "vestigial feudal thought." In spite of the concern, strenuous efforts do not seem to have been made to combat this lingering tradition, apart from accelerating the "family revolution" and "women's liberation." This is easily explainable: In the urban-industrial sector, a social security system—labor insurance and retirement pensions, etc.—was institutionalized as early as the mid-1950s, but there is still no comprehensive, much less adequate, social security arrangement for the rural-agricultural sector. Given this situation it makes little sense for the government to try to persuade the peasants not to have "too many" children, especially male children.

Prospect of Fertility Decline

Snow reported that during his last trip to China in 1970–71 he was told "authoritatively" that by 1966 the natural rate of increase had been brought down to below 2 per cent. During the Cultural Revolution, however, the rate "shot up" again. "Millions of Red Guards went on a 'long march,' when the sexes more freely intermingled; many early marriages helped boost the birth rate."[44] Since most of the conditions accounting for the revival of high fertility have now been brought under control, the rate has presumably once again dropped to below 2 per cent. As is to be expected, the birth control campaign has not achieved equal success in all places, and urban-rural fertility differentials persist.[45]

The reported decline in the natural increase rate can hardly be attributed to a temporary rise in mortality in the mid-1960s. Mortality probably rose in the early 1960s in the immediate aftermath of the Great Leap, but certainly not in the mid-1960s. Since there was steady improvement in nutrition and in medical and health care in the 1960s, mortality probably declined steadily during that period. In view of this the decline in the natural increase rate has to be attributed to overall fertility reduction.

The decline cannot be accounted for in terms of economic development, since there has been no substantial increase in the

GNP or per capita income. Nor can it be attributed to increasing urbanization or to a significant change in the composition of the labor force, or, for that matter, to other conventional indicators of development. If anything there has been a deurbanization process, with the government vigorously implementing a policy aimed at stabilizing the urban population at the 110 million level.[46]

It seems more likely that most of the factors accounting for the fertility decline have been created by specific changes and programs initiated by the government since 1949, such as the acceleration of the "family revolution"; the "liberation of women"; collectivization of agriculture; improvement in the literacy rate and expansion of the education system; explosion in mass media and social communication; great improvements in health care and environmental sanitation resulting in lower mortality—especially infant mortality; the Cultural Revolution that has resulted in increasing erosion in and replacement of traditional familial norms by modern and socialist familial norms; and the organized action program to spread and facilitate birth control.

Many of these changes and programs must have had a profound psychological impact on Chinese in all walks of life, especially the young who comprise more than 50 per cent of the population. Although they may still be poor by Western or Japanese standards their new feelings of personal efficacy and their newly gained confidence must have delivered them from the "culture of poverty" and fatalism. While some of the cultural and institutional changes initiated under Communist auspices have pronatalist consequences, most have the effect of removing or undermining many of the forces and norms that traditionally sustained high fertility practices. Furthermore, the government's vigorous efforts to bring culture, education, and health care to the masses, and to bridge the rural-urban gaps—by such programs as the *hsia-fang* (downward transfer) system and rustification of urban intellectuals and educated youth— have the "unintended," or perhaps "intended," consequences of assisting it to inculcate the small family norm and to make birth control knowledge, means, and technical service easily accessible to the broad masses in the vast rural areas.[47]

The experience of the advanced countries that have completed their demographic transition is no model for what may be taking place in China today, or, for that matter, although to a lesser extent, in other less developed countries with high fertility rates.

First, the pace of mortality decline from the high level characteristic of a preindustrialized society to the low level typical of an advanced society has accelerated over the past century, thanks to the breakthroughs in medical science and public health techniques. Substantial mortality reduction has occurred without profound socioeconomic structural transformation.[48] This has been the case for many less developed countries and for China in particular.

Second, many reliable, inexpensive, and convenient contraceptives became available only after the early 1960s.

Third, fertility rates declined in Europe and elsewhere without the benefit of large-scale, organized efforts to promote birth control. With the possible exception of postwar Japan, birth control measures spread and fertility dropped in a climate hostile to such practices.

Fourth, the government of China has created a physical-cum-human network of social communication, linking the average peasants in rural villages to the outside world and political centers, making them aware of the possible alternatives to the traditional way of life, and reshaping their attitudes toward the family, the status of women, the role of the individual, and life in general.[49]

Fifth, the disadvantages the Chinese government may find in its attempt to spread birth control methods in a preindustrialized society may be compensated for to some, albeit undeterminable, extent by its organizational ingenuity and the control it has over the lives of its citizens.

The extent to which the government has been able to reach its citizens, to rearrange their daily lives, to change and replace their old values and norms with the new "socialist" values and Mao Tsetung thought, to manipulate rewards and punishments to induce compliance and deter defiance, and to mobilize and unleash the people's latent energy[50]—all of these were unheard of in the presently developed countries during their comparable stage of development. (The only possible exceptions are the Soviet Union in the 1930s and 1940s and North Vietnam during the second Indochina war. For obvious reasons I have no intention of drawing parallels.)

Because conditions are drastically different, the past is definitely no guide to what is possible at present and in the future, particularly with respect to China. It follows that any serious attempt to predict the pace of demographic transition in China or to assess the government's capability of realizing its stated policy goal must take these differences into account.

Concluding Remarks

So far in history there has been no instance in which a major fertility transition took place as a result of an organized promotional program. Nor has there been a case in which such a major transition took place without concomitant or prior profound social and economic transformations in the society involved.[51] In the West and elsewhere fertility transitions have occurred as a result of the initiative taken by millions of married couples in response to opportunities and pressures, for example, the desire for a better life and upward mobility for themselves and their offspring, arising in the course of socioeconomic transformation or "modernization."

While there can be little doubt that for a society at her present level of "modernization" (industrialization and the concomitant social change), China most probably has effected a significant reduction in the fertility level, and that she will continue to reduce it in the near future, there is legitimate doubt that she will be able to accomplish a major demographic transition without a further substantial degree of "modernization." If she accomplishes this feat China will win the distinction of being the first nation to have done so.

NOTES

1. Entitled "Sixth Critique of the White Paper," Mao Tse-tung's writing originally appeared as an editorial in *Jen-min Jih-pao* (September 17, 1949). When the fourth volume of his *Selected Works* was released, this article was included, with the title changed to: "The Bankruptcy of the Idealistic Conception of History." (*Selected Works of Mao Tse-tung*, vol. 4 [Peking: Jen-min Publishing Co., 1960]: pp. 1515–16.)

2. "Import Ban on Contraceptives," *Survey of China Mainland Press*, no. 545 (April 5–7, 1953): 8. Semiofficial views of the period were expressed in the following writings: Editorial, "How Does the Malthusian Theory of Population Serve Imperialism? What Functions Does It Perform in the Realpolitics of International Political Life?" *Hsueh Hsi*, Peking, 3, no. 5 (December 1, 1950): 16–17; Alexandrov (transliteration of a Russian name), "The Ideological System of American Imperialism Is a Cannibal Ideological System," *Hsueh Hsi Yi Chung*, Peking, no. 6 (1952); Rekina (transliteration of a Russian name), "Critique of Neo-Malthusianism," *Wen Shih Tse*, Peking, no. 8 (August 1955); Yang Shih-ying, "Fundamental Knowledge: Malthusianism," *Hsueh-Hsi* no. 10 (October 1955): 24–25.

3. Chen Ta, "New China's Population Census of 1953 and Its Relations to National Reconstruction and Demographic Research," *Bulletin de l'Institut International de Statistique* 36, part 2 (1958): 266–68; "Census and Registration Work Completed in Areas with Sixty Per Cent of Population," *Ta-kung Pao* and *Jen-min Jih-pao* (March 11, 1954). This news release also revealed a sample survey conducted in two *hsiang* (Ai Ling and Sheng Li) in Kiang Ning *hsien*, Kiangsu, by the Population Census of Registration Office of Kiang Ning *hsien*. The only findings reported were a birth rate of 33.6:1,000, a death rate of 19.3, and a natural increase rate of 14.3.

4. Editorial, "Birth Limitation Should be Appropriately Practiced," *Jen-min Jih-pao* (March 5, 1957).

5. Shao Li-tze, "On the Problem of Disseminating Knowledge about Contraception," *Kuang-ming Jih-pao* (December 19, 1954).

6. "Communique of Results of Census and Registration of China's Population" *Jen-min Jih-pao* (November 1, 1954); "Pai Chien-hua, 600 Million People— A Great Strength for the Socialist Construction of Our Country," *Jen-min Jih-pao* (November 1, 1954).

7. John S. Aird argues that the 1953 census represented a genuine effort on the part of the government to count the population of China, and that the results probably understate the true population size by 5 to 15 per cent. See Aird, "Present and Prospective Population of Mainland China," in *Population Trends in Eastern Europe, the U.S.S.R. and Mainland China* (New York: Millbank Fund, 1960): pp. 94–116; Aird, "Population Growth," in *Economic Trends in Communist China*, Alexander Eckstein et al. (Chicago: Aldine, 1968): pp. 183–328. D. H. Perkins, though agreeing with Aird on the nature of the 1953 census taking, doubts that the margin of error could be as high as 15 per cent. "Such an error would imply that the census takers missed two persons in every three families investigated, or perhaps failed to register as many as one in seven families. . . . It is difficult to see how such an enormous number of mistakes could be made." See Perkins, *Agricultural Development in China*, 1368–1968 (Chicago, 1969): p. 201. John Durand, though willing to accept the official figure, questions the government's claim of the accuracy of the enumeration by pointing out the methodological and operational deficiencies. See Durand, "The Population Statistics of China, A.D. 2–1953," *Population Studies* 13 (March 1960): 246. Ho Ping-ti also points out the procedural defects of the census, but accepts its results as being "closer to the truth than any previous population figures" without hazarding a guess at the margin of error. See Ho, *Studies on the Population of China, 1368–1953* (Cambridge, 1959): pp. 93–94. John L. Buck believes that "the Communist 1953 census figure . . . is undoubtedly more nearly correct than that of any previous census, and there is no reason to suspect the 1953 Communist census figure as being too high." See Buck et al., *Food and Agriculture in Communist China* (New York, 1966): p. 40. Of all the demographers who have studied the 1953 census returns, Irene Taeuber and Nai-chi Wang are the most critical. They point out the "strikingly consistent patterns of similarities and differences" between the 1953 provincial registration figures and those of the 1850s and 1920s, which were "defective and unreliable," and suggest that there had probably never been "either field enumeration or a controlled registration of the population of all China." See Taeuber and Wang, "Questions on Population Growth in China,"

in *Population Trends in Eastern Europe, the U.S.S.R. and Mainland China* (New York, 1960): pp. 263–302. Some Western-trained Chinese social scientists have also politely questioned the "scientific" quality of the 1953 census. At a symposium sponsored by the State Statistical Bureau of China on May 27, 1957, in connection with the Hundred Flowers campaign, Chen Ta criticized the processing of data by tallies at successive levels, and recommended that a second census be taken in 1960 and that a pilot project be first set up in a *hsien* with a population of less than 300,000, not too far away from Peking, in order to field-train cadres of the State Statistical Bureau. See Chen Ta's remarks, *T'ung-chi Kung-tso*, no. 12 (1957): 1–2. Ma Yin-ch'u also suggested that the actual vital rates were probably higher than those reported by the State Statistical Bureau, and recommended that a second nationwide census be taken in the near future. See Ma, "A New Theory of Population," *Jen-min Jih-pao* (July 5, 1957).

8. *Jen-min Jih-pao* (September 18, 1954).

9. *Jen-min Jih-pao* (March 5, 1957).

10. Tsai Ch'ang, "Actively Cultivate and Promote Female Cadres," *Jen-min Jih-pao* (September 25, 1956).

11. For evidence and documentation, see Pi-chao Chen, "Policy Making as a Collective Learning Process: The Case of Evaluation of Population Planning Policy in the People's Republic of China, 1947–72," *Caltech Occasional Papers on Population Series*, forthcoming.

12. "Speech by Li Teh-chuan," *Jen-min Jih-pao* (June 19, 1956).

13. *Jen-min Jih-pao* (September 19, 1956).

14. *New York Times* (June 13, 1957). According to the official version of his February 27 speech at the Supreme State Conference, Mao did not specifically discuss the question of birth control, but evidence strongly suggests that he did indeed speak on behalf of birth control in the course of his speech. See Mao Tse-tung, *Selected Readings from the Works of Mao Tse-tung* (Peking: Foreign Languages Press, 1967): p. 375. Evidence and analysis are given in the study referred to in Note 11.

15. *Jen-min Jih-pao* (March 5, 1957).

16. For their speeches, see *Jen-min Jih-pao* (March 1957).

17. *Liaoning Jih-pao* (Shenyang, June 9, 1958).

18. *Yang Cheng Wang-pao* (Canton, August 17, 1962).

19. A Japanese journalist traveling through China in 1966, however, reported that "meetings to familiarize the people with methods of birth control were held frequently in various parts of the country despite the fact that the Cultural Revolution was going on at full blast." See R. Trumbull, ed., *This Is Communist China* (New York: David McKay, 1968): p. 191.

20. "Edgar Snow's Five-Hour Interview with Chou En-lai," *The Washington Post* (February 3, 1964): p. A-12; Edgar Snow, "An Interview with Premier Chou En-lai," *Asahi Januaru* (Tokyo, March 7, 1965): 16.

21. Some of the more detailed studies are: H. Yuan Tien, "Birth Control in Mainland China—Ideology and Politics," *Milbank Memorial Fund Quarterly* (July 1963); H. Yuan Tien, "Sterilization, Oral Contraception, and Population Control in China," *Population Studies* 17, no. 3 (March 1965): 215–35; Leo Orleans, "Evidence from Chinese Medical Journals on Current Population Policy,"

China Quarterly no. 40 (October–December 1969): 137–46; and P. C. Chen, China's Birth Control Action Program," *Population Studies* 24, no. 2 (July 1970).

22. For a description of the labor-intensive mass movement approach to public health, see Joshua S. Horn, *Away with All Pests . . . An English Surgeon in People's China* (New York: Monthly Review Press, 1969): Chapters 9 and 10.

23. Editorial, "Mao's Revolution in Public Health," *Current Science* 6, no. 7 (May 1, 1968): 1.

24. Editorial, "The Mao-Liu Controversy over Rural Public Health," *Current Science* 7, no. 12 (June 15, 1969): 17. This charge was made by the Red Guards during the Cultural Revolution; there were no figures to substantiate the charge.

25. Horn, *Away with All Pests*, Chapter 13.

26. Ibid., p. 135; "Mao's Revolution in Public Health," p. 4; see also E. Grey Dimond, "Medical Education and Care in People's Republic of China," *Journal of the American Medical Association* 218, no. 10 (December 6, 1971): 1555.

27. Han Suyin, "Family Planning in China," *Japan Quarterly* 17, no. 4 (October–December 1970): 440.

28. Ibid., p. 440.

29. Orleans, "Evidence from Chinese Journals," p. 144.

30. Edgar Snow, "Letter from Peking, January 14, 1971," in the Victor-Bostrom Fund and the Population Crisis Committee, *Population and Family Planning in the People's Republic of China* (Washington, D. C., 1971): p. 5.

31. Han Suyin, "Family Planning in China."

32. Ibid.

33. Conversation with Carmelita Hinton and members of the Hinton Students Team who visited China in 1971.

34. Orleans, "Evidence from Chinese Journals," pp. 140–41.

35. Snow, "Population Care and Control," p. 21; Huang Yu-chuan, *Birth Control in Communist China* (Hong Kong, 1967), p. 102; "Fewer and Better," *Far Eastern Economic Review* (Hong Kong, October 14, 1965).

36. *Jen-min Jih-pao* (March 20, 1957).

37. Chi-ping Tung and Humphrey Evans, *The Thought Revolution* (New York: Coward-McCann, 1966), p. 157.

38. Lu Yang, *The Correct Handling of Love, Marriage and Family Problems* (Chinan, Shantung: People's Publishing House, 1964), trans. in *Chinese Sociology and Anthropology* 1, no. 3 (Spring 1969): 28; Chou Hsin-min, "On the Question of Promoting Marriage," *Kung-jen Jih-Pao* (November 15, 1962).

39. The Myrdals, however, reported that in the village they visited in the late 1960s, the age of marriage for girls had been raised from eighteen to twenty-two or twenty-four, or so. See Jan Myrdal and Gun Kessle, *China: The Revolution Continued* (New York: Pantheon, 1970): pp. 132–33.

40. Ansley Coale and C. Y. Tye, "The Significance of Age Patterns of Fertility in High Fertility Populations," *The Milbank Memorial Fund Quarterly* 39 no. 4 (October 1961): 631–46; Norman Ryder, "The Conceptualization of the Transition in Fertility," *Cold Spring Harbor Symposia on Quantitative Biology* 22 (1957).

41. Robert Worth's data appear in Janet Salaff, "Institutionalized Motivation for Fertility Limitation in China," *Population Studies* 26, pt. 2 (July 1972): 233–62. The data he and Salaff collected in the mid-1960s show that the stated size of the family remains well above replacement level. However, "the relatively

young rural women had lower ideal family size than older women. For those aged eighteen to forty-four model preferences were four children as first choice and two as second choice. In contrast, the bimodal distribution for women older than forty-four was six and four children." This observation is hardly surprising, for in the much more "developed" Taiwan, as of 1970 the average woman wanted 3.9 children. See Oliver D. Finnigan, III, and T. H. Sun, "Planning, Starting, and Operating an Educational Incentive Project," *Studies in Family Planning* 3, no. 1 (January 1972): 2.

42. See, for example, Jan Myrdal, *Report from a Chinese Village* (New York: Random House, 1965): pp. 226–27; and Myrdal and Kessle, *China: The Revolution Continued*, pp. 132–33.

43. Edgar Snow, "A Conversation with Mao Tse-tung," *Life* (April 30, 1971): 47. Mao was quoted as having remarked to Snow: "In the countryside a woman still wanted to have boy children. If the first and second were girls, she would make another try. If the third one came and was still a girl, the mother would try again. Pretty soon there would be nine of them, the mother was already forty-five or so, and she would finally decide to leave it at that. The attitude must be changed but it is taking time." A provincial official in Canton made more or less the same remark: "Seldom did I find such earnestness as when provincial officials talked of their birth control efforts. A cloud came over a lively banquet in Canton when the 3 per cent rate was announced. 'It's the old problem,' explained a senior editor of the *Nanfang Jih-pao* (Southern Daily), 'Peasants have a daughter. They think that's no good. So they keep going till they get sons.' " See Ross Terrill, "The 800,000,000," *Atlantic Monthly* (November 1971): 110. A prominent woman in modern China, Madame Sun Yet-sen, wrote recently: "As farmers want to add to the labour force in their families, the birth of a son is expected while that of a daughter is considered a disappointment. This repeated desire to have at least one son has an adverse effect on birth control and planned births." See Soong Ching-ling, "Women's Liberation in China," *Peking Review* 15, no. 6 (February 11, 1972): 7. Visitors to China in 1971, however, presented a somewhat different picture. "As we traveled, we asked the people how many children there were per couple in each place. . . . Most couples agree that three children are too many, they told us, but the problem is that most women want one daughter and most men want one son, so if the couple's first two children are of the same sex, they frequently try for a third. After the third they give up, if they still have children all of the same sex." See Committee of Concerned Asian Scholars, *China: Inside the People's Republic* (New York: Bantam, 1972): p. 286

44. Snow, "Population Care and Control," p. 21.

45. "In Kwangtung, the birthrate figure given me was 3 per cent. In Hunan, 1.5 per cent (in Changsha it was down to 0.97 per cent last year)." See Terrill, "The 800,000,000," p. 110. The surprising low fertility rate for Changsha, and presumably large cities in general, cannot be explained entirely in terms of the conventional theory of demographic transition. Nor can it be accounted for by delayed marriage alone, which is definitely more widespread in cities. The resumption of the *hsia-fang* (downward transfer) system and the rustification program since 1968, by separating urban married couples and postponing marriage, must have contributed significantly to the reduction of fertility levels in the cities.

46. For a study of the deurbanization policy and the rustification program, whereby millions of urban school graduates have been resettled in the country-side, see P. C. Chen, "Overurbanization, Rustification of Educated Youth, and Politics of Rural Transformation: The Case of China," *Journal of Comparative Politics* (April 1972): 361–86.

47. The arguments summarized here are elaborated in an article of mine entitled "Prospects of Demographic Transition in a Mobilization System: The Case of China," in *Research in the Politics of Population*, ed. Kenneth Godwin and Richard L. Clinton (Lexington, Kentucky: D. C. Heath and Co., 1972: pp. 153–82. Janet Salaff has also dwelt on the probable effects of agricultural collectivization on fertility in the rural areas. See Salaff, "Institutionalized Motivation." In a provocative article, B. Maxwell Stamper has tentatively attributed the recent fertility decline in Cuba to the Castro revolution. "It seems likely, however, that many of the factors affecting this decline have resulted from specific governmental programs carried out in the context of a socialist revolution." See Stamper, "Some Demographic Consequences of the Cuban Revolution," *Concerned Demography* (1971): 19–23.

48. George Stolnitz, "A Century of International Mortality Trends: I," *Population Studies* 9, part I (July 1955): 24–55, reprinted in Charles B. Nam, *Population and Society* (Boston: Houghton-Mifflin, 1968): pp. 124–51.

49. To measure the extent of social communication in China by such conventional indicators as the number of radio and television sets or newspaper circulation rate per 1,000 population is utterly inadequate. Through the ubiquitous small groups that meet frequently and into which virtually all urban population are organized, the ubiquitous production teams into which virtually all peasants are organized, the mobile movie, culture, and propaganda teams which bring entertainment and the government message to even the most remote villages, inaccessible by cars or other modern means of transportation, and person-to-person communication, the Chinese government has been able to reach and communicate to its population in a way and to a degree that governments of other preindustrialized societies could hardly imagine. What the society lacks in material resources, the government compensates for by intensive mobilization of human resources in order to reach and communicate with its people. See Alan P. L. Liu, *Communications and National Integration in Communist China* (Berkeley: University of California Press, 1971). Also, Martin Whyte's forthcoming study of small groups to be published by the University of California Press.

50. See, for example, James Townsend, *Political Participation in Communist China* (Berkeley: University of California Press, 1968); Franz Schurmann, *Ideology and Organization in Communist China* (Berkeley: University of California Press, 1966); Doak A. Barnett, *Cadres, Bureaucracy, and Political Power in Communist China* (New York: Columbia University Press, 1967); Robert J. Lifton, *Thought Reform and the Psychology of Totalism* (New York: Norton, 1961): parts II and III.

51. For some studies of recent cases of demographic transition see, for example, Irene B. Taeuber, "Japan's Demographic Transition Re-examined," *Population Studies* 14, no. 1 (July 1960): 28–40; and Jerzy Berent, "Causes of Fertility Decline in Eastern Europe and the Soviet Union, Part II," *Population Studies* 24, no. 2 (July 1970): 247–92.

VII. Concluding Remarks

Present Status and Future Perspectives

TSUNG-YI LIN AND MYRON E. WEGMAN

Taken as a whole the information presented at the conference helped to develop a general contour of public health in the People's Republic of China, although the data were imprecise and sketchy in many aspects and there were a great number of lacunae and areas of ignorance.

Some Findings and Observations

What impressed the conference most was the prominent position and high priority occupied by health issues and health programs in national politics and administration. This is a unique development, unparalleled not only in Chinese history but in the history of many developed and developing nations. A combination of factors —political, historical, and practical—seems to have contributed to this departure from the more common picture of subordinating health programs to other considerations.

First was a political decision at the highest level, apparently originating from Mao Tse-tung's philosophy that the new China could be constructed and developed for the people, particularly for the hitherto neglected and deprived peasants. To him and to the new nation, health represented a most immediate, direct, and massive challenge on which much of both national and personal prestige was at stake; the state of health of the Chinese people would be a most visible indication of the success or failure of the policy Mao had proclaimed. The experiences in Yenan and the neighboring countryside during the revolutionary war provided him with an excellent opportunity to try out some of his ideas, and convinced him and his comrades of the essential role health care could play in maintaining a robust and well-motivated society for a sustained revolution. This historical development in philosophy

259

and experience was thus carried over to the postrevolution era and put to a wider application. The overall slogan "serve the people," interpreted as constant efforts to put the common good first, rather than individual or class advancement, found a natural focus in the broad field of the health of the public.

Second, there was a practical necessity for the new China to pay special attention to its human resources. For a preindustrial nation such as China, healthy workers were a prerequisite to agricultural reconstruction and national development; it would clearly be necessary to rely on human labor rather than on machinery for much of the nation's production for some time to come.

Papers and discussions at the conference made clear that a characteristic feature of Chinese public health was that it constitutes an integral part of the overall social system. Thus there has been a high degree of intermeshing with other national developmental programs, such as education, welfare, and agricultural and industrial production. Repeatedly throughout the conference the importance of mass involvement, not only in learning about health but in action for health, was emphasized. Directly related is the interrelation of health activities with other forms of social action and the repeated adjuration that one cannot understand progress in health without seeing it in the total social and political context. The ingenious use of schoolchildren and peasants for environmental sanitation, the development and training of peasants, during their leisure time, into a new category of health worker, barefoot doctors, are but selected concrete examples.

An equally striking feature is that health programs and health conduct are highly political activities. Political pressure or coercion, implicit or explicit, of varying degrees, calling on the political conscience of the people and demanding loyalty and self-sacrifice seems to be present in all phases of the execution of the programs. The degree of cooperation with health programs and the reported change in health conduct of the people are amazing considering the briefness of time—twenty-five years since the revolution—and the vastness of the country in terms of both its geography and its population.

In many countries with shortages of resources and personnel trained in modern medicine there is great variation in utilization of indigenous folk healers. The conference was impressed with the apparently orderly combination of traditional and Western medicine in China, and the evidence of plans for division of responsibility and mutual support. This development is at least in part related to national pride and to the habits of the people, especially of the peasants. While the correlated program seems to have come about rather reluctantly at the beginning, the momentum and enthusiasm for a full-fledged integration seems to be at hand. This includes the provision of curative and preventive services, health education of the masses, the teaching of medical students, and the training of all kinds of health personnel. Joint clinical research on specific treatment modalities, such as acupuncture and pharmacological study of herbs, is also in progress. Objective assessment of the potential of the methods and remedies of traditional practitioners in China and better understanding of how the scope of their activities can be limited to their competence will have great significance for developing countries.

Of major importance is the evidence of how much the local community at the commune, brigade, or neighborhood level has assumed responsibility for its own health programs. This local participation is an instance of "mass-line approach" which makes it possible for the local community to select its own method of implementation, often making ingenious use of local resources and circumstances and drastically reducing health care costs. Precisely because of this there is great expectation that the effects of a particular health program in the community may be maintained for a long period, and that there will be beneficial changes in the health conduct of the people. A useful device to facilitate general involvement has been the national conference or broadly attended meetings to spread promptly the information and methods of health programs advocated for general adoption.

The phrase, "walking on two legs," interpreted as combining mass involvement and participation of the people, with skillful guidance by informed and creative professionals, is particularly adaptable in public health.

Though self-reliance and national interest are the guiding principles for designing and implementing public health programs at all levels, and the specific features described emanate from Chinese concepts and traditions, certain important elements of Western origin, especially from socialist philosophy and socialist approach, can also be identified. They are: (1) emphasis on equality and universality; (2) emphasis on prevention and on integration of preventive and curative services; and (3) emphasis on quantity and a massive increase of human and natural resources.

The apparent determination with which the principles of equality and universality applied to health programs are emphasized, particularly since the Cultural Revolution, is evident from the intensive and nationwide effort to make health services comparable for urban and rural populations. This principle is reinforced by concentration on improving the quantity of services and by the massive increase of resources, manifest in intensive efforts to train subprofessional health workers as well as in the apparently thorough reorganization and shortening of medical education. The emphasis on prevention as an integral and essential part of health services is an impressive new development, particularly welcome to public health professionals who see in prevention the major avenue for reduction of societal costs of disease and disability. The chief evidence of the effect of preventive activities is the general observation that there has been a substantial decline in major infectious and parasitic diseases, apparently dependent as much on individual and community participation as on carefully organized programs and technological advances.

Using venereal disease as an example, in one session it was noted that a fruitful way of looking at Chinese progress, particularly in preventive programs, is as a progressive application of eight steps, even though all cannot be identified in every program.

The first is direct intervention for obvious disease, e.g., treatment of prostitutes; second, long-term social engineering, e.g., finding other employment for them so the brothels could be closed; third, resolution of technical controversies as to tactics, e.g., concentration on techniques and trained manpower for syphilis serology versus the use of limited available resources to identify sources and carry out secondary prevention; fourth, experimentation, e.g., trying to identify high risk individuals through a questionnaire; fifth, field trials of the experimental technique; sixth, validation of results, such as measuring results in a stratified sample; seventh, use of national conferences for prompt dissemination of the results and their implications for public health programs; eighth, wide extension to other areas, with maintenance of maximum local autonomy.

Public health professionals will note the absence of one cherished step—careful assessment and quantification of the problem so that one can have an accurate appraisal of progress. It has, however, been demonstrated in many developing countries with very high incidences of major disease problems that more immediate benefit will come from prompt inauguration of a program and direct intervention, and that long-term results will not be jeopardized provided the quantitative phase is not overly delayed. It appears that China has followed this path deliberately, but published data are not yet available to judge the timeliness of instituting assessment procedures.

Some Unanswered Questions

The Dearth of Data

The first group of questions stem from insufficient informational data on results and on the working of the health system in China.

Unavailability of certain essential data and lack of information on completeness and validity of the health and population data that were presented at the conference were enough to convince a few participants that it was unwise to publish these data. For example, it was not clear whether reported rates of population increase represent the actual situation or a target figure of the policy proclaimed by the government. Furthermore, absence of secure population data based on either census or scientific random sampling of a specific population makes it hazardous to discuss decline of mortality or variations in birth rate. Understandably, under such restraints objective assessment is made difficult and evaluation becomes almost impossible. The data presented in this volume must therefore be regarded as rough estimates based on the best available information. Nevertheless, accumulation of similar observations in certain situations, along with evidence that consistent trends of events can apparently be traced, permits some causal relationships to be inferred. Still, nothing can take the place of factual, reliable, and consistent data, which, it is hoped, will be forthcoming in the near future.

Second, much-needed information on the structure and working of the medical care organization was not available. For example, how are maternal and child health services and school health programs organized? How are they related to the general preventive and curative services for the whole population? What roles are played by physicians, nurses, and other personnel in health supervision? How much is carried out in a clinic setting and how much at school or in the home? How much health instruction is carried out in groups and how much is individual? How are hospitals and health facilities related to ambulatory services; for example, the follow-up of newborn and premature infants? How are preventive services and curative services correlated? Is there a system for relating health records on well children and adults to hospital or clinic records? Similar questions might be raised on the organizational and working relationships between the health facilities at various levels—national, big city, county, commune, brigade— particularly as to methods of referral and division of responsibilities.

Third, much clarification is needed on the decision-making process in health matters and on how these decisions and other health information are transmitted to the various levels. How much of the information and data collected at the local level are fed to the body in the hierarchy responsible for evaluation, and how are such evaluative data used for future policy decisions? An understanding of these steps would be of significant assistance in understanding the process and quality of health planning in the PRC.

Fourth, the conference was struck by some apparent contradictions in relation to health programs of documented efficiency. Two examples involve human motivation: the individual worker's use of protective techniques against silicosis and efforts to reduce cigarette smoking. Environmental measures are used against silicosis and special provision is made for patients with silicosis through extra food and extra rest, but observations of mines and foundries reported no attempt to use masks, filters, or other techniques to cut down individual exposure to dust. As to cigarette smoking, it may be that Chinese health authorities are not convinced by the evidence, but most epidemiologists would agree that we have reached the stage where the burden of proof is on the health agency that does not take steps to reduce cigarette smoking.

Another curious omission was information on health programs for school children. With the emphasis on education, one would think that the school, so readily adapted to preventive measures and to education on health matters, would be a natural focus for intensive public health activities. Yet visitors interested in child health had nothing to report on this phase.

A number of other health activities and health problems were not covered at the conference, either because of lack of time or a paucity of available information at hand for useful discussion. Examples include medical education and training programs for various health personnel, industrial and occupational health programs, programs for control of chronic diseases, including mental illness, and programs for control of drug abuse. It is difficult to have a proper perspective and a sense of the direction of public health in China without information on these and other aspects of health activities.

The second group of questions has to do with the future of public health in the PRC.

The Future of Public Health

Will health continue as an important critical force in China?

The prominent social status and political attention that health and medicine are enjoying is unprecedented and unparalleled in Chinese history. Maintenance of their present status seems to depend on how policy makers judge their usefulness for the people and the nation, rather than on the strength or weakness of public health as a profession, as a system, or as a scientific discipline. Health programs are making two major contributions to the nation: (a) control and prevention of certain diseases improve the health and work capacity of peasants and workers; and (b) health services constitute an integral part of a social system through which social reorganization is being worked out, channels of communication, political and otherwise, maintained, and the power structure of the society strengthened. It is therefore conceivable that to the extent the health system might become a less significant factor regarding these contributions, health would have lower priority in the eyes of the policy makers.

The likelihood that public health will in fact cease to be of importance in improving the work capacity of the people in China is slim indeed, at least in the foreseeable future, for progress is urgently needed in many areas of disease control and prevention. As regards the political usefulness of the health system, it is also difficult to foresee that another system, for example, education or the organizational structure for industrial and agricultural production, may replace it in a short period of time. In fact, these various systems seem already to be intermeshed to so high a degree that the singling out of the health system for diminished influence would be difficult. It seems fair to conclude that as long as public health serves to improve and increase the work capacity of the workers and farmers, its political usefulness will likely be taken advantage of by the policy makers, assuming that health costs stay within reasonable limits and do not interfere with or cause sacrifice of other high priority social or economic investments.

A related question may be raised: Have other social investments or economic investments been sacrificed in China because of investment in health? This will be an area of considerable importance in examining the health policy in China. It may be rephrased as: Has the investment in health been complementary and an essential ingredient to raising other aspects of the society? As seen in Chapter II, the health expenditure of the central government has been relatively small, while the local investment has been quite heavy in terms of human effort. The latter is very difficult to quantify in numerical terms, particularly when one recalls that the major expenditure is during the farmers' so-called "leisure time." It would be highly desirable to have some notion of how health status and health investment are related to agricultural or industrial productivity by obtaining factual data from one community or several communities—to compare, say, health costs with total effective working days and production of goods. Other short-term analyses might be devised; a longitudinal study of such data in a single community might provide useful clues. In some respects these data might be collected more easily in China than in other countries, and they would have great significance for all the countries of the world, both less developed and developed.

Will there be a shift of emphasis in the public health programs from the control of infectious diseases to chronic disease control, following the pattern of industrialized nations? If so, what would the approach be like?

With the exception of cancer control, information on the public health approach to chronic diseases in China is extremely limited. Even here, it is still difficult to assess how much has remained from the anticancer campaign in the mid-1950s and the ensuing ambitious Five-Year Plan, as no recent reports are available about the continuity of function of tumor or cancer clinics, the Tumor Institute, and the local committees on cancer research. It seems fair to say that chronic disease control as a whole has not figured much in the order of priority in current Chinese health planning. This is understandable in view of the tremendous involvement of the government and local communities in the nationwide campaigns against the widespread serious infectious and parasitic diseases and in the projects of prenatal and postnatal care of mothers and infants. Right now, these activities will clearly save more lives and prevent more disability, at lower cost, than more complicated and less "efficient" chronic disease programs. As communicable diseases are brought under control and environmental sanitation perfected, it is to be expected that there will be a shift of emphasis and reallocation of resources to the activities against chronic degenerative diseases such as cancer, heart disease, hypertension, diabetes, and mental illness, as has happened in other industrialized societies.

Compared to campaigns against various infectious or parasitic diseases, chronic disease programs usually show less visible dramatic effects in reduction of mortality or morbidity and require a long-term investment of larger manpower and material resources. Assessment of chronic disease programs is further complicated by the fact that the cause and effect relationship of the procedures adopted and the results obtained are usually difficult to demonstrate; quite often the procedures are difficult to standardize in specific simple terms. In the late 1950s, for example, a campaign was launched involving education of the public, mass screening for cancer of the cervix, development of a registry, utilization of various forms of therapy, and intensification of research. Data on the extent and results of this campaign are not available and it therefore remains to be seen whether or not the experience was successful enough to influence formulation of future policy aud control programs.

As is known from the experiences in the West, the health behavior of the people plays a crucial role in combating chronic diseases. The Chinese people's reported change of health behavior, their susceptibility to health education, and their willingness to perform health-related tasks certainly would speak favorably for the prospect of chronic disease control. It would, however, be premature in our view to categorically accept the change of health behavior in the Chinese as conclusive and permanent. Even twenty-four years of social experiment, no matter how intensively and systematically conducted, would seem to be too brief a period to effect a permanent change of concepts and attitude, unless perhaps previous cultural patterns were in fact more adaptable to the kind of change reported than had previously been thought. A more extended period of observation and analysis is in order before reaching conclusions in either direction.

One factor in the decision as to the best timing for intensification of chronic disease control programs is the stage of development of a substantial and sophisticated system of basic curative services. Since such a system is usually regarded as essential for tackling the problem, it may be that the PRC will elect to delay major steps in the direction of chronic disease programs until these resources are well in hand. Nevertheless, the novelty and ingenuity of China's approach to communicable disease, combining technical knowledge with human organization, raise hopes that, when the time comes, a similarly innovative approach will be developed in combating chronic diseases.

What are the trade-offs between quantity and quality in the Chinese approach to health?

Egalitarianism appears to be a dominant principle pervading every aspect of Chinese society and its value systems, particularly since the Cultural Revolution. Health is no exception, as is evidenced by the emphasis on leveling-off urban-rural services, the deemphasis on professional elitism, the mass production of low-level health workers, and the emphasis on service over theory in medical education. The effects of such philosophical changes on the health scene, in contrast to the past, seem extensive. For the first time in Chinese history the Chinese mass seems to be assured of some medical attention when ill and to have become imbued with the notion that they themselves can do something for the improvement of their own health.

The question may well be raised as to how much such a leveling-off process deprives the medical and public health institutions of the stimulus for creative function that is essential for maintaining and elevating technological standards. Some believe that it is essential to provide extra facilities and resources to some institutions so they will have a better chance to develop new ideas, try out innovations, and establish new outposts of knowledge and techniques. Available information is insufficient for a sound judgment in this matter. If the enthusiasm for service should result in a serious decrease in the interest of the health profession in scientific endeavor, and, moreover, should such a popular movement carry with it an atmosphere of anti-intellectualism, there would be serious hazards to long-term progress in health programs.

What will be the long-term balance of traditional medicine and Western medicine in China?

The position of traditional medicine in the Chinese health system has gone through a number of changes, largely reflecting the political ideological climate of the time. It would seem fair to say that use of traditional medicine was intensified at the time of the revolution, primarily as a stopgap to meet the enormous medical needs of the peasants until modern resources could be developed. Then came the 1954 campaign to raise the status of traditional medicine, which included denunciation of medical leaders and modern medicine, followed by the establishment of many special schools for training traditional doctors. It was later proposed that the then existing two-track health system be integrated through a higher medical synthesis at the theoretical and the practical level. Traditional medicine was to be included in the modern medical curriculum. A research institute of traditional Chinese medicine was to be established, and hospitals and clinics were to be built for both traditional and modern doctors. The recent Cultural Revolution seems to have added further momentum and dimension to this direction, especially through the popular use of barefoot doctors, who are largely trained in the use of traditional herb medicine. Judging from available information, however, it seems premature to conclude that a true integration has taken place. The relationship between the two seems to be an uncertain and occasionally uneasy one, existing for convenience; there does not seem to have developed as yet any scientific synthesis as the basis for solid technical cooperation.

Rational assessment of the value of traditional medicine in China differs little, logically, from many other developing countries with insufficient modern resources. For the many ills in which modern medicine influences the course of disease relatively little, symptomatic relief and recovery come about as much by physician-patient relationships as by any special therapy. Herbs and traditional medicines may be as effective or ineffective as some modern drugs. The essence of rational and effective use of the traditional physician would seem to be through instilling enough knowledge for direct handling of minor diseases in which the natural history tends toward recovery, while encouraging prompt utilization of modern resources for diseases for which such resources are needed. Careful planning for the availability of these limited resources is essential.

Available information suggests that a rationale of this order is behind the organization of traditional and Western medicine in China. Given such a distribution of responsibility, along with recognition of the vital educational function the barefoot doctor can play, one can see a useful long-term role. Furthermore, the stage is then set for systematic evaluation of the pharmacology of the vast collection of herbs, and identification of those that are effective therapeutically. Understandably, much still depends on the political climate, which seems to hold the key to such cooperative large-scale experimentation, and on the quality and quantity of scientific results and practical uses to be made as a result of such cooperation.

How can the Chinese model be utilized to advantage by other countries?

Reports on Chinese experiences seem to have brought a kind of "fresh air" and a glimpse of hope to the public health and medical profession in both developing and developed nations in their current search for feasible new ideas, methods, and models for reformulating their health policies and restructuring their health care delivery systems. For example, one common viewpoint expressed is: "If China has made such remarkable achievements in health with so few resources, and with almost no outside aid, in such a short period of time as reported, why cannot other nations of similar social and economic development with similar health problems do the same by taking advantage of some of the Chinese experiences?"

An examination of Chinese experiences in the last fifty years poses important questions of health development strategy. Earlier in this century, particularly in the second quarter and mainly under the Nationalist administration, the Chinese looked mostly to a model for developing their medical care system patterned after the Western (or American) approaches, as described in Chapter I, called by some the PUMC or quality model. An argument can well be made for such high-quality training of a very small cadre at an early stage of national health planning, on the theory that once an acceptable standard has been developed the plan can then multiply itself relatively rapidly as necessary resources are provided in an orderly manner.

The more recent approach utilized by the PRC, after attaining power, emphasized quantity and self-reliance, using the "two legs" concept of combining mass involvement with existing and expanding technical expertise. The results appear to have been dramatic. One should not forget, however, that the second experiment took off from whatever was left of the first experiment, and therefore there was continuity of at least technological or certain material resources, if not continuity of ideology and professional ethics. With availability of more complete data a more extensive study of the Chinese experience may provide insight into what would be an optimum strategy, or an optimum trade-off between quality and quantity, in the early stage of health development of a developing nation.

The Chinese experience raises another important issue in health planning: The reported improvements in the health status of the population does not seem to have been a function exclusively of either economic development of the society or of health technology. Although health enjoys a high priority in national development policy, the allocation of resources to health has in fact been rather limited. Furthermore, the overall economic development of China in the last two decades, at least as measured in per capita income, does not in itself seem to be sufficient to account for the improvement in the health status of the population. One is drawn toward considering that extraeconomic, most probably political, factors were highly influential to the extent that they dictated the distribution of human and material resources and the mobilization and motivation of the people for health activities.

Still another significant factor was the deliberate attempt to simplify health technology in general, or at least to so adapt what was known as to increase its availability to larger segments of the population.

In the United States, as well as in many other developed countries, there is greatly increased interest in "consumer" involvement in health, that is, meaningful participation by the general population in decision making about health programs affecting them. The success of the mass line in China is directly apropos, as is the thesis that health programs can be most productive when they walk on two legs—active and informed support of the people combined with proven technology. The limited information currently available suggests that recent experience in China has important implications for other countries, both less developed and developed. As further and more precise data become available, these lessons will be clearer and their influence proportionately greater.

Addendum:
Some Firsthand Observations:
June 15-July 6, 1973

MYRON E. WEGMAN

As we were correcting the galleys of this volume, I had an un-
expected opportunity to visit China for three weeks, beginning on
June 15, 1973, as a member of the medical delegation sponsored
by the Committee on Scholarly Communication with the People's
Republic of China.

Visits to hospitals, medical schools, factories, and communes in
Kwangchow (Canton), Peking, Shenyang, Anshan, Fushun, and
Shanghai confirmed the basic validity of the main conclusions of
this conference report, although specific data are still not readily
available—there is obviously considerable variability, and patterns
are by no means fixed. Some additional information was obtained,
however, as well as confirmation and clarification of the significance
of two points made at the conference: the importance of motivation
(the "New Man"), and of the post-Cultural Revolution interaction between professionals and the mass.

Motivation

As a permanent factor of life in China, motivation is manifest
in many ways, not solely in relation to health. My experiences
over many years in densely populated and crowded countries in
all continents of the world had not prepared me for the sight of
masses of people in the streets, showing in their every action not
the apathy I had come to expect but a sense of movement, of
direction, of purpose, that is hard to convey in words. Of course,
even in prerevolutionary days the Chinese people had a justified
reputation for industry and hard work. Now, however, the constantly reiterated motto, "Serve the People," seems to permeate
the atmosphere and to foster the group activity, so evident in the

273

fields and on the streets, that clearly must have a positive influence on health awareness.

The motivational factor is reinforced by another axiom of Chinese life today: self-reliance. The repeated adjuration, "We must depend on our own resources and our own strength," can succeed only with maximum involvement of the consumers—the general population. Health achievements, not only in the control of venereal and other infectious diseases, but in areas such as pre-natal and child supervision are directly dependent on this kind of participation and motivation, which are in turn favored by worker and peasant participation in decision making.

As reported by other visitors, the cleanliness of the streets is striking, in small towns and rural areas as well as in the large cities. Cleanliness seems to be almost an obsession, but in a society where a great deal of disease incidence has been directly related to environmental contamination a constant preoccupation with hygiene is highly salutary. One example cited by all visitors is the marked change in concern for the living environment—the process-ing of human excreta, the control of garbage, agricultural wastes, and other environmental factors that promote flies and other insects, and the general level of sanitation. At one commune I had an opportunity to study a model that illustrated what appears to be an effective method of collecting and storing human feces to destroy microorganisms and make the material safe for use as fertilizer; the model is being used to educate commune members.

Not all is perfect, to be sure. In one of the better communes we saw unprotected and uncovered latrines with several flies buzzing around. While infant diarrhea has by no means disappeared, mothers apparently know where to take their children for treat-ment and appear to do so promptly. Deaths from this worldwide scourge appear to be few; in the Shanghai Children's Hospital, for example, of the 5,182 inpatients in 1972, there were 190 admissions for diarrhea and dehydration, but only four deaths. Other children were successfully treated on an outpatient basis in "rehydration centers" similar to those used extensively, apparently with less success, in Latin America.

In all the medical institutions we visited there was constant repetition of two of Chairman Mao's thoughts: emphasize preven-tion, and stress the rural areas. Although the need for these two emphases has long been recognized and endorsed by health workers in many parts of the world, what is unique in China is their advocacy as public policy by the nation's greatest and most revered leader; thus vigorous implementation as a national health policy has been assured. Evidence that prevention is indeed being stressed is manifest through attention to environmental measures, insistence that *all* children receive standard immunization procedures,* great emphasis on health education, an extensive scheme for home visits (which unfortunately we did not observe in practice), and a medical care system that provides everyone with ready access to some level of diagnosis, treatment, and rehabilitation. In the rural areas the communes take pride in their organization of basic health services, which are generally available to all.

Occupational Health

In a worker- and peasant-oriented society one would expect great emphasis on occupational hygiene. There was much talk of this, and some control measures were observed in factories we visited. The Institute of Hygiene in Peking and its counterparts in each province concentrate on the working environment. Nevertheless, in some of the large factories objective evidence of worker protection against all hazards was not striking, and only in the past year has work begun on revising standards for working conditions and for the general environment.† Little attention apparently is being paid to noise abatement or to the dense air pollution at the steel foundry we visited. On the other hand there does seem to be great emphasis on reducing the incidence of silicosis among miners.

Schools of Public Health

One important development is that the six schools of public health in China are being reactivated. Located on a regional

---

* Immunization routines parallel, although not precisely, United States practices, with some important differences: (1) all infants receive BCG twenty-four hours after birth, at one year, and at four years; and (2) all children are immunized against meningococcus meningitis and Japanese B encephalitis.

† A new draft of these standards, last promulgated in 1964, is scheduled for completion in July 1973 and for review at ministry and governmental levels prior to issuance.

basis, there is one in Harbin for the northeast, one in Peking for the north, one in Taiyüan for Shansi Province, one in Wuhan for the middle-south, one in Changtu for the southwest, and one in Shanghai for the east. The latter is the only one currently enrolling students, who recently completed the first year of instruction.

Prior to the Cultural Revolution the schools of public health had a six-year program, modeled roughly on the Russian pattern. Since the Cultural Revolution the course has been reduced to three years and the curriculum has still not been settled. In general, the first year will be concerned with premedical subjects, including anatomy, physiology, chemistry, physics, mathematics, and English; the second year will consist of a somewhat abbreviated general medical program: medicine, pediatrics, surgery, and obstetrics; and the third year will concentrate on public health, including biostatistics and vital statistics, epidemiology, environmental health, occupational health, food sanitation, and the health of young people. The latter is defined as essentially covering the school years, as it is assumed that maternal and child health care will have been covered during the second year in the obstetrics and pediatrics courses. Administration is not taught as a separate subject, but is included in the teaching of the epidemiology of the various specific topics.

Health Organization

One reason for the lack of emphasis on administration is that it is almost impossible to interpret Chinese health organization and structural patterns in Western administrative terms. The provision of health services is tied in much more closely to the general social system, and the exact locus of health care facilities varies according to work place and residence. Since all the people, including mothers, work, this obviously affects both the place and the manner in which maternal and child health supervision is provided. The latter is a good example of how responsibility for health care may be divided. Prenatal care may be given originally either at the factory or local health center level, and later by the maternity hospital where the mother will be delivered. After delivery the hospital usually provides early postnatal care and the first immunizations. Following the mother's return to work, early child care is given in the factory clinic. At eighteen months, at the early kindergarten level, the place of supervision varies according to where the mother lives or works. The several steps are of course modified in the commune, which is much more self-contained.

These variations are paralleled in other health care situations and illustrate what appears to be a pattern based on each social unit providing essential services to its own group. Bilateral contracts, such as those between rural commune hospitals and more sophisticated urban hospitals, expand the kind of overlap that helps assure general availability of health services to all. The scheme appears to work well, even though it does not constitute a neat and orderly administrative package. It is also clear that, in general, organizational matters in the People's Republic are still in a state of post-Cultural Revolution flux.

Traditional Medicine

There is constant emphasis on another of Chairman Mao's dictums on health policy: Western and Chinese medicine should be combined. There are several reasons for this, including the greater availability of traditional medical personnel and the readiness with which the people accept their ministrations. It is reasoned that, by using the technical expertise developed by Western medicine, traditional diagnosis and therapy may be made more precise and effective. Clearly much may be learned from a sympathetic but analytical examination of traditional methods, and Western medicine can well use a critical review of some of its practices. On the other hand, while considerable potential exists in the vast array of traditional Chinese medicines and procedures, in my view the emphasis on using them tends to exaggerate the importance of the concept that there is "a drug for every symptom." It seems to me that insufficient attention is being given in China to teaching an understanding of the natural history of disease and of the self-limiting character of many diseases.

One of Chairman Mao's basic principles, we were told, is that there should be constant experimentation with new ideas. Unfortunately, the reaction against critical statistical analysis that took place during the Cultural Revolution is still impeding the proper evaluation of such experiments. Inadequately planned and evaluated trials can in fact be harmful to the people, through the incorrect popularization of superficially attractive, yet basically ineffective, remedies. We were told that a trend toward reinstituting reasonable statistical analyses is appearing; one hopes devoutly that this will be intensified, to the benefit of all.

Vital Statistics

Nationwide demographic data relating to health are still scarce, but there are interesting contrasts between some limited data from Kwangchow and some startling figures from Shanghai. In a report on child health care, published by the Chinese Medical Association in May 1973,[1] the infant mortality rate in Shanghai (presumably the city proper, which has an estimated population of 5.6 million) was given as 150.0 in 1948, 38.9 in 1959, and an almost incredible 8.7 in 1972. I expressed great skepticism that the rate in even one section of Shanghai could be almost 25 per cent lower than in Sweden, and some days later Vice-Premier Li Hsien-nien told us we should be skeptical of such reports. Nevertheless, health technicians in Shanghai insisted that standard definitions are used, particularly the WHO definition of a live birth, and that the reporting is complete. Details were, however, unavailable on what areas of the city were involved, or on how sustained the reported figure is.

It is clear that there are important population factors to be considered, especially the current late age of marriage in China and the effect of the highly successful family planning campaign. Almost no women become pregnant before the age of twenty, and relatively few before twenty-five; two children are now considered the family norm. These two factors help to explain, partially at least, the reported 1972 crude birth rate of 10.6 for Shanghai municipality, with a population of over 10 million, and 6.4 for the city proper. The crude death rate for the city proper was reported as 5.6, which would mean a natural population increase of 0.8 per 1,000 population. Such low rates are of course also related to the changing age distribution of the population, and particularly to the recent steady increase in the survival rate of children and young adults, which is temporarily and disproportionately augmenting the nonchildbearing age groups.

While it is difficult to accept these remarkable rates readily, an important contributing factor to the low infant mortality rate is the relatively small proportion of low-birth-weight infants, which is probably related to the essential absence of teenage pregnancies. Since low-birth-weight infants have far higher mortality rates, a decline in their numbers results in a lower overall rate. Table 1 presents a combination of data kindly provided by the Provincial Hospital in Kwangchow and the International Peace Maternity Hospital in Shanghai, and some roughly comparable data for California gathered by Puffer and Serrano as part of an international study of child mortality.[2]

While the data from Shanghai are striking, it is significant that the hospital fatality rate for "mature" infants, those over 2,500 g., is not as good as the neonatal mortality rate in the California study (see note 3 in Table 1). By contrast, the fatality rate among immature infants, those under 2,500 g., is far lower in Shanghai, a difference that might be accounted for, at least in part, if there were a much lower proportion of very small infants among the premature infants born in that city. We were told that this was the case, and in the many maternity hospitals we visited tiny infants were in fact a rarity; we saw many empty modern incubators.

Although the detailed birth and hospital fatality data from Kwangchow cover a small number of births, they are more similar to reports from other parts of the world. The 3,110 g. median birth weight compares with the median of 3,295 in California, and the proportion of babies with birth weights below 2,500 g. is higher than others reported in China. Fatality rates in Kwangchow also reflect a vast improvement over earlier years, even though they are far higher than those reported in the Shanghai hospital. Shanghai has of course traditionally been a medical center of great prominence, and even today its resources are probably superior to those of Kwangchow.

Some other data from the Shanghai International Peace Maternity Hospital were consistent with the total picture. Of the twenty-four newborn deaths in 1972, twelve took place in the first day and twelve in later days. There were in the same year thirty-five fetal deaths: twenty-one prior to the onset of labor and fourteen during delivery, the respective fetal mortality ratios being 7.8, 4.7, and 3.1 per 1,000 births. These ratios are not easy to interpret, but they might seem a little high in relation to the re-

Table 1. Newborn Weight Distribution and Death Rates: Kwangchow, Shanghai, and California

Weight at Birth (in grams)	Provincial Hospital[1] Kwangchow (Canton), 6/1/71 to 5/30/73				International Peace Maternity Hospital[1] Shanghai, 1/1/72 to 12/31/72				California[2] (44,740 births)	
	No. Born Alive	Percent in Weight Group	No. Died Before Discharge	Hospital Fatality Rate (per 1,000 live births)	No. Born Alive	Percent in Weight Group	No. Died Before Discharge	Hospital Fatality Rate (per 1,000 live births)	Estimated Percent in Weight Group[3]	Neonatal Death Rate[4] (per 1,000 live births)
Under 1,000	12	0.45	7	583.3					0.45	940.0
1,000–1,499	13	0.49	6	461.5					0.62	434.8
1,500–1,999	38	1.43	5	131.5					1.48	106.9
2,000–2,499	170	6.40	16	94.1					5.10	28.2
Under 2,500	233	8.77	34	145.9	193	4.3	7	36.2	7.62	129.9
2,500–2,999	823	30.97	14	17.0					19.11	5.4
3,000–3,499	1,215	45.73	10	8.2					39.48	2.5
3,500–3,999	332	14.53	3	13.0					33.79	2.4
4,000 and over	54		2							
2,500 and over	2,424	91.23	29	12.0	4,279	95.7	17	4.0	92.38	3.1
Total	2,657	100.0	63	23.7	4,472	100.0	24	5.4	100.0	12.7

(1) Personal communication; (2) data from San Francisco and sections of Alameda, Contra Costa, and San Mateo counties, June 1969–May 1970 (Ruth R. Puffer and Carlos V. Serrano, Patterns of Mortality in Childhood [Washington, D. C.: Pan American Health Organization, Scientific Publication no. 262, 1973]); (3) birthweight distribution for San Francisco and for Alameda, Contra Costa, and San Mateo counties for 1969. (Ibid.); (4) in contrast to hospital fatality rates, which reflect only hospital stay in the new-born period, neonatal mortality rates are based on deaths during the first twenty-eight days of life, regardless of place of occurrence.

ported liveborn fatality rates. All the figures are remarkably low, however, probably reflecting again the great significance of delayed marriage and the absence of teenage pregnancies.

These data are clearly not sufficient to allow an analysis of the relative significance of China's vastly improved health services, great environmental improvements, and demographic and statistical factors. One may expect that more detailed and comparative data will become available as the People's Republic participates more actively in the World Health Organization. The essential fact now is that there has been enormous improvement in child health indices.

Contact with the People

One of the major factors said to have led to the Cultural Revolution was the criticism that a new separation of classes was developing, and that professionals were becoming far too removed from the mass of the people. An outsider has difficulty in understanding the changes that occurred as a result of this criticism, but they have been far reaching.

General policy now stipulates that professional men and educators must have continuing and meaningful contact with the workers and peasants in Chinese society. Thus university professors, for example, spend a half-day a week in some form of manual labor, perhaps on a construction project on their campus or in some area nearby. At intervals they spend months in the rural areas, either working in the fields or carrying out less strenuous activities commensurate with their physical condition.

My immediate reaction on hearing of this policy was, "What a waste of highly skilled talent!", but one comes to understand that the advantages may well outweigh the shortcomings. Those professionals with whom I spoke insisted that continuing communication with the people they are serving makes their work much more meaningful and effective, and that the transitory loss of time in using their professional skills is more than compensated for by the increased effectiveness of their performance after the experience of working with their hands among the people.

I can sum it up by simply paraphrasing a comment made by Professor Yang, an engineer who is head of the School of Public Health in Shanghai, who said that after many years of teaching about water supply and sewage disposal, the time he spent on a commune made him far more aware of the importance of water to the people of China.

This visit, then, reinforced the conclusion drawn at the Ann Arbor conference: that the advances in public health in China since 1949 have been outstanding, but that, while there are many aspects that may be applied effectively elsewhere, far more study is necessary in order for us to understand the rationale, methods, and results of the Chinese achievements.

NOTES

1. *Child Health Care in New China* (Peking: Chinese Medical Association, May 1, 1973).

2. Ruth R. Puffer and Carlos V. Serrano, *Patterns of Mortality in Childhood* (Washington, D. C.: Pan American Health Organization, Scientific Publication no. 262, 1973).

Annotated Bibliography

🐦

Introduction

This annotated bibliography was prepared as an attempt to list
published material on public health in the People's Republic of
China that is available outside of its frontiers. As all serious students
of China are painfully aware, useful scientific information and data
on health and related fields have been scarce, fragmented, and
scattered. It is hoped that this bibliography will perhaps serve
as a step toward filling the gap of scientific communication in the
health field between China and the other countries of the world.

A brief description on the process of compiling this bibliography
may help the reader to understand its usefulness, as well as its
limitations.

1. The period covered is from the establishment of the new
regime in 1949 up to 1971.

2. The search progressed in three major directions:

(a) A study was made of major medical journals in Chinese,
Japanese, English, and French; the WHO library list of
references on Chinese medicine; and the *Chinese Medical
Journal*, which was the major source;

(b) A major reference source on Chinese studies was the Public
Affairs Information Service; the list prepared by the National
Academy of Science was also most useful;

(c) Chinese newspapers, popular magazines, and other published material were read, as well as the *Quotations from
Chairman Mao Tse-tung*.

3. Purely technical medical articles were excluded from this
list, although the distinction between medical and public health
papers was not always clearcut.

4. Repetitive articles were omitted. Two categories of papers
are included in this category:

(a) Those concerned with policy statements made by various health or political officials and editorials;
(b) Similar local reports on results of certain health measures; for example, many reports made at a conference on schistosomiasis control in various provinces were combined as one reference.

5. Several fields in public health were not included in this bibliography as they are not the immediate concern of the present conference, for example, mental health, child development, etc.

6. No attempt was made to review monographs; only their titles are noted.

7. The list of the published references is arranged in accordance with the year of publication in each of the fields:

I.   Historical Material and Visitors' Reports (Pp. 284–99)
II.   Disease Control (Pp. 299–321)
III. Population Planning (Pp. 322–27)
IV.   Nutrition and Food (Pp. 328–38)
V.   Health Services Organization and Manpower (Pp. 329–38)
VI.   Other (Pp. 338–39)

I. Historical Material and Visitors' Reports

1953

Fang, S. S. "Effects of War on the Health of the People." *Chinese Medical Journal* 71 (September): 321–27.

During the Japanese aggression the mortality rate was 30:1,000 population; at least 50 per cent of the deaths were due to infectious diseases. Infant mortality was increased markedly—in one district in Peking it was 140–190:1,000 during the war, and 55:1,000 in 1952. The principal causes of death during the war, other than casualties of the conflict, were malnutrition, prematurity, tetanus neonatorum, and pneumonia. Plague and cholera broke out every year during the Japanese occupation. Malnutrition also affected the physical development of children: 60–80 per cent had a marked retardation of development in weight and height. Striking differences in people's health can be observed in peacetime: cholera and plague are completely under control; many regions are free of kala-azar; and ample vaccinations are given to children.

Since 1952 free medical care has been extended to all government employees, workers in public institutions, and university students.

Fu, L. C. (President, Chinese Medical Association.) "An Address to the Members of the Medical Profession among the Delegates to the Peace Conference of the Asian and Pacific Regions." *Chinese Medical Journal* 71 (January): 1–6.

The achievements of the health program during the last three years include:

1. Prevention of epidemics. Over 45 per cent of the population have had smallpox vaccinations. The extermination of rats and fleas has had marked effect on the prevention of plague. Cholera has not occurred since 1949. The morbidity rates of malaria, kala-azar, schistosomiasis, and other infectious diseases have declined markedly.

2. Maternal and child health. The number of maternal and child health institutes has increased sixfold since Liberation. Such health stations are being set up in counties and mining districts where there were none before. The dissemination of information on the theory and practice of painless labor, introduced from the U.S.S.R., has been successfully accomplished in the larger cities.

3. Industrial health and the health of the minorities. Health hazards and occupational diseases dropped from 6.4 per cent in 1949 to 1.6 per cent in the first half of 1951. Medical teams are sent out to give free health care to workers and minorities.

4. Medical education. Enrollment in medical and pharmaceutical schools increased by 190 per cent between 1949 and 1950, and further increased by 62 per cent between 1950 and 1951. The number of new medical students enrolled in 1950–51 alone constituted more than 60 per cent of the total number of medical students graduated in the previous sixty-nine years.

5. Patriotic Health Movement. Environmental sanitation has greatly improved: over 15 million tons of garbage and 25,000 km. of sewage have been removed, and 1.5 million public latrines have been repaired or rebuilt. The extermination of disease-carrying insects and animals has resulted in the reduction of infectious diseases and in "flyless" cities. In rural areas large amounts of manure are being collected and stored for fertilization purposes. Large-scale purification of public food and water supplies has also been carried out.

1953 *(Continued)*

Kung, N. C. "New China's Achievements in Health Work." *Chinese Medical Journal* 71 (March): 87–92. (Material covered is the same as in the foregoing article of L. C. Fu.)

Needham, J. "Chinese Science Revisited." *Nature* 171 (February 7): 237–39.

On November 1, 1949, the Chinese National Academy of Sciences (Academia Sinica) was reactivated with Dr. Kuo Mo-jo as president. It underwent a complete reorganization. Many research institutes with overlapping and uncoordinated fields of interest were reorganized into different institutes, each with its own responsibilities. The academy is also responsible for the editing of journals, the centralization and reorganization of libraries, and the translation of modern scientific terms into Chinese. The Bureau of Scientific Instruments was set up by the academy to produce apparatus needed for particular research projects. The universities were also reorganized: Peking, Yenching, and Ch'ing Hua universities were amalgamated into one institution. Many research institutes were set up not only by the academy, but under the Ministry of Health.

The achievements in public health are extraordinary. The campaign against flies and mosquitoes has made Peking freer of flies than most European cities. Formerly, vaccinations were given only to the privileged few (7.3 million a year), but since 1949 307 million people (more than half the population) have been vaccinated. Traditional Chinese doctors have been instructed in Western medicine and act as inoculators and give first-aid. Health education "reaches into the remotest corners of the country."

The budget for all scientific research institutes in 1953 is forty times higher than in any year in the Kuomintang period. "The close union between science and the people in New China is a fact which must impress every Western Visitor."

1954

"Chinese Medicine and the Communists." *Far Eastern Economic Review* 17 (December): 814–15.

It is accepted that "the task of bringing into play the medical legacy of the country can be gradually accomplished only through long periods of cooperation between Western and traditional Chinese medicine." It is significant to note that the Ministry of Health concentrated its effort on modern health prevention work, using vaccinations and inoculations. Sanitation and modern preventive methods against epidemic diseases brought about spectacular results. There are now thirty-one medical and pharmacological colleges with over 29,000 students, and 220 secondary medical schools with over 47,000 students. The minister of health has stated that future health policy should be based on four principles: "To serve the workers, peasants, and soldiers; to aim chiefly at prevention; to unite the strengths of native and Western medicine; and to integrate health work with mass movement."

Kilborn, L. G. (Former dean of medicine and director, College of Medical Science, West China Union University in Chengtu, Szechwan, and now professor of physiology at the University of Hong Kong.) "Medical Education in Communist China." *Journal of Medical Education* 29, no. 4: 21–27.

The claim that the Communist government is doing much to promote the health of the people is untrue. In fact, the health program can only lead to an opposite effect. In the following three aspects the actions taken are actually backward:

1. "The rejection of the traditional system of ethics which has governed the activities of the profession in most areas in which scientific medicine has prevailed." The physician's first duty to a patient is "the diagnosis, not of his disease, but of his status." Only if the patient is qualified as an important person does he deserve treatment. Thus "the medical profession is being made into an instrument for the enforcement of official policy, a policy which has decreed the elimination from society of certain groups or classes whose existence is obnoxious or is believed to constitute a danger to the new order."

2. "The repudiation of the scientific spirit, and the substitution for it of authoritarianism . . ." Examples are given from the conference reports in 1951 on tissue therapy, and the forceful acceptance of Pavlovian concepts in physiology. The author feels that the scientific spirit of honesty in observation as well as in the assessment of results, a critical attitude toward authority, and complete objectivity in the evaluation of scientific work have been completely discarded. In its place the government dictates the direction of

1954 *(Continued)*

methods of treatment, and government findings are accepted without question in spite of the doubtfulness of the results; only official opinion can be tolerated.

3. "The enforced lowering of standards of medical education." At a convention in 1950 the government indicated that "quality in medical education was to be relegated to a subsidiary position, in order that the number of doctors might be multiplied enormously." The medical curriculum has been reduced to five years, one of which is spent in taking political courses, one as an intern in a specialized field, and only three in studying premedical and medical subjects.

A further requirement that instruction be in Chinese has resulted in mass translations of Western texts, which are full of inaccuracies and much abridged. Sizes of classes have been enlarged without an accompanying increase in equipment or teachers. The emphasis on ideology rather than professional attainments, and the inclusion of students and servants as voting members of faculty committees have resulted in the rejection of brilliant students from medical schools because of their political unreliability.

It is true that many students are eager to help the common people. Isolation from scientific progress in the West and the glorification of the achievements of the Soviet bloc have, however, upset the aim of delivering medical services to the common people.

1957

Cox, L. B. "Chinese Medicine Today." *The Medical Journal of Australia* 44, no. 2 (October): 554–56.

There are thirty-seven medical schools, thirty-three of which teach Western medicine and four traditional Chinese medicine. Graduates of the former type number 400. Traditional Chinese doctors serve the needs of the peasants. The older Western-trained doctors form the backbone of medical research today. In order to produce enough doctors the medical curriculum was shortened to four years but later extended by one year. The students now have the choice of English or Russian as a foreign language.

The public health program has made the most important contribution to community health. "Cholera, typhoid, typhus, and smallpox have been materially suppressed." Training midwives in hygienic practices has resulted in a reduction in mortality. The birth control campaign is now underway.

Editorial. "Medicine in Red China." *Journal of Pediatrics* 51: 360–62.

The *Chinese Medical Association* has reported that the Chinese physician trained in modern medicine does not find it easy to co-operate and learn from the traditional Chinese doctor. "A second difficulty seems to lie in a conflict between his scientific integrity and the acceptance of the materialistic medical philosophy of Pavlov, which dominates Soviet medicine, as the final supreme authority."

Fox, T. F. "The New China: Some Medical Impressions." *Lancet* 2: 935–39, 995–98, 1053–57.

It is hard to know how much importance Chinese doctors trained in Western medicine really attach to traditional medicine. The author believes that students study traditional medicine more for patriotic or political reasons than for scientific purposes.

The majority of the people still cannot afford medical care. In Peking the doctors charge the equivalent of U.S. 15 cents for the first visit and 10 cents for the second. The cost of drugs is relatively high; operations often run as high as $70—equivalent to the monthly wage of a moderately skilled worker.

China is in urgent need of doctors. To achieve this the number of medical schools has increased, as have student enrollments. The medical course has been reduced to less than five years and attendance at lectures is usually as high as 200. While the author realizes that the need for doctors is great, the downgrading of medical schools is a step backward. Four to six medical students share a room in a dormitory. They pay a nominal amount for their education. In Peking, of 5,000 curriculum hours, 2,400 are devoted to lectures and 270 to political studies. As in Russia, examinations are not so important. At Peking University 80 per cent of the tests are oral and 20 per cent written; usually only 5 per cent of the students fail to qualify.

The graduate becomes a specialist and is assigned to a post by the head of the medical college, although the wish of each graduate is taken into consideration. Postgraduate opportunities are rare.

1957 *(Continued)*

Many doctors other than medical school faculty are engaged in research. A central committee under the Ministry of Health formulates a general plan and then asks the institutes and colleges what they will contribute. Freedom to pursue one's own research is obviously limited.

Chinese doctors work eight-hour days, six days a week, for a wage of $500 a month. Many self-examination meetings are held by party members for medical professionals. The author believes that the regime makes such remarkable achievements because it is still "capable of changing not only what people do but also what they think."

A street committee looks after a section of a district. Its main functions are: "(1) to administer welfare service; (2) to explain the policy of the government; and (3) to reflect and transmit the opinion of the residents." The health group of a street committee disseminates information about sanitation, immunizations, and health propaganda generally. The slums are usually clean and free of flies, rats, and mosquitoes, but people have very little privacy. The Red Cross helps to organize health teams in the neighborhoods and gives first aid.

Three levels of medical care are recognized: (1) the doctors, traditional and Western trained; (2) hospitals run by a city, district, or county; and (3) hospitals run by a city, province, or medical college. Primary medical care is given to factory workers and their families. In the countryside the people depend mostly on the traditional doctors, but they also receive care from nurses and feldsher-type workers who come to the countryside.

While hospitals are increasing in number and at great speed, the need for more is great. Specialized medicine is practiced only in hospitals run by medical colleges or by provinces. Mental hospitals are especially scarce. Many beds are not in use because of the lack of staff. Administration of the hospitals seems to be primarily the task of the doctors; the superintendents of each hospital are there only occasionally.

The Chinese use a lot of open ether; nitrous oxide is scarce. They still have to import drugs such as streptomycin and aureomycin from Japan, Denmark, Poland, and Britain.

Instead of going to a hospital, a patient may go to a clinic, health office, or laboratory set up by antiparasitic institutes. These institutes have greatly facilitated the delivery of medical service to the mass of the people.

Despite the achievements in many fields, some of the major diseases are still far from being prevented.

1. Schistosomiasis: 11 million people are infected.

2. Tuberculosis: although the death rates in Peking fell from 2.3 in 1949 to 0.69 in 1956, new cases are still being reported.

3. Dust and smoke: not enough use has been made of the lesson learned in the West about the hazards due to dust and smoke in factories.

About 60 per cent of births take place in hospital. Midwives have been given special training in sanitation and child health, and as a result maternal mortality in 1956 was 0.3:1,000, compared to 2.0 in 1949. Infant mortality in Peking fell from 117:1,000 in 1949 to about 37 in 1956. The immunization program is extensive in cities, for example, 90–97 per cent of the infants get BCG at age ten to twelve days, immunization against whooping cough at six months to two years, and against diphtheria at two to eight years.

Fu, L. C. (President, Chinese Medical Association.) "Learn from the Advanced Soviet Medical Science with Resolution and Persistence." *Chinese Medical Journal* 75 (December): 869–72.

Since Liberation the Soviet Union has supplied China with technical and material aid and has accepted a large number of Chinese students for special training in the Soviet Union. A large amount of Soviet medical literature has been translated and published. China has followed the Soviet's experience in sanitation and prevention. It has established more than 600 specialized prevention centers and stations, and more than 1,500 antiepidemic stations, teams, and groups. Under the guidance of the Soviet Union, medical stations have been set up in industries and special emphasis is placed on prevention.

Ho, P. "Development of Hygiene and Health Work During the First Five-Year Plan." *Chinese Medical Journal* 75 (December): 953–57.

Many epidemic diseases have been eliminated. Not one case of cholera has occurred in the past eight years; smallpox and plague have been virtually eliminated; the mortality rates of measles and scarlet fever have dropped from 8.6 to 1.6 per cent and 17.8 to 1.65

1957 *(Continued)*

per cent, respectively, in the last six years. Up till 1957 more than 760,000 cases of schistosomiasis and 600,000 cases of kala-azar have been treated. Antimalaria campaigns have eliminated the disease in many provinces. Cases of acute gonorrhea and primary and secondary syphilis are rarely seen. In industrial hygiene the incidence of heat stroke in iron and steel factories has been reduced to 10 per cent of the 1953 figure. The silica dust content has been lowered by 60–80 per cent by the use of encasements, dust suction, wet drilling, grinding, and ventilation, etc. Both maternal and infant mortality rates have been reduced considerably as a result of the reeducation of old midwives and the training of new ones. Health education of the masses has been successful. Garbage dumps and stagnant ponds have been moved and parks and public recreation grounds established. Medical education has improved considerably. In 1956, 10,386 medical students were graduated, compared to 1,700 in 1947. Twelve hundred and sixty antiepidemic stations have been set up, and maternal and child health stations have soared from nine to 4,564 since Liberation. Traditional medicine has also developed tremendously. Over 80 per cent of the drugs used are manufactured in China, whereas before 1953, 70–80 per cent had to be imported.

Jones, F. A. "A Visit to China." *British Medical Journal*, Part 2: 1105–07.

Traditional doctors had generally served the needs of China's 600 million people. In an effort to increase the number of Western doctors, over 8,000 students were enrolled in 1956. Eight hundred and sixty new hospitals have been built since 1949. The X-ray equipment in the hospitals is mainly inadequate, and anesthetics are less advanced than in the West. Relaxant drugs are used, but on a small scale.

The doctors trained in modern medicine generally work in hospitals, public health stations, and polyclinics; very few have their own practices. The pattern of medical research is determined by the government.

Tuberculosis and cancer of the esophagus and liver are more frequent in China than in the West. Much work has been done in eliminating snails, which harbor the cercariae. The control of malaria and filariasis has been successful.

Williams, H. "Child Health in China." *Medical Journal of Australia* 44, no. 2 (October): 588–90.

The problem of raising the standard of child health in China is colossal, as there are approximately 200 million children under the age of fifteen years and a rising birth rate, now in the region of 47:1,000. The mass of the people are peasants who live in small villages with primitive housing, sanitation, and hygiene. Food is just sufficient in quantity, but suboptimal in protein content. Parasitic infestations, infectious diseases, and poor nutrition are the major problems. Preventive pediatrics is soundly based, and living standards are being steadily raised by the development of agriculture and industry and by education of the people in simple hygiene. Immunization against the common infectious diseases is now under way in the cities, but there is no reliable information about its extent in the country as a whole. Curative pediatrics is being dealt with by the development of health stations and new children's hospitals, but trained nursing and medical staffs are far too few to cope with present needs. The training of pediatricians is not thorough, but it has been designed to meet the urgent need to provide limited health services for the people. While little or no research is being carried out in children's diseases, the Chinese government is taking a sound and realistic approach to the enormous problem of child health.

1958

Fu, L. C. "Learning from Advanced Soviet Medicine." *Chinese Medical Journal* 77 (July): 241–47.

Every year from 1947 to 1949 the Soviet Red Cross and Aescent societies sent plague-prevention teams to northwest China to assist in the antiplague campaign. The teams included specialists, nurses, and other personnel, who brought with them equipment, medical supplies, and even clothes and bedding for the sick. The teams gave instruction about scientific methods of prevention, and trained Chinese health workers as preventive personnel.

The Soviet Red Cross Hospital in Peking has served as a model of hospital administration and treatment, and of attitudes toward caring for the people's health.

1958 *(Continued)*

"Outstanding Achievements in Health Work in 1958." *Health Bulletin.*

After a year's struggle against the four pests, 1,590 million rats, 1,650 million sparrows, 100,980 kg. of flies, and 11 million kg. of mosquitoes were destroyed. The health campaign resulted in the disposition of 5,800 million tons of garbage and the collection of 56,100 million tons of manure. "The total length of irrigation ditches drained covered 1.5 million km., 62.7 million public latrines were built. . . ."

Many people received treatment for the five major parasitic diseases, and the health of industrial workers reached a new height, with the reduction of silica density to 2.0 mg./m.3.

Traditional medicine has introduced new methods of treatment in the area of surgery and bone fractures. A network of rural health stations has been organized, and there are now 47,000 hospitals and 45,000 health protection stations or bureaus in the rural areas, as well as medical teams on workers' construction sites.

Along with the advances in health work, medical education has forged ahead. In one year, sixty-one medical colleges and 117 medical schools were established. Enrollment in the medical colleges has quadrupled.

Antibiotics such as aureomycin, tetramycin, tetracycline, and erythromycin are being produced successfully in China.

Yudkin, J. "Medicine and Medical Education in the New China." *Journal of Medical Education* 33: 514–22.

There are 17,000 people officially engaged in dealing with schistosomiasis, which affects 12 million people. Treatment centers are set up, and the control of snails is taught to people in the endemic area. The mass of the people is genuinely concerned and involved in the campaign to eliminate the disease. Cholera has not been seen since 1949, and smallpox since 1950. In Peking infant mortality fell from 117:1,000 in 1949 to 37 in 1956.

Seventy thousand doctors are being trained in Western medicine. Before Liberation the instruction was usually in English or in another European language, and the method of training was based on the British and American patterns. Since Liberation, however, the language of instruction in all medical schools is Chinese, and the training is based more on the Soviet pattern. The number of medical students has increased three to four times since 1949, the length of study has been reduced to four or five years, and the lack of qualified teachers is more acute than ever. Upon graduating the students are assigned to posts by school authorities.

1959

Li, T. C. "Ten Years of Public Health Work in New China." *Chinese Medical Journal* 79: 483–88.

"The key tasks of public health work have been elimination of the four pests (mosquitoes, flies, rats, and grain-eating sparrows), the promotion of social and personal hygiene, and the fight against disease for health improvement and socialist construction." As a result of the Patriotic Health Movement many cities and villages are free of pests.

Since Liberation, plague and smallpox have been virtually wiped out, and not a single case of cholera has been seen. The mortality rate from measles and scarlet fever has dropped markedly. Short courses on treatment and prevention of the five major parasitic diseases are given to the people in order to facilitate the campaign. Environmental sanitation and personal hygiene have been paid great attention. In the villages, the changing and airing of bedsheets and clothes and nail paring have become habits with the people.

By the end of 1958 there were over 300,000 medical institutions in the country, ninety times as many as in 1949. To improve medical services, a system of hospital networks has been worked out on a district basis in the cities, while medical teams and health stations have been set up in the communes, production brigades, teams, factories, and mines.

Western-style doctors are encouraged to study traditional medicine, and there are now thirty classes with 2,000 students in each class. On the other hand, traditional doctors are being instructed in simple, basic Western medicine, and research in traditional medicine is encouraged.

Workers and their families receive medical care at almost no cost. Hospital services to pregnant women are free, and particular attention is paid to the needs of women workers in industrial plants and mining enterprises.

Over 80 per cent of Western medicines and medical equipment,

1959 *(Continued)*

such as penicillin, chloromycetin, X-ray tubes, refrigerators, and ultrashortwave diathermal sets, are manufactured in China.

Den, C. S. "Success of the Patriotic Health Movement for 1958." *Journal of Microbiology, Epidemiology and Immunobiology* 30, no. 10: 17–22.

The fight against pests is usually combined with agricultural measures. For example, "in the village of Shun-pu 66,000 persons simultaneously started to dig from opposite sides, turning over the soil to expose its undersurface before sowing the land." The rodents thus exposed were killed. By sealing up sewer outlets and burning sulphur in the sewers, hordes of rats have been killed. Masses of people were mobilized to make as much noise as possible to frighten the sparrows. After a few hours of this continuous noise, the birds were unable to eat and died on the wing from fatigue. As a result of the elimination of pests, cases of kala-azar (90 per cent of the foci) and schistosomiasis (65.4 per cent) are declining. Malaria has been wiped out in 722 counties, and malaria morbidity has dropped from 71 to 0.2 per cent.

Maternal health care centers have been set up in the communes, and infant mortality has decreased because of better sanitation.

Rogozin, I. I., and Mikhailov, I. F. "Advances in Epidemiology in the Chinese People's Republic." *Journal of Microbiology, Epidemiology and Immunobiology* 30, no. 10:1–7.

In 1950 the Ministry of Health created the Central Anti-Epidemic Team which founded several mobile medical teams with a total of 6,000 medical workers. More than 1,000 antiepidemic groups were formed within the local health bodies.

The production of the most modern range of vaccines, sera, antibiotics, and disinfectants is now underway. The Patriotic Health Movement has not only exterminated the four pests, but, by the beginning of 1959, 1,660,000 km. of canals had been cleaned out, more than 600 million m.^{2} of pits and ponds—the hatching grounds for mosquitoes—filled in, and more than 4 million wells reconstructed. Smallpox, plague, and cholera have been eradicated, and success is being achieved in the fight against schistosomiasis, kala-azar, and malaria.

1960

Hsueh, Kung-chuo. "Medicine in China." *British Medical Journal* pt. 2: 1875–76.

The integration of traditional and Western medicine is stressed by the party. Health care in China since 1949 has been reaching the mass of the people rather than the privileged few. By the end of 1969 there were 390,000 health care institutes—100 per cent more than in 1949. "Since the establishment of peoples' communes, a system of collective medical care has been practiced. By paying a nominal fee annually every commune member is entitled to free medical care."

The number of maternal and child care centers has doubled since 1949. Many child care workers have been trained, and scientific methods of child care have been brought to the masses. Women are allowed fifty-six days maternity leave with full pay; 48 million children were in the care of nurseries run by rural communes in 1959.

By 1959 there were 1,360,000 medical personnel, of whom 86,000 were Western-style physicians, 400,000 intermediate-grade health workers, 500,000 traditional doctors, and 400,000 junior-grade health workers. China now manufactures 90 per cent of the drugs needed in the country.

1961

"Science in Communist China." *Bulletin of the American Association for the Advancement of Science* (March).

There is a shortage of highly-trained research scientists in China —fewer than 400 in mathematics, and at the doctoral level in the natural sciences no more than 1,200 are engaged in full- or part-time research. These numbers are changing quickly, however. The Chinese have made tremendous progress in the field of geology: 21,000 geological workers are engaged in discovering mineral deposits, as compared to 200 in 1949. Weather reporting stations have increased, and China is third in the world in the number of such facilities.

While electric power production has increased by 800 per cent since 1952, production in 1960 was only 90 kwh./capita, compared to 4,250 kwh. in the United States. Physics as a whole is in a state

1961 *(Continued)*

comparable to that of the Soviet Union in the 1930s. "In electrical engineering, China is about fifteen years behind the United States, but on a high-speed chasing curve."

Science and scientists must serve the state and the masses. Since the end of 1959 the number of Chinese scientific and technical periodicals reaching the United States has dropped sharply. Increasing scientific isolation of Communist China is also evident in its withdrawal from international scientific associations.

1963

Penfield, W. "Oriental Renaissance in Education and Medicine." *Science* 141: 1153–61.

During the forty- to fifty-year pre-Liberation period, only 18,000 qualified doctors were trained in China. During the past thirteen years, 102,000 physicians have been graduated from modern medical schools; 450,000 qualified nurses, technicians, and midwives have also been graduated.

The organization of medical teaching is as follows: One college calls for a curriculum of eight years—the Chinese Medical College in Peking. It is planned to train teachers and research workers. Each physician should have mastered two foreign languages before graduation from this college. Of the other medical colleges, one-third now provide a six-year curriculum, and less than two-thirds, a five-year curriculum. A very few schools have a three-year course which is intended to prepare manpower for the practical needs of factories, mines, and farms. The medical school calendar is as follows: The academic year starts in September, there is a four-week vacation in January, and one of six to eight weeks in July and August. Every student is expected to devote eight weeks each year to manual labor.

Schistosomiasis is the most serious medical concern. Infectious hepatitis, measles, poliomyelitis, and encephalitis are also problems. Tuberculosis and leprosy are treated with drugs and isolation. Syphilis and opium and heroin addiction have disappeared.

As a result of better health among the people, the annual birth rate has increased to 2 per cent. A birth control campaign is underway, with emphasis on late marriage and small families.

1967

Christie, R. V. "Medicine and Medical Education in China." *Journal of Medical Education* 42 (May): 463–66.

Great emphasis on preventive medicine was observed during the exchange professorship between McGill and Peking from 1961 to 1966. Even during the height of the famine in 1961–62 there was no evidence of malnutrition or starvation among the people. The government launched campaigns against the four pests, and emphasized the importance of public hygiene. Smallpox, plague, cholera, kala-azar, and venereal disease have almost disappeared.

There are about eighty medical colleges. While the usual length of the medical school course is five or six years, that at the Chinese Medical College in Peking is eight years. The first three years are devoted to premedical studies, followed by two years of preclinical study, two years of clinical study, and a one-year internship. Formal lectures, rather than seminars or group discussions, are given. There are about 100,000 doctors trained in modern medicine, and 500,000 who practice traditional medicine.

II. Disease Control

1957

Ch'iao, S. M. "Intranasal Vaccination of BCG Against Respiratory Infection of Tuberculosis in Guinea Pigs." *Chinese Medical Journal* 75 (January): 61–73.

One hundred guinea pigs were divided at random into ten equal groups. BCG vaccines were given to eight groups intranasally, intracutaneously, or orally. The animals were inoculated one or more times. The two groups not vaccinated were used as controls. Seventy-two days after vaccination all the animals were challenged with an H37Ru strain of mycobacterium tuberculosis intranasally to simulate the natural course of tuberculosis infection. Medium survival time, body-weight change, and pathological findings on necropsy were obtained to compare the protecting effect of BCG.

The experiments showed that there was a significant difference between the vaccinated and nonvaccinated groups. The effect of intranasal administration of BCG vaccines was found to be about equal to that of intracutaneous and oral administration in protecting guinea pigs from intranasal infection of virulent tubercle bacilli.

1957 *(Continued)*

Among the different methods used for intranasal inoculation, intranasal dripping seemed to be the most simple and practical. There was no untoward effect in the groups repeatedly vaccinated.

Fang, T. C. et al. "The Effect of Thyroidectomy and Antithyroid Drugs upon Antimony Potassium Tartrate Toxicity." *Chinese Medical Journal* 75 (October): 783–91.

    Although antimony potassium tartrate (APT) has been used extensively in the treatment of *Schistosomiasis japonica*, it has a very high toxicity. From experiments on rats it was found that APT toxicity is decreased by thyroidectomy and antithyroid drugs—thiourea, methylthiouracil, and sodium *p*-aminosalicylate—and intensified by desiccated thyroid and dinitrophenol. The mechanism is thought to be the inhibition of thyroid function and the lowering of metabolism. Antithyroid drugs administered twenty-four hours previous to APT can reduce acute APT toxicity.

Huang, M. H. "Schistosomiasis Dwarfism." *Chinese Medical Journal* 75 (June): 448–61.

    Dwarfs are frequently encountered in the endemic areas of schistosomal infection. In three villages in Chiang Pü, Kiangsu Province, where surveys were done, 4 per cent of the people were dwarfs. From close observation of ten cases of schistosomiasis dwarfism it was concluded that the underlying mechanism of dwarfism should be ascribed to depression of the pituitary function; sexual infantilism, retarded maturation of the skeleton, and dysfunction of the adrenal cortex are secondary characteristics. The pituitary dysfunction is probably due to the influence of dynamic disturbances of the central nervous system induced by the toxic products of the parasites and by reflex mechanisms of the local lesions. Other factors, such as metabolic disturbances induced by cirrhosis of the liver and gastrointestinal dysfunction, are also contributory.

    The only effective treatment for this form of dwarfism is to eradicate the parasites from the body. Successful results were obtained with antimonial treatment. Follow-ups of patients indicated that there was "a growth of six to eight cm. in height, with development of the sex organs and secondary sexual characters, as well as marked improvement in physical strength."

Kemiya, Y. "A Recommendatory Note for the Control Problem of Schistosomiasis in China." *Japanese Journal of Medical Science and Biology* 10: 461–71.

The Japanese delegation to China discovered that the endemic foci of schistosomiasis are distributed over twelve provinces with a population of 10 million. The habitat of vector snails is rich in variety compared to that of Japan. The snails are found on the banks of almost all creeks, ditches, and fish ponds, and on leaves and stems of reeds in the shallow water of marshy lakes.

The use of sodium antimony tartrate is preferable to potassium salt because it has fewer side effects. The use of skin tests to diagnose carriers is very useful for mass application. Control work should be emphasized more, however; in particular, the environmental control of snails by: "(a) burying snails with soil; (b) blocking the margins of creeks with stone; (c) cementing ditches; and (d) developing marshy areas. Physicochemical control of vector snails using the "molluscicidal technique, with hot water, direct burning, utilizing a flame projector, sodium pentachlorophenate, calcium arsenite, benzene hexachloride (BHC), and calcium cyananide," should be applied simultaneously with the environmental control.

Shao, P. J. et al. "Studies on the Artificial Infection of Oncomelania Snails with Miracidia of *Schistosoma Japonicum*." *Chinese Medical Journal* 75 (March) 189–211.

From experiments with laboratory infection of more than 300,000 Oncomelania snails with the miracidia of *Schistosoma japonicum*, it was found that larval development was greatly influenced by temperature and rearing conditions. Up to 32–33° C., the higher the temperature the quicker the development, and vice versa. The shortest development cycle observed from miracidia to cercariae was forty-four days, the longest was 186 days. After a satisfactory shedding of cercariae, an interval of one week in summer and two to three weeks in cold weather was required before sufficiently large numbers of cercariae could be expected. The longest period for an infected snail to shed cercariae without being reinfected was thirty-two months. Under identical rearing conditions, the death rate of infected snails was much higher than that of normal ones, especially in the hot season.

With miracidia obtained from Puchen, Nanking, as the infective source, it was found that the infection rate of snails collected from

1957 *(Continued)*

various parts of China differed greatly; those from Nanking and a neighboring city were most easily infected, while those from remote provinces were refractory to infection. Under experimental conditions the incidence of infection was higher among male than female snails, and among adult than young snails, although larval schistosoma developed more quickly among the young.

1958

Chang, H. T., and Liu, C. C. "Rheumatic Fever in Peking: A Clinical Study." *Chinese Medical Journal* 76 (April): 328–43.

The clinical materials of 168 cases of acute rheumatic fever in Peking were analyzed. Because of the complexity of clinical manifestations and the natural variation of the course of the disease, the reliability of clinical diagnosis was far from satisfactory. There is at present no specific therapy; salicylate should be used for ordinary cases, and cortisone and ACTH for specially indicated cases. Benzathine penicillin is at present the most useful weapon in the prevention of rheumatic fever.

Chiang, Y. T., and Ch'en, T. H. "Reaction and Immune Response to Typhoid and Paratyphoid Vaccines of Different Dosage and Routes of Injection." *Chinese Medical Journal* 76 (January): 47–58.

Fifteen hundred and seventy-four young recruits aged eighteen to twenty were randomly divided into three groups and given different vaccine dosages through different routes. The inoculations were as follows: (1) 0.5, 1.0, 1.0, subcutaneous; (2) 0.25, 0.5, 0.5, subcutaneous; (3) 0.1, 0.1, 0.1, intracutaneous.

Two samples of blood were taken from 350 recruits for mouse protection and serum agglutination tests, as indications of the immunity level of the subjects. It was found that reduction of the standard dosage of the triple vaccine by half, lowered the percentage of general and local reactions by nearly 40 per cent, while the increase in the protection titers remained the same. Intracutaneous vaccine inoculation of three doses of 0.1 ml. each reduced the reaction by 70 per cent. The protection antibody showed the same increase. Ten months after completion of the initial vaccination the protection titers of these individuals, irrespective of differences in dosage of vaccination and routes of inoculation, diminished to almost the same level. It was also found that higher postvaccination temperature is associated with higher preinjection temperature. Based on this fact it would be advisable to postpone vaccination for those with oral temperatures over 37° C.

Chien, H. C. "Summary of Mass Technical Experiences with a View to Expediting Eradication of the Five Major Parasitic Diseases." *Chinese Medical Journal* 77 (December): 521–32.

Achievements in attempting to eradicate the five major parasitic diseases over the past nine years are these: Schistosomiasis affects nearly 10 million people in China today. The disease is most serious on both sides of the Yangtze and in twelve provinces in the south; altogether 197 prevention and treatment stations have been established across the country, with a total of 17,000 specialized workers and forty-two research institutes. Treatment at the early stage of schistosomiasis consists mainly of intravenous injections of trivalent antimony tartrate; at the late stage it consists of both traditional and Western methods with a shortened course of treatment. As a result, 400,000 people were treated in 1956, 500,000 in 1957, and 2.8 million during the first nine months of 1958. For prevention, the burying of Oncomelania snails has been found to be most effective. Another preventive measure is the chemical treatment of waters. Chemically treated footgear and puttees are worn in lakes, ponds, and rice paddies to prevent cercarial infection.

Malaria has an endemic history of thousands of years and is spread over the whole country. Thirty million people are stricken annually. Western drugs such as atabrine, paludrine, neopaludrine, pyrimethamine, chloroquin, and plasmoquin, as well as acupuncture, are used in the treatment of the disease. In prevention, ditches and canals are dredged and cleaned, and pits and marshes are filled in. It is claimed that the pest elimination campaign has killed over 13 million kg. of mosquitoes.

The filariasis endemic in China is of two types—*bancrofti* and *malayi*. It affects 20–30 million people. Currently, hetrozan and carbarson are used in treatment, both of which have been found to possess filariacidal properties. As a result of shortened therapy, to one dose of 1 gm., more than 660,000 patients were treated in the first ten months of 1958.

The main endemic areas of kala-azar are the provinces north of the Yangtze River. Injections of sodium stibogluconate and the spraying of DDT or "666" on sandflies have greatly reduced the incidence of the disease. If cases of kala-azar in the early post-

1958 *(Continued)*

Liberation period were taken as 100, then it would be 6.6 in 1955, 5.4 in 1956, 4.7 in 1957, and 0.5 in 1958.

Ancylostomiasis is endemic throughout the country. In the treatment of the disease both Chinese-produced tetrachloroethylene in one dose and 1-bromo-2 napthol are effective. Some traditional drugs such as *chih huang wan* and *ch'u chung san* are also used. Methods used to destroy the ova include mixed storage of feces and urine, packing manure into bricks, and chemicals.

Ho, E. A., and Tien, S. M. "The Endemicity and Periodicity of Cholera in China." *Chinese Medical Journal* 76 (March): 266–75.

Cholera was introduced into China from India during the first epidemic in 1820–23. Cholera is not an endemic disease in China, however, because of the following facts observed in Shanghai and other parts of China.

Epidemic years have alternated with quiescent years during which not a single case has appeared. In epidemic years cases occur only in the warm season and disappear entirely in the cold season. Chronic carriers of cholera have not been found among convalescent patients or the general population in Shanghai. Examination of water samples collected from rivers, creeks, and ponds in Shanghai were negative for *Vibrio cholerae*, and there is no evidence to show that *V. cholerae* can survive long outside the human body. Not a single case of cholera has been reported in China since 1949. Outbreaks of cholera in China have occurred irregularly in the past, contrary to the belief that it occurred with epidemic cycles every four or five years.

Editorial. *Jen-min Jih Pao* (September 2). "Let the Technical Revolution in Medicine, Pharmacology, and Public Health Blossom and Yield Fruit." Trans. in *Chinese Medical Journal* 78 (January): 1–3.

Over 800 counties or cities have been freed of the four pests. With the government's recognition of traditional Chinese medicine, the importance of combining it with Western medicine is stressed.

Lin, L. C., and Ch'en, K. K. "Certain Epidemiologic Features of Filariasis in Foochow." *Chinese Medical Journal* 76 (May): 490–96.

An epidemiologic study on filarial infection and its reaction to fluorosis was undertaken in Foochow between September and

November 1956. *Filariasis bancrofti* was responsible for the filarial infection found in the city. The rate of infection was highest in the urban area, lower in the rural areas, and still lower in the mountainous areas. The reasons for this uneven rate of infection lie chiefly in the difference of density of *Culex fatigans*, the abundance of domestic animals, and the population density in these areas.

Both sexes were more or less equally infected. The infection rate was lowest among children under nine years and highest in the age group twenty to forty-nine. Factory workers were most prone to infection, farmers were next, and schoolchildren third. The protection afforded by mosquito nets had a definite bearing on the rate of infection, especially in the rural areas.

C. fatigans was the chief natural vector involved in *F. bancrofti* infection. The human infection rate was not directly proportionate to the mosquito infection rate, but was proportional to the number of microfilariasi harbored in each mosquito. Where the average fluoride content in drinking water amounted to a high proportion of 2.42 ppm. in certain districts of the city, fluorisis reached 38.25 per cent. *F. bancrofti* infection is present both in fluorosis and non-fluorosis districts. In the former districts the occurrence of filariasis seems to have no relationship to the fluoride content of the drinking water or to mottled teeth.

Shih, P. T. "The Use of Concentrated Typhoid Vaccine for Intradermal Immunization." *Chinese Medical Journal* 77 (July): 27–29.

The results of immunization of 112 subjects by intradermal inoculation of a concentrated typhoid vaccine, and 112 by subcutaneous inoculation of the usual vaccine were compared. No appreciable difference was noted in the rise of agglutinin titers. The side reactions after intradermal inoculation were much less than those after subcutaneous inoculation.

Hu, C. K. et al. "The Control of Venereal Diseases in New China." *Chinese Medical Journal* 77 (July): 248–58.

The ban on prostitution was one of the first measures taken in the antivenereal campaign. In Peking over 300 houses of prostitution were closed and more than 1,303 inmates freed. The women received training, and after the educational program they were given work and a chance to lead a normal life. Thorough medical treatments were given without charge. Penicillin with the addition

1958 *(Continued)*

of arsenic/bismuth was used in the treatment of syphilis and gonorrhea. Of the prostitutes in Peking, 96.5 per cent had venereal infection: 84.9 per cent had syphilis, 53.8 per cent had active gonorrhea,
and 28.7 per cent had positive Frei reactions. Venereal diseases
were most serious among the minorities. Free medical care was
given to minority women with great success.

Tai, T. Y. et al. "Typhoid and Paratyphoid Fevers Occurring in
Cases of Schistosomiasis." *Chinese Medical Journal* 76 (May):
426–35.

From a study of sixty-two cases of typhoid and paratyphoid
fevers associated with schistosomiasis, it was found that their clinical
pictures differed in many respects from those observed in simple
typhoid or paratyphoid infections; the onset was mostly sudden—
67.7 per cent compared to 27.2 per cent in simple typhoid cases.
The fever was of the remittent or intermittent type in 71.0 per cent
of the cases, while in simple typhoid cases the fever was mostly of
the continuous type (63.3 per cent); hepatomegaly and spleno-
megaly were more pronounced and more frequent (85.5 per cent
and 90.3 per cent). In 95.1 per cent of the cases, the eosinophil
count was less than 2 per cent during the height of the disease, a
condition also observed in simple typhoid infections. It rose rapidly
as the fever subsided, with an average increase of 15.6 per cent as
compared with an average of 4 per cent in simple typhoid cases.

Although the course of fever was prolonged considerably, there
was no apparent increase in the severity of the disease, nor in the
fatality rate. In the present series only one patient died; the cause
was intestinal perforation. The therapeutic effect of chloramphenicol or synthomycetin was apparently lessened in such cases; in
more than half of them the temperature rose again upon discon-
tinuation of treatment or reduction of dosage. Corticotropin or
antimony may be used in conjunction with chloramphenicol or
synthomycetin, as the condition indicates.

Wei, P. H., and Kuo, N. K. "Intradermal Reaction in Ancylostomiasis." *Chinese Medical Journal* 76 (June): 556–60.

Intradermal reaction is of value in the diagnosis of ancylostomiasis. It has been shown to detect light infections that had been
missed by microscopic examination. Of two methods for the preparation of antigens—pancreation digestion and cold extraction—

the latter is considered to be the best because it is simpler in procedure and the antigen produced is highly specific. Intradermal reaction is valuable in mass diagnosis of hookworm infection.

Wei, W. P. "New Victories on the Antischistosomiasis Front." *Chinese Medical Journal* 77: 107–10.

In Hupei Province a lake bed was ploughed three times and the snails were buried and destroyed. As a trial, 840 *mou* of land were planted with cotton; the annual yield from 220 *mou* was more than 120 kg. of ginned cotton per *mou*. Similar results of the antischistosomiasis campaign have been observed in other provinces. In the spring of 1958 alone, 350,000 patients were treated with the three-day course of therapy by mobile units. The slogan "kill three birds with one stone" in the fight against schistosomiasis, means to drain the water, dredge the earth, and use it as fertilizer, to improve the system of irrigation, and to exterminate snails.

Wu, C. C. "Some Achievements in the Study of Kala-azar in New China." *Chinese Medical Journal* 77 (October): 307–309.

The examination of 113,393 dogs showed that those with the leishmania parasite were common in northwest China; it was rarely seen in east China. There are two types of leishmania infection—that in the northwest resembles the Mediterranean type, while the one in east China resembles the Indian type. Sodium antimony gluconate is effective for the treatment of kala-azar, although less so in the northwest than in the east.

Surveys were made of sandflies in 193 *hsien* in twenty provinces; eight species were discovered. *Phlebotomus chinensis* is the predominant species in kala-azar-endemic areas. Seventy per cent of the sandflies released were found within 30 m. of the releasing center. *P. chinensis* are known to feed preferentially on donkeys, cattle, and other animals. Though DDT has a longer-lasting effect than gamma 666, the combination of DDT and gamma 666 Co. 69 g., and 0.064 g., 1 m.^{2}, respectively, is most effective for destroying sandflies.

1959

Hou, T. C. et al. "Achievements in the Fight Against Parasitic Diseases in New China." *Chinese Medical Journal* 79 (December): 493–520.

1959 *(Continued)*

Since Liberation 5,000 reports have been published about the fight against parasitic diseases. The following is a summary of the important findings:

Achievements in epidemiologic studies

1. The geographic distribution of parasitic diseases in China can be categorized as: (a) Parasitic diseases such as ascariasis, oxyuriasis, trichuriasis, amebiasis, and trichomoniasis vaginalis have no geographical predilections; (b) the area with the greatest varieties and prevalence of parasitic diseases is bounded by 32° N, in the east in the coastal region, and in the west by 97° E. All the important parasitic diseases except kala-azar, that is, schistosomiasis, malaria, filariasis, ancylostomiasis, clonorchiasis, and fasciolopsiasis, are concentrated in this area; (c) kala-azar, paragonimiasis, and taeniasis are the diseases with special geographical distribution. Kala-azar is endemic in hilly regions of the Yellow River and the Huai River areas. *Taenia saginata* is concentrated in the southwest and northwest.

2. Epidemiologic data useful in the destruction of disease vectors are as follows: (a) Oncomelania snails. It was found that the snails are distributed in paddies, ditches in hilly regions, and along the banks of rivers, creeks, and lakes. Water flowing over 0.14 m./sec. is unsuitable for the breeding of the snails. Animals such as oxen, sheep, pigs, and dogs are naturally infected and serve as sources of infection; (b) kala-azar. Two types of kala-azar are found in China: the presence of canine leishmaniasis in endemic areas where the patients are young adults; and the absence of canine leishmania, to which older people are most susceptible. *Phlebotomus Chinensis* is the most important vector in the transmission of kala-azar; (c) 43 different species of anopheline mosquitoes have been found in the study of malaria and filariasis. Four varieties of melania snails are the primary hosts of paragonimus; crayfish are found to be secondary hosts in northeast China.

3. Studies on factors causing the prevalence of parasitic diseases found that, in general, places with warm temperatures and higher humidity are suitable for the spread of parasitic diseases. For example, sandflies are not found where the temperature is below 20° C.; flooded fields do not transmit ancylostomiasis: for

mosquitoes the optimal temperature is 21.1–33.3° C., and humidity 70 per cent. The infection rates of the diseases are highest among the twenty-year age group, diminishing gradually with an increase of age (an exception is kala-azar in northwest China). The infection rate of schistosomiasis is highest between the ages of twenty and thirty years, becoming markedly lower after fifty; the infection rate of malaria in persons under twenty is 70 per cent, for those over twenty it is 39.8 per cent.

Clinical and therapeutic treatment

1. Symptomatology: (a) The main features of acute schistosomiasis are fever, acute toxemia associated with leukocytosis, and marked oesinophilia; (b) the most important late manifestation of schistosomiasis is cirrhosis of the liver and schistosomal dwarfism; disturbances in growth and development are also common in long-standing malaria or kala-azar; (c) the most common form of the parasitic diseases of the brain is cerebral paragonimiasis (about 5–10 per cent of all cases); (d) aside from dermatitis caused by hookworm larvae and schistosome larvae, the most common forms of skin involvement in internal parasitic diseases are lymphangitis, erysipeloid dermatitis, and elephantiasis of filarial origin.

2. Achievements in diagnostic procedures: (a) Stool examination. By means of the 40° C. warm-water hatching method, and the method of hatching tissue-paper-wrapped stool in diluted sodium hydroxide solution, the efficiency of hatching schistosome ova was raised over ten times. For diagnosis of ancylostomiasis, the positive rate by the test-tube hatching method was seven times higher than that by the use of slides. For schistosomiasis, rectal mucosal biopsy for schistosoma ova showed 4.2 per cent of 1,213 apparently negative cases to be actually positive. For diagnosis of paragonimiasis in children, examination of the centrifuged gastric juice sediment was found to be a very useful method; (b) for immunodiagnosis, the intradermal test and serum complement fixation test are the two most widely used methods; (c) in the diagnosis of kala-azar, the Leishman-Donovan bodies may be identified in 85–90 per cent of cases through bone marrow puncture of the ilium, the sternum, or the spinous process of the vertebra. Cases negative by bone marrow examinations may show L-D bodies in lymph gland smears. Special straining methods for the rapid diagnosis of microfilaria have been devised; (d) for radiographic diagnosis, in the

1959 *(Continued)*
early stage of schistosomiasis miliary or small fluffy shadows may be observed in X-ray films of the chest.

3. Since people are generally the greatest sources of infection, the elimination of such sources rests in the treatment of the patients. For schistosomiasis the three-day treatment with tartar emetic at a total dose of 12 mg./kg. body weight is most effective. For kala-azar the six-day treatment with antimony sodium gluconate (total dose 1.2–2.4 g.) is mainly used, with a cure rate of 99 per cent and a relapse rate of 7.4 per cent in two years. For ancylostomiasis, tetrachloroethylene and 1-bromo-2-naphthol are used mostly. For filariasis, a moderate treatment of hetrazan (200 mg. three times a day for seven days) produces a cure rate of 80 per cent. For personal protection against schistosomiasis, liquid extract of 1:5,000 *Camellia oleosa* (tea-cake) is sufficient. The wearing of foot puttees and cloth stockings in water is also useful. Traditional Chinese medications such as areca nut are very effective in cases of schistosomiasis, taenia infestations, and ancylostomiasis; pumpkin seeds cause the fever to disappear rapidly in schistosomiasis; *Veratrum nigrum* is used for *Schistosomiasis baucea*, amebic dysentery, and malaria. Acupuncture and moxibustion have been used successfully in the cure of toxic reactions during antimonial treatment.

The combination of preventive and curative measures is the most effective way of eradicating diseases. The following are the preventive measures used: Fecal controls are done by collecting and storing feces in assigned places; centralizing control of animal excreta; separating water sources used for cleaning human fecal containers from water for domestic use; promoting hygienic habits; and building public latrines.

For destruction of ova in stools, the following four methods are used: (a) The urine-feces storage method is most suitable in the south where, if the urine and stool mixture is sealed at a volume ratio of 4:1, the schistosome ova are killed in three days in summer and seven days in winter; (b) compost heaping in packages is suitable for use in the north where dried feces are used as fertilizer; within a week all the ova will be killed; (c) ovicidal effect during manufacture of methane from human excreta; the manufacture of methane from feces not only affords a cheap supply of heat and power, but also kills ova in two to three weeks; (d) chemicals such as urea, acid ammonium carbonate, calcium cyanimide, and

Derris powder are used; wild plants such as *Talirum japonicum* seeds and *Buddleia japonica* are also used in the rural areas.

Eradication of intermediate hosts and insect vectors: (a) snails can be eradicated by land cultivation, burial, conversion of paddies into dry fields; burning or scalding the snails; the use of calcium arsenate and sodium pleutachlorophenate, etc.; (b) mosquitoes' habitats can be destroyed by the elimination of small pools of water, and by the raising of fish in large bodies of water; spraying with DDT or 666 is not as effective in the control of mosquitoes as it is in control of sandflies.

The factors that made the achievements in the control of parasitic diseases possible are due to the "superiority of the socialist system." The organization of communes played an important part. The collective ownership of the means of production on a greater scale made possible such projects as filling up old ditches and digging new ones to destroy snails; centralized fecal control; and the planned use of fertilizer without loss to the peasant. Moreover, the higher degree of collective living and the extensive establishment of nurseries and primary schools have promoted hygienic habits among children. With improved dining hall hygiene, gastrointestinal diseases are being controlled. Finally, the improved living conditions of the peasants, and their higher cultural level, have facilitated the thorough application of antiparasitic measures.

Scientists from abroad, especially those from the Soviet Union, have contributed greatly to the control of diseases.

Wang, C. T., and Wu, C. C. "Studies on Kala-azar in New China." *Chinese Medical Journal* 78 (January): 55–71.

In 1951 the average infection rate of kala-azar was 10–50:100,000 population—a total of 500,000—90:10,000 for males and 60:10,000 for females. Two types of kala-azar are believed to exist in China: In east China the disease resembles that of India, occurring mainly in older children and young adults, and rarely in infants and dogs; in the northwest the disease is similar to that of the Mediterranean basin and Central Asia in that it occurs chiefly among infants and very young children and is frequently associated with canine leishmaniasis.

Apart from *Phlebotomus chinensis*, the chief vector of kala-azar, *P. nankingensis* and *P. barrandi* were also discovered. It was found that *P. chinensis* has limited flying power and activity, usually

1959 (*Continued*)

within 30 m., and that it feeds preferentially on the blood of humans, cattle, and donkeys. *P. chinensis* has a long life cycle, with only one generation in a year. The combined use of DDT and gammaexane (0.69 g. and 0.064 g./m.^{2}, respectively) for spraying is most effective. The middle or latter part of May, at the beginning of the sandfly season, is the best time for spraying.

The main symptoms of the disease are fever and enlargement of the spleen, frequently associated with general weakness, anorexia, night sweating, coughing, and bleeding of the gums. Enlargement of the liver occurred in 40.2 per cent of 4,269 cases examined, and the white blood cell count was usually low. For the diagnosis of kala-azar, ilium and spinous process punctures are most commonly used. Bone marrow punctures are more accurate than either liver or lymph gland punctures, but the latter is most simple in technique and devoid of risks. Antimony sodium gluconate is effective for the treatment of kala-azar.

Wang, C. Y. "Studies on Ancylostomiasis in New China." *Chinese Medical Journal* 78 (March): 257–266.

The incidence of hookworm infection is as high as 80–90 per cent in the rural areas; it is quite common to find 50 per cent of the population infected with the parasite. The transmission of hookworm disease is closely related to the cultivation of sweet potatoes, corn, mulberries, tobacco, and coffee. For hookworm control, the storage of night soil with human or horse urine is a simple and economical method for disinfecting the hookworm ova in the stored stool; 1–2 per cent of urea destroys the viability of hookworm ova in one to three days. Calcium cyanamide, lime, and urea are widely used in preventive work. Tetrachloroethylene (3–4 ml.) is most commonly used for the treatment of ancylostomiasis. Since 1-bromo-2-naphthol (dosage 6.0 mg. x 2) is less toxic than tetrachloroethylene, it is more suitable for children, aged people, and pregnant women.

1960

Feng, L. C. et al. "Research on Parasitic Diseases in New China." *Chinese Medical Journal* 80 (January): 1–20.

Little work was done on parasitic diseases before Liberation. After Liberation, in order to strengthen such research, the Institute of Parasitic Diseases was established under the Chinese Academy of Medical Sciences, and similar institutes were organized in the provinces and municipalities. Nationwide surveys showed that there is only one type of human schistosomiasis in China; the causal organism is *Schistosoma japonicum* and the intermediate host is *Oncomelania hupensis*. The endemic regions of schistosomiasis are canals, hills, lakes, and marshes. The snails thrive in environments where the temperature is not too high, where there is humidity, and shade. Clinical investigation shows that schistosomiasis dwarfism is of pituitary origin; during the acute stage of schistosomiasis the lung and the brain are most frequently involved in ectopic lesions.

More than 500 drugs belonging to twelve categories have been tested for the treatment of schistosomiasis. For eradication of infective sources, the storage of night soil with ammonia, urea, ammonium bicarbonate, and calcium cyanamide are effective in killing the ova. The removal of breeding places of snails by constructing embankments and drains and cultivating swamps in the lakes and in the marshy areas is very helpful.

Different malaria regions may be summarized as follows: In the region south of 25° N, the chief transmitters are *Anopheles minimus* and *A. jeyporiensis candidiensis; A. leucosphyrus* is also of considerable importance in wooded areas.

In the region between 25° and 32° N, the chief carrier is *A. hyrcanus sinensis*, of which the small type is especially important; in hilly districts *A. minimus* is also of importance.

In the area north of 32° N, *A. hyrcanus sinensis* is generally the transmitter, but north of 41° N, in the northwestern provinces and in the northern part of Sinkiang, *A. messeae* is an important transmitter.

Western drugs such as chloroquine and primaquine are used in the treatment of malaria. BHC is being mass-produced in China for killing mosquitoes, and wild plants have been found effective as fumigants or watery extracts against adult mosquitoes and their larvae. To prevent mosquitoes from breeding, holes and pits have been filled, ditches and water courses drained, stagnant water in small ponds diverted into larger ponds, and large water surfaces freed of vegetation.

There are two types of filariasis: *Filariasis bancrofti* is distributed in the low-lying plains, and its main transmitters are the dirty-

1960 *(Continued)*

water-breeding *Culex pipiens pallens* and *C. pipiens fatigans; Filariasis malayi* is chiefly found in the water-rich, hilly districts of south China. *A. hyrcanus sinensis*, especially the small type, is the chief carrier.

The most effective method of treating filariasis is by means of a one- to two-day course with a total dosage of 1.5–3 g. of hetrazan. DDT and BHC are used to kill the mosquitoes.

The epidemiology of kala-azar is different in various localities. *Phlebotomus chinensis* is the only transmitter in this country. A nodular dermal type of infection is common among kala-azar patients. Antimony sodium gluconate is effective for treatment. DDT is just as effective as BHC in killing sandflies, and it lasts even longer.

Hookworm disease is mainly caused by *Ancylostoma duodenale* and *Necator americanus*. Footwear painted with tung oil is protective against hookworm larvae. Urea is lethal to 90 per cent of hookworm ova in one to three days. These are examples of research findings on parasitic diseases.

Huang, M. H. "Schistosomiasis Dwarfism." *Chinese Medical Journal* 80 (May): 437–40.

The incidence of dwarfism in the general population was about 4 per cent. In 1958 it was reported that dwarfism occurred in about 1.5 per cent of all schistosomiasis cases, and in about 5.8–8.1 per cent of late cases.

The ratio of male to female dwarfs was about 2:1. Most of the patients were sixteen to twenty years of age, and they rarely lived longer than age thirty.

A few characteristics were found common to all dwarfs: (1) Their stature was definitely small, weight and height being equivalent to those of children eleven to fifteen years of age; (2) no maturation of sexual organs could be found; (3) skeletal growth and maturation were suppressed; (4) the dwarfs were unusually mentally alert and sensitive; (5) 17-ketosteroid values in twenty-four-hour urine were markedly lower than normal.

The characteristics agreed well with pituitary dwarfism. Further, only gonadal deficiency could explain the delayed maturation of their bones, and that suppression of skeletal growth, which was of primary importance, was the result of deficient secretion of the growth hormone of the pituitary gland. The pituitary hyperfunction is due to the influence of the dynamic disturbances of the central nervous system induced by the toxic products of the parasites and ova, and by the reflex mechanism from local lesions.

After tartar emetic treatment for one year, the ten patients had gained in height by 6–8 cm. and in weight by 5.5 kg. Similar effects were observed in the development of the sex organs and secondary sexual characteristics. The dwarfs showed no adverse effect after treatment with antimony potassium tartrate.

Teng, C. H. "Adenovirus Pneumonia Epidemic among Peking Infants and Preschool Children in 1958." *Chinese Medical Journal* 80 (April): 331–39.

Between October 1958 and February 1959 a serious epidemic of infantile bronchopneumonia broke out in Peking. Most of the patients were infants between six months and two years of age. Many cases presented with bronchiolitis with severe anoxemia, often complicated by congestive heart failure. The WBC was normal or a little low in most of the cases. Autopsy revealed necrotic and proliferative peribronchial pneumonia, often associated with hemorrhages. In some of the cases intranuclear inclusion bodies, similar to those seen in tissue culture cells into which adenovirus had been inoculated, were found in the bronchial and alveolar epithelial cells. Adenoviruses types 3 and 7 were isolated from the pharyngeal secretions of many patients, and from the pulmonary tissues of some fatal cases.

Serologic studies showed increase of titers of adenovirus antibodies in the convalescent serum. The course of the disease was about two to three weeks. The fatality rate was 15.5 per cent. It was concluded that adenovirus was chiefly responsible for the epidemic.

1962

Hsu, C. W. "A Study of Rapid Diagnosis of Influenza." *Chinese Medical Journal* 81 (June): 394–97.

During an outbreak of Asian influenza in Shanghai in 1958, 410 patients were examined using Pikarevski's method. From the study it is believed that the nasal imprint method is a practical and rapid one for the diagnosis of influenza, especially during a suspected outbreak. The study also shows that the positive finding of inclusion bodies seems to be very significant and constitutes a definite diagnostic aid.

1963

Cheng, T. H. "Insect Control in Mainland China." *Science* 140 (April): 269–77.

Research in entomology was started in 1953–57, during the first Five-Year Plan. Since then, entomological research has advanced with amazing speed and new generations of entomologists are being trained by universities and agricultural institutes. Elementary training in entomology is offered even to members of the communes.

Between 1950 and 1955 insect control measures were dependent on human labor. Since 1956 insecticides of foreign and native origin have been used frequently. DDT and benzene hexachloride are the mainstays in chemical control, and it was reported in 1958 that 17,478,000 tons of insecticides were used, 70 per cent of which was produced in China. In 1960 no less than thirty-eight basic chemical compounds were manufactured. Sprayers of the compressed-air type and insecticides were distributed to farmers. The mass production and circle application of BHC in exterminating the major pests has been successful. The wide use of organic phosphorus compounds as systematic insecticides has resulted in an increase in yield of 30–40 per cent in eighteen provinces.

Biological controls are used in addition to chemical controls: *Trichigramma evanescens*, a minute wasp, is able to parasitize the eggs of sugarcane borers; *Dibrachys carus* is harmful to pink bollworm; *Zenillia roseanal*, a tachierid fly, is an effective parasite of the many rice insects. Fish and birds have also been employed in the control of insects.

Cultural control, such as the late sowing and transplanting of rice and the selection of insect-resistant varieties of crops, is also an important aspect of insect control in China.

Mechanical and physical control using new irrigation facilities to eliminate infestation centers for rice borers and locusts, and the submersion of rice roots for five to seven days, have proven to be useful methods of eliminating insects.

Ordinary farmers and commune members have been taught to forecast the insect outbreaks. The most important contribution of Chinese entomologists has been their work on migratory locusts. In the past farmers were helpless in the face of an outbreak of locusts, but since 1950 many measures have been taken. Initially, manual destruction was used; trenches were dug to bury the young hoppers, and thousands of farmers killed them with bamboo sticks. More recently the use of benzene hexachloride has largely replaced this method. For permanent solution, the breeding grounds of waterlogged locust areas have been transformed into rice paddies, forest hills, and livestock pastures.

Chu, C. M. et al. "Immunity in Influenza: Response to Live and Inactivated Influenza Vaccines." *Chinese Medical Journal* 82 (January): 9–17.

Both virus and host factors are believed to influence the response of man to live influenza vaccine. Antibody response is, in general, better and more uniform with the use of inactivated vaccine. It is also more stable, more readily standardized, and suitable for combination with many virus strains or with other immunizing agents. On the other hand, the live vaccine has the chief advantage of easy, economical production and administration, and is particularly suitable in the emergency of an impending pandemic.

Jen, K. F. et al. "A Study on the Interfering Effect of Asian Influenza Virus on Type 3 and Type 7 Adrenoviruses." *Chinese Medical Journal* 82 (January): 18–23.

In the experiment with human embryonic kidney cells, it was found that the multiplication of Types 3 and 7 adrenoviruses was significantly suppressed by Asian influenza virus, and that the kidney cells were not quite sensitive to the virus. It has been suggested that there existed a negative correlation between the incidence of Type A and Type B influenza viruses in sequential years due to interference. It is therefore tempting to conclude that from the demonstration of interference of adrenoviruses by Asian influenza virus, such an event might also occur in nature.

Ku, F. C. "Mass Vaccination against Polio." *China Reconstructs* 12 (July): 28–30.

In the summer of 1955 a polio epidemic broke out in China for the first time. The disease is most common in the summer and autumn, mainly among children from six months to seven years. During the past three years, over 20 million children have been given free oral vaccination (live polio vaccine) which has been produced domestically.

1963 *(Continued)*

Worth, R. M. "Health in Rural China: From Village to Commune." *American Journal of Hygiene* 77: 228–39.

In the 1930s the population density in cultivatable farm areas was about 730 per square mile (nineteen for the United States, 478 for Japan). Farm families, with 5.65 persons per household, were scattered out in small villages with populations of between seventy and 700. "Enteric infections were among the major causes of childhood morbidity and mortality, including typhoid, the other salmonelloses, and shigellosis." Other diseases transmitted by the fecal-oral route included cholera (every summer in the Yangtze delta); 40–90 per cent of the people in widely scattered areas showed the presence of a tremendous variety of intestinal parasites in their stools. The causes were largely due to shortages of fuel for adequate cooking, the use of human feces for fertilizer, and the contamination of water supplies. Diseases transmitted by the respiratory route included tuberculosis, smallpox, streptococcosis, meningococcal-meningitis, diphtheria, and pertussis. Tuberculosis was probably the greatest single cause of mortality in adults (10–15 per cent of adult deaths). Diseases with an extrahuman cycle included malaria, which was prevalent throughout the country, and kala-azar, which occurred mainly in north and central China. "Among the parasitic diseases with an extra-human cycle, *Schistosomosa japonicum* was a major problem related to the fecal contamination of rivers and lakes from human and other animal sources." Other important diseases included tetanus neonatorum (a major cause of infant mortality), trachoma, hookworm, venereal diseases (especially in cities), leprosy (more in the south than north), and opium smoking.

The war with Japan brought on serious outbreaks of malaria, cholera, and plague in crowded wartime groups or postwar groups. After Liberation the Communists instituted a land reform policy that caused profound changes for Chinese farmers. The land reform passed through three stages: (1) In each area, the Communists took land from large owners and redistributed it to peasants who had little or no land; they were urged to form cooperative teams for production and marketing purposes; (2) beginning in about 1955, a program was instituted to encourage formation of collective farms of about 350 households each, with private ownership of garden plots, tools, and animals, but with common fields for major crops; profits were shared after the deduction of the state allotment; (3) beginning in the summer of 1958, there was a big push to form rural "communes" of 1,000 to 10,000 households each, and to abolish private property. The massive centralization of farmers into communes facilitated health education efforts, immunizations, medical care, and environmental sanitation. Gastrointestinal and arthropod-borne infections were reported as being brought under control.

The author believes that "gastrointestinal infection . . . will assume the form of severe local epidemics due to accidents in central dining halls. The chronic degenerative diseases of old age should eventually emerge to a position of importance as the population ages . . . and, due to the formation of large population aggregates, tuberculosis will assume paramount importance during the next few years."

1965

Worth, R. M. "Health Trends in China Since the Great Leap Forward." *The China Quarterly* 22: 181–89.

From observations of eighty young children aged five, six, and seven years, recently arrived in Macao from neighboring rural districts of China, and 120 children of the same age group from farming villages in Hong Kong, the following conclusions were made: (1) Both groups had a high percentage of vaccination scars, demonstrating adequate preventive medical service; (2) the proportion of young children from China who had had mumps was significantly higher than among those in Hong Kong, an indirect evidence of crowding among children in China; (3) with regard to nutrition, only a marginal protein intake could be observed in both groups of children.

1971

Cheng, T. H. (Department of Biology, Pennsylvania State University.) "Schistosomiasis in Mainland China: A Review of Research and Control Programs since 1949." *The American Journal of Tropical Medicine and Hygiene* 20 (January): 26–53.

In 1949, before any action had been taken on the treatment of schistosomiasis, it was estimated that 10,470,000 were suffering

1971 *(Continued)*

from the disease, and that another 100 million were constantly exposed to infection. Many peasants left their native villages in the endemic area and some of the best ricelands lay waste. The disease was most serious in the region between the middle and lower Yangtse River.

After Liberation the antischistosomiasis campaign got underway. By 1958 it was estimated that about 330 research workers had been engaged in schistosomiasis studies in China. More than fifty research institutes and hospitals and numerous medical colleges were involved in the studies.

To extend the antischistosomiasis program into a mass movement, mobile medical teams were sent into endemic areas in the countryside to demonstrate preventive measures and the use of drugs. At the same time, special training in prevention and cure was given to thousands of people. Popular interest in the campaign was sustained largely through the formation of agricultural producers' cooperatives in many endemic areas where "work and treatment" programs reduced the loss of productive labor to a minimum.

In the countryside, barefoot doctors who render medical services and disseminate antischistosomiasis information are becoming very popular. In the cities, factory workers participate in training programs in hospitals, and are also useful members of the antischistosomiasis campaign.

Active prevention is the most important aspect of the program. Extermination of the snails through "change of the snail's environment—by burying and reclaiming marshlands for crop production" has been very effective. Chemicals such as sodium pentachlorophenate have exhibited high toxicity to the snail and its eggs. Calcium arsenite and benzene hexachloride are also effective. A teacake, the residue of the fruit of *Camellia oleosa* after extraction of oil, not only destroys snails but is valuable as a fertilizer. Storage of schistosome eggs in human feces with ammonia, or treatment with urea, ammonium bicarbonate, and calcium cynanasride, at 1 per cent, 0.5 per cent, and 0.25 per cent, respectively, kills eggs of *S. japonicum* within twenty-four hours.

Change in cultivation from rice to other crops in hilly regions, use of improved tools for gathering rushes in marshlands, removal of wild vegetation from, and repair of, banks of rivers and canals are effective preventive measures. It was claimed that by 1958 about 40 per cent of snail-infested areas, totaling 8 billion m.^{2}, were free of snails.

Treatment of *Schistosomiasis japonica* is based on the combined use of traditional Chinese and Western medicines. Pumpkin seeds and *Veratrum nigrum* are the herbal drugs used by the traditional Chinese doctors. In addition, the three pills used in combination, *Chia Chien Wei Ling*, *Han Pa Chiang Fan*, and *Chou Ch'e*, have been responsible for the cure of 93 per cent of schistosomiasis patients suffering from ascites.

In 1958, a three-day period of therapy, with 12 mg. per day of body weight with a 1 per cent solution of tartar emetic, was effective. "Because of well-recognized hazards involved in use of remedies containing antimony," however, efforts were concentrated on finding new nontoxic substitutes. In 1965 a nitrofuran compound effective for the treatment of schistosomiasis was discovered—N-isopropyl-(5-nitro-2-furyl)-acrylamide. Recently two other members of the nitrofuran series have been discovered: N-(ethyl glycinyl)-(5-nitro-2 furyl) acrylamide and B-(5-nitrol-2 furyl) acryl (N-piperidinyl-l-ethyl) amide hydrochloride.

While contributions by Chinese scientists are in large measure responsible for effective prosecution of the drive against schistosomiasis, the undertaking owes its progress to the wholehearted support of the Central Government by the peasantry. The cure of 3.5 million patients claimed in mainland reports is tantamount to an increase in the labor force of 1 million people. Death rates have fallen and birth rates have soared in endemic areas; 300,000 acres of infested land have become suitable for farming. Betterment of environmental sanitation, repudiation of superstition, and promotion of public education through release of scientific information are the fringe benefits of the campaign.

The author believes that China's struggle against schistosomiasis has not been won, and that her seven-year plan of nationwide schistosomiasis eradication has fallen behind schedule because of the Cultural Revolution. Relying on her huge manpower to carry on the struggle, however, China will be rid of schistosomiasis in a decade or so.

III. Population Planning

1957

"China's Birth Control Campaign." *Far Eastern Economic Review* 22 (April): 421–22.

With improved conditions and care, cases of infanticide have dropped, and an annual average of 5 million more infants survive compared with pre-Liberation years. The population has been increasing at a rate of 2.2 per cent, the highest in the world. The livelihood of the people has improved, however, because industrial and agricultural production have been increasing at an annual rate of 10 and 5 per cent, respectively. To accelerate the improvement in living conditions, birth control has assumed nationwide dimensions. Methods of birth control are: (1) Promoting late marriages; and (2) making all forms of contraception readily available to the mass. Along this line, the minister of health has indicated that abortion and sterilization will "be performed on request without restriction."

Women workers in China have risen by 20 per cent and now total 3 million. Equal opportunities and pay are given to women. Over 100 million women are members of agricultural cooperatives. Their involvement in the production of the country is perhaps the decisive factor in the birth control campaign.

1960

Orleans, L. A. "Birth Control: Reversal or Postponement?" *The China Quarterly* 3: 59–73.

In 1953 the Chinese population was reported to be 582.6 million, and the government appeared to be confident at the time. Concern over the size and rate of population growth began to grow in 1954, however, and in the next few years the controlled fertility campaign got underway with the following justifications: "To improve the health of mothers and infants; to advance the education of children; to allow mothers more time for work and study; and, in general, to provide a happier life for all young men and women." In 1956 the birth control policy was officially accepted by the state and reached a peak in March 1957. Hospitals and clinics were set up with special facilities to give advice on birth control. Abortion and sterilization were encouraged by the Ministry of Health. The suggested marriage age was raised to twenty-six in connection with the campaign. Despite these efforts the natural increase rate approached 2.5 per cent.

The failure was due to the low economic status of the population, the early age of marriage, the general educational level, and the overwhelmingly rural character of the country. The problem was accentuated by the traditional attitude of the Chinese toward large families and the lack of government resources to sustain the program. Unemployment and underemployment also caused concern.

The government reversed its policy: it abandoned the birth control program, organized a new propaganda campaign stressing the shortage of labor, created communes, and launched the "Great Leap Forward." Since 1958 the birth control campaign has been pushed into the background and the population policy seems to be oriented "toward a more realistic and less forceful approach to the problem of birth control . . . informal persuasion directed toward planned parenthood."

1964

Freeberne, M. "Birth Control in China." *Population Studies* 18 (July): 5–16.

China's first birth control campaign started in 1956 and ended in 1958 with the establishment of the communes and the creation of the "Great Leap Forward." Optimism prevailed in China and "the question is not so much overpopulation, as shortage of manpower." Between 1958 and 1962, while the birth control campaign was never actually abandoned, it was forced underground. The revival of the campaign of 1962–63 was accompanied by two approaches: (1) The raising of lawful marriage ages; and (2) the dissemination of family planning information. It has been suggested that the optimum age for men to marry is between twenty-five and thirty, and for women between twenty-three and twenty-eight. Propaganda campaigns on the use of contraceptives, induced abortion, and sterilization have been launched. It is believed, however, that China's population is likely to reach 1,000 million by 1980 or 1985.

1964 *(Continued)*

Lal, Amrit. "Fertility Management and Concern with Overpopulation in Mainland China." *Eugenics Quarterly* 11 (September): 170–74.

Since the time of Confucius, growth in population has represented increments in the social capital of the nation, and this belief continued until the present Communist government. In 1956 a birth control campaign was launched with the backing of many influential personages such as Shao Li-tzu, and was adopted as party policy in September 1956. Health organizations were requested to give technical guidance on contraception. The period between 1957 and 1959 saw a slack in fertility control management "because of dogmatic compulsions to the contrary and functional difficulties in implementing the scheme on a large scale." Then, in 1962, the campaign against early marriage reached its peak and an exhibition of planned parenthood materials was held in Canton. China imported contraceptives in large quantities. By 1964 China was sincerely committed to birth control as a means to raise her people's living standards.

1965

Tien, H. Y. "Sterilization, Oral Contraception, and Population Control in China." *Population Studies* 18 (March): 215–35.

Surgical methods for the prevention of conception in China were not limited to sterilization; they included acupuncture and cauterization as a combined method for fertility control. Sterilization remains the major method, however. Initital success in the production of oral contraceptives in China was reported in 1957. It is possible that abortions on a massive scale will become a major policy of population control.

1966

Wu, P. C. "The Use of Vacuum Bottle in Therapeutic Abortion: A Collective Survey." *Chinese Medical Journal* 85 (April): 245–48.

Since 1958 the vacuum suction method has been used in abortion. In 1964 the first vacuum bottle was designed and used. It is a 250 or 400 ml. bottle with a suction canula attached to a connecting tube. The vacuum inside the bottle can be produced by an electric pump, a hand pump, or by the combustion method (a modification of the traditional Chinese cupping)—a vacuum is produced inside the bottle by the sudden combustion of the alcohol inside.

Since the bottle produces only suction force, it is safer to use than an electric vacuum pump which, in case of mechanical trouble, may reverse from sucking to blowing and result in a fatal air embolism. In an electric pump the pressure is kept at a high level, while that in the bottle (initially at 400–500 mg. hg.) is reduced simultaneously during the operation so that blood loss and chance of injury are minimized. In a study of 203 cases, 29 per cent of 103 cases using the electric pump lost more than 20 ml. in the 100 cases using the vacuum bottle. A shorter time is required for the operation. Added advantages to using the vacuum bottle are that it is less painful and less irritating. It is recommended for wide use, especially in the countryside.

1969

Field, R. H. "A Note on the Population of Communist China." *The China Quarterly* 38: 158–63.

The official statistics of January 1, 1958, claimed a total population of 646,530,000 persons. In 1966 it was said to be 700 million, and in 1968, 750 million. Compared to the estimates prepared by Dr. John S. Aird of the United States Bureau of the Census, the official figures of the 1950s correspond closely to Aird's high series, while that of the 1960s are closer to the level of his low series. The figures of 700 million and 750 million should not be taken to represent the population of China in 1964, because there are many differences between those figures and the official projections for the 1950s, which are too large to be accounted for by rounded figures and boundary changes.

The size of the Chinese population cannot be estimated accurately. It is therefore advisable to use "the full range of reasonable alternatives" covered by Aird's series rather than any single estimate.

Orleans, L. A. "Evidence from Chinese Medical Journals on Current Population Policy." *The China Quarterly* 40: 137–46.

The birth control campaign has become much more action-oriented in the 1960s. Mobile medical teams are primarily responsi-

1969 *(Continued)*

ble for the dissemination of birth control information. Propaganda meetings and birth control exhibitions, including films, are held in the communes. Over a four-month period, one medical team in one commune distributed 3,475 birth control kits, and performed 547 IUD insertions, forty-eight abortions, eight sterilizations of women, and ten sterilizations of men. China's birth control is at present centered around artificially induced abortion. Three methods are usually used: syringe suction, electrical suction, and uterine curettage. In a study of 600 abortions it was concluded that the syringe suction method is superior because there is less loss of blood, quicker shrinkage of the womb, less pain, and above all it can be taught quickly to lower-level personnel. Sterilization and all forms of contraceptives, including pills, are available to the mass of the people. The IUD is the most popular contraception among women and medical personnel.

1970

Chen, P. C. "China's Birth Control Action Program, 1956–1964." *Population Studies* 24 (July): 141–58.

"The Chinese leaders had indicated that the target of birth control campaigns was to lower the natural growth rate to 2 per cent in the near future and to below 1 per cent before 2000 A.D." The birth control organizational setup could be divided into four levels—national, provincial, county, and village. At the national level, the Ministry of Health is responsible for planning the campaigns, and supervising the training of birth control personnel. At the *hsien* level, the health bureau is the unit responsible for its fertility control program, while the tasks of delivery, maternal care, *and* birth control are assigned to the same group of health personnel at the village level, Lectures, films, traveling exhibitions, face-to-face contacts, small group discussions, and cultural entertainments are organized to persuade the mass to adopt fertility control measures. In 1962 China adopted "extremely frank sex education" measures. Methods of contraception are taught to college students. Condoms are the most popular contraceptive, though the IUD has apparently gained popularity. Foam tablets, diaphragms, and jellies are manufactured and distributed. Despite resistance from the Chinese Medical Association, since 1962 the government has encouraged induced abortion, and great emphasis has been placed on vasectomies. Another measure taken by the party in 1963 to encourage fertility control was the recommendation of the "optimal marriage age of thirty for men and twenty-two for women."

The strategy used by the party has been *tien hsien man how*—start with a point and then extend outwards. For implementation of the birth control policy, this strategy has had three specific implications: (1) Efforts were initially concentrated in metropolitan areas, then spread to smaller urban areas, and finally to rural areas; (2) the initial efforts were directed toward the educated section of the population, such as cadres, intellectuals, skilled industrial workers, and professionals, and then extended to cover the uneducated peasants and unskilled workers; and (3) some pilot projects were carried out and the experience gained from them was applied to larger areas.

Tien, H. Y. "Marital Moratorium and Fertility Control in China." *Population Studies* 24 (November): 311–23.

Postponement of marriage is used by the Chinese as a mechanism for demographic control. The Marriage Law of 1950 stated that the legal age of marriage for men was twenty, and for women, eighteen. It was recognized that the Marriage Law should be amended in order to make postponement of marriage compulsory. Other means to stimulate delayed marriage are through social and economic measures. The government adopted the latter policy.

In the campaign for delayed marriage, two central themes were amplified: "(1) Condemnation of early marriage in the form of confessions of personal miseries or self-reproach; and (2) recommendation of marriage at suitable ages in terms of individual well-being, self-enrichment, and personal achievement."

"The fertility dispute within China has been carried on in a context of revolutionary change, and to involved persons who have conceived and implemented deep-reaching programs of social and economic recognition, . . . a decision to delay marriage is in itself antithetical to tradition. In this sense a full scale marital moratorium cannot but be more than a partial assault on the hold that the family has over its offspring."

IV. Food and Nutrition

1953

Jain, J. "New China Solved Her Food Problem." *China Monthly Review* (April): 30–34.

In the course of a few short years China has turned from a major food importer to an exporter. Under the leadership of the government, the average yield of rice has increased from 2.25 tons per hectare (about 2.5 acres) to 7.5 tons in 1951. The reasons for this increase in production is due to: (1) The introduction of land reform throughout the country—peasants are now able to own land; (2) exceedingly low-interest loans are available to the peasants to buy farming equipment and better seeds; (3) the government's many irrigation projects have constituted a great aid to land cultivation; and (4) cooperatives supply markets where the farmers can dispose of their produce at a guaranteed price.

1960

Huang, K. W., and Hang, C. P. "The Low Incidence of Atherosclerosis and Its Relation to Certain Dietary Features among Chinese." *Chinese Medical Journal* 80 (May): 455–58.

Out of 2,032 autopsies there were 536 cases (26.4 per cent) of different grades of atherosclerosis, the highest incidence being in the fifty-one- to seventy-year age groups. Overall, the incidence was higher among males (27.1 per cent) than females (24.3 per cent), but the reverse was true in the age groups between forty-one and seventy years. In comparison with Soviet and American statistics, the incidence of atherosclerosis among Chinese is definitely lower.

Good results have been obtained when patients are treated with a cholesterol-free diet, and it was found that the Chinese diet is very low in cholesterol. The low incidence of atherosclerosis is thus explained by this feature of the Chinese diet.

1961

W. K. "The State of Nutrition in Communist China." *The China Quarterly* 7: 121–27.

Between January 1958 and June 1959, that is, before and after the introduction of communal eating services, samples ranging from twenty-eight in 1958 to 558 in 1959 were used in five nutritional surveys. The first three surveys showed that male peasants "doing heavy work had a daily food intake equivalent to 2,692 calories, or 89.3 per cent of the requirement of 3,000 calories for a peasant doing medium heavy work. . . . The corresponding data for females were 2,245 calories, or 80 per cent. . . ." The fourth survey, carried out in the initial stages of the commune, revealed food intakes of 4,070 and 2,864 calories, respectively, for the categories surveyed previously; by the spring of 1959, however, food intakes of 3,363 and 3,150 calories, respectively, were registered. In 1959 twenty-seven persons, or 5 per cent of the sample, were reported to suffer from edema. The food supply is believed to be sufficient "to keep the Chinese people in reasonably good physical and working condition."

V. Health Services Organization and Manpower

1959

Chang, P. "Health and Safety for Workers." *China Reconstructs* 8 (October): 50–52.

During the first Five-Year Plan considerable funds were used to improve ventilation, drainage, and temperatures in the mines, as well as to reduce dust and prevent dangerous fumes in the factories. More than 90 per cent of the coal digging and transportation is mechanized, and miners get free artificial sun treatments. The wet-working process has greatly reduced the incidence of silicosis.

In the factories, women workers have equal pay and opportunity. They may take fifty-six days maternity leave with full wages. When they return to work, the factory nursery usually cares for their babies.

Hsu, Y. P. "Great Victories for Health." *China Reconstructs* 6 (March): 25–28

The targets of the twelve-year National Program for Agricultural Development was elimination of the four pests and the prevention of diseases. These have been accomplished with great success and the sanitation of both the urban and rural areas has improved, as 29,900 million tons of garbage were disposed of, 3,970 wells made clean and safe, and ditches and marshes dredged and filled. The extermination of snails and the treatment of 3.6 million

1959 *(Continued)*

patients in 1958 eliminated schistosomiasis from many provinces. Cholera, plague, and smallpox have basically disappeared. Mortality from measles fell from 8.6 to 1.5 per cent between 1950 and 1957, while that from scarlet fever fell from 17.5 to 1.3 per cent. Research on the prevention of parasitic diseases and the manufacture of antibiotics is being carried out.

China now has at least one hospital in each county; each district has a community-run hospital; each rural commune a clinic; and each agricultural work team a health worker and midwife.

Wu, S. L. "Problems of Rural Health Organizations in China's Commune System." *Jen-min Pao-Chien (People's Health)* 8 (August): 764–68.

To cope with the shortage of medical doctors and health workers in communes, each county should set up short courses to train sufficient numbers of secondary school graduates for health work. Since most of the communal health stations are ill-equipped, the county hospitals should have more specialized equipment such as X-ray generators and laboratories.

Yang, K. S. "Organization of Health Service under Communist China's Commune System." *Jen-min Pao-Chien (People's Health)* 1 (January): 82–85.

In Heilunkiang province, the health service in each commune is set up according to its economic resources and population. In general, every commune has about eighty-one health stations, 800 health workers, and 520 midwives. Typically, the fee for a doctor's visit is about one-tenth of a *yüan*. Free nurseries are available for the convenience of working mothers. A junior health worker, usually a graduate of a secondary school, performs first aid and disseminates information about health and sanitation in the fields. Regular medical checkups are given to the people in the commune. The health policy in the communes emphasizes preventive medicine and the extermination of pests.

1960

Chien, H. C. "Research in Labor Hygiene and Occupational Diseases: Its Achievements and Perspectives in Socialist Construction." *Chinese Medical Journal* 80 (March): 197–207. (This article also includes material described by Liu, S. C. et al. in "Industrial Health and Prevention of Occupational Diseases in New China," see p. 334.)

In the future, priority should be given to preventing and treating the most serious and common occupational toxicosis in industrial and agricultural production. Mass-scale education must be carried out in the prevention of toxication, the use of nontoxic substances as substitutes for toxicones, physical examination of workers, sanitation of working sites, and purification of industrial wastes. Town planning should take into account the possible harmful substances from factories nearby, and allow for a safe distance between the plant sites and residential areas.

Hsu, Y. P. (Vice-minister of public health.) "Advance the Great Work of Protecting the People's Health." *Chinese Medical Journal* 80 (May): 405–14.

The achievements in the improvement of mass health can be seen from the treatment and prevention of schistosomiasis, endemic in twelve provinces; the number of patients reached 4.9 million. Remarkable development can also be observed in health organization in the communes, where 270,000 hospitals and health centers are in operation. By the end of 1959 there were 14.6 million specialized medical and health workers; enrollment in medical and pharmaceutical colleges reached 90,000. Close coordination with industrial and agricultural production; extermination of the four pests; observance of the rules of hygiene; and elimination of the major diseases are the objectives of health work in 1960.

Orleans, L. A. *Professional Manpower and Education in Communist China*. Washington, D. C., U.S. Government Printing Office.

From 1949 to 1958 the number of medical students increased by only 223 per cent, barely keeping up with the rise in total university enrollment. In rural areas the government relies on subprofessional personnel to do the tasks of health improvement and sanitation.

Chinese traditional doctors, on whom the great majority of the Chinese had depended in the past, were estimated to number half a million in 1958. Physicians trained in Western medicine are required to study traditional Chinese methods, while herbal doctors

1960 *(Continued)*

are "instructed in short study courses and are acquainted with the principles of anatomy, physiology, and pathology."

Most medical schools are divided into medical (therapeutic), public health, oral medicine (dentistry), and pharmacology departments: a five- to six-year course of study for the first two categories, and a four-year course for the last two. In 1957 there were thirty-eight medical institutions; 40 per cent of the students were women. Although efforts have been made by the government to disperse medical and health personnel to the rural areas, at least 75 per cent of all qualified doctors are in the cities, where 15 per cent of the population resides.

"Urban Sanitation Pace Setter—Foshan." *Chinese Medical Journal* 80 (June): 564.

The people of Foshan in a matter of sixty days built and repaired the whole drainage system, using materials from torn-down shrines and cement substitutes. Thirteen hundred narrow streets and lanes were reduced to 500 in one year. The creation of 200 children's playgrounds or small gardens was also carried out.

1961

Chen, W. Y. "Medicine and Public Health." *The China Quarterly* 6: 153–69.

Before 1949 there were only 12,000 doctors, 500 hospitals, and 500 medical graduates every year in China. Eighty-four per cent of the population in the rural area was unable to pay for medical care.

In the past ten years 40,000 graduates have come out of medical and pharmacological schools. Graduates of secondary medical schools and secondary public health schools, which provide only two to three years' training, number more than 153,000. Integration of traditional and Western medicine, and the need for eight weeks of practical fieldwork by the doctors, is stressed. China has achieved great success in preventive medicine and sanitation: in 1959 over 1 billion sparrows, 1.5 billion rats, 100 million kg. of flies, and 1 million kg. of mosquitoes were eliminated.

Doctors and health workers are not free to practice where they wish, but are government employees, paid set salaries. The trend in medical care at present is to provide more hospitals in order to render more free care. At present the medical care system is divided into three levels, starting with the municipal clinics in the cities and health centers in the rural areas, then better-staffed and better-equipped county or district hospitals, and finally, the highly specialized hospitals or health institutions operated by large municipalities, provincial governments, or medical colleges. Each commune has its own health center clinic, and maternal and child health nurse. Nurseries and kindergartens are provided to people in the communes at nominal fees.

Ho, P. "Health Work Aids Agriculture." *China Reconstructs* 10 (February): 23–25.

The establishment of communes in 1958 has helped to improve health in the countryside. A network has been established, consisting of county hospitals and their branches in the communes. There are commune-run hospitals, clinics, and health stations in each production brigade, and a health room and medical attendant in each small work team. "The basic measures to strengthen rural health work are mass movements centered around elimination of the 'four pests' (rats, flies, mosquitoes, and bedbugs), improvement of sanitation, and wiping out the most prevalent diseases."

The communes make it possible to give all-round treatment to the rural population in an organized fashion. The costs of collective medical and health care in the communes is borne in the main by commune public welfare funds. This system will eventually be changed to one of free care. To aid agricultural production, medical teams and health workers work in the fields with commune members.

Each year about 200 county hospitals with 100 beds are built or expanded. They are equipped with X-ray and other modern equipment and serve as centers for technical direction and training personnel. Sixty per cent of the hospitals have set up health schools and short-term courses.

1962

Li, C. C. "Health Work in Our Mine." *China Reconstructs* 11 (August): 36–38.

In lowering the dust density in the air, the medical team in Nantung mines has encouraged the use of wet drills and moisture

1962 *(Continued)*

sprayers along transport lines. More sprinklers, fans, and other ventilation equipment have been installed to reduce cases of heat stroke. In the winter, better heating in the changing rooms is provided to prevent workers from getting cold, and regular medical checkups are given. Many miners are instructed in how to treat fractures, cuts, and gas poisoning. The medical team not only works in the pits and in the workshops, it also serves to improve the sanitation in diningrooms, the quality of the food served, and environmental sanitation of the workers' quarters.

Liu, S. C., et al. "Industrial Health and Prevention of Occupational Diseases in New China." *Chinese Medical Journal* 81 (January): 1–8.

Since Liberation ten institutes have been established to teach and do research in industrial health. Dust concentration has been brought down to a healthy level (2 mg./cu. m. air) through the combined measures of wet processing, ventilation, enclosure of machines, better personal protection, inspection and repairing of the dust density, and regular medical examinations of workers. Severe cases of heat stroke have dropped owing to the improved heat insulation and the increased use of natural ventilation. Beverages containing salt (0.2–0.5 per cent) and nutritious food are provided to workers. It has been found that CaEDTA is the best drug in promoting lead excretion, and the most suitable for mass treatments. At factories, mechanization and control at the source have reduced the lead concentration. Ninety per cent of the printing shops in Peking are equipped with lead-fume exhaust hoods. No specific remedy has yet been found for chronic benzol poisoning, however.

1965

Chang, T. K. "The Development of Hospital Services in China." *Chinese Medical Journal* 84 (June): 412–16.

There were three times as many hospitals in 1964 as in 1947. Today every one of China's 2,000 counties has a fairly well-equipped and staffed hospital. In addition, hospitals in marketplaces and industrial areas are set up to better serve the peasants and workers. To stress medical service in the countryside, urban medical teams go to the rural areas.

Treatment of the most common diseases is emphasized; for instance, between 1958 and 1964 the Peking Children's Hospital treated 6,937 cases of toxic dyspepsia, 30,178 cases of pneumonia, 3,988 cases of toxic dysentery, and 6,728 acute abdominal surgical cases.

Hsueh, C. P. et al. "An Experimental Study of the Organization of Urban Child Health Services." *Chinese Medical Journal* 84 (September): 563–70.

Thirty-seven hundred children under the age of seven were distributed in two districts, A and B, with different health organizations. In A, each assistant physician (junior medical staff) took care of 500–600 children, "carrying out the work of overall medical care with special emphasis on early prevention and treatment." He was also required to provide: (1) Health services for non-communicable diseases; (2) periodic health evaluation; (3) neo-natal care; (4) control of communicable diseases; (5) health guidance in nurseries and kindergartens; and (6) health education. In district B each assistant physician took care of 800–1,000 children, with emphasis on the overall prevention of diseases; the six items of routine work mentioned were simplified. There was no local clinic. It was shown that while both organizations are practical and feasible, the district B pattern is perhaps more suitable for working on a wider scale.

Huang, C. S. "Our Medical Teams in the Countryside." *Chinese Medical Journal* 84 (December): 800–803.

Thirty doctors and nurses, eleven of them over the age of fifty, went to the countryside for four-and-one-half months and received a warm welcome from the people. Whenever possible cheaper sulfa drugs were used instead of antibiotics in the treatment of dysentery, ascariasis, tuberculosis, bronchitis, and asthma. Minor and even some major surgery was performed. In the event of limited facilities and the lack of expensive drugs, common drugs such as sulfa-thiazole were used in the treatment of bacterial infection; a stomach tube was employed to introduce common salt and sugar water, together with sodium bicarbonate, in the correction of dehydration and acidosis. As a result of a successful experiment, the doctors

1965 *(Continued)*

found that 15–20 g. of gammexane powder could keep a latrine free of larvae for seven to ten days. The team discovered that "the best way to convince the peasants of the significance of prevention is to do propaganda through treatment."

In order to train local medical personnel, a two-year medical course was started. Thirty-six people enrolled in one school. The mobile medical team is certainly a new direction for Chinese medicine and health work.

Pen, Y. "Red Cross and Public Health." *China Reconstructs* 14 (February): 28–30.

The Chinese Red Cross was reorganized in 1950 and its membership reached 5 million. Most of the members acquired knowledge of first aid, the prevention of contagious diseases, and home nursing care. They then applied this knowledge in their neighborhoods to improve the personal health habits of their neighbors. Health habits, hygiene, and the prevention of diseases are taught to its junior members in school.

1966

Ch'ien, H. C. "Prelude to the Great March of Orienting Health Work towards the Rural Areas: Some Questions Concerning the Work of the Rural Mobile Medical Teams." *Chinese Medical Journal* 85 (April): 209–22.

The role of the medical team, as seen by the minister of health, is "to promote a new upsurge in agricultural production and in the construction of a new socialist countryside." The tasks of the team are the prevention and treatment of the common diseases in rural areas; the training of medical health workers for the countryside; the improvement and reinforcement of existing rural health organizations; the improvement of hygienic conditions in the rural regions; and the dissemination of hygiene information.

"Health Work Serving the Peasants." (An interview with Chang Kai.) *Chinese Medical Journal* 85: 143–49.

Health work has turned its attention to the rural areas because over 80 per cent of the population, about 500 million people, are peasants. To strengthen rural health, two measures have been taken: (1) The mobilization of existing medical forces and facilities to serve the peasant masses; and (2) the training of rural health workers. During the first half of 1965 alone, an estimated 30,000 health and medical workers went to the countryside. More than 200,000 people have been trained for health work by participating in the yearly medical courses in special "slack season" classes in the countryside, and/or in three-year courses in some medical colleges for students who will become doctors in the rural communes.

The overall achievements in health work since Liberation are: the elimination of the "four pests" and diseases such as smallpox, plague, cholera, kala-azar, and venereal diseases; curing more than 3 million people of schistosomiasis; the reduction of silicosis, and improved insulation and ventilation in industry; the setting up of one clinic for every commune, and of hospitals in more than 2,000 counties. In medical education, "the number of graduates from medical college since Liberation is more than ten times the total number of graduates in the twenty years before Liberation. Secondary medical school graduates total eight times the number of graduates from similar schools in old China." In the area of research, attention has focused primarily on the most harmful diseases. Methods have been devised for the prevention and treatment of schistosomiasis, kala-azar, and malaria, and for the production of live measles virus vaccine, which has been successfully tested on 100,000 children.

1967

Collier, H. B. "Teaching and Research in the Basic Medical Sciences in the People's Republic of China." *Journal of Medical Education* 42 (May): 467–69.

Compared to his visit in 1937, in 1965 Dr. Collier was most impressed by the lack of dirt, smells, beggars, and mangy dogs on the streets of China. Medical education has greatly expanded since Liberation: there are now eighty medical colleges in the country. The standards of the schools vary from the Chinese Medical College in Peking, which is comparable to those in the United States, to large provincial schools with enrollments of 2,000 (about one-third female). The government provides completely for the students while in school, and upon graduation they spend their first year in a rural clinic. The schools usually have three faculties: Western

1967 *(Continued)*

medicine, hygiene, and traditional medicine. Active research is being carried out, with emphasis on traditional drugs, cancer research, and parasites.

1968

Fan, Y. "Revolutionary Medical Workers Go to the Countryside." *China Reconstructs* 17 (December): 35–37.

Two medical teams from Peking went into the northwestern province of Kansu to give medical aid to peasants and herdsmen. They went to patients' homes, construction sites, and communes to give treatment and perform surgery. With limited facilities they performed 9,100 successful operations for such disorders as ulcers, appendicitis, hernia, trichiasis, and tumors. Due to the great demand for doctors and health personnel in the countryside, the teams gave refresher courses to 1,600 health workers who not only work in the fields but give medical treatment in their free time. Since last spring, medical teams from Shanghai, Kweichow, and many other cities have also gone to the countryside.

1969

"The 'Barefoot Doctors.' " *China Reconstructs* 19 (March): 34–37.

The Chiangchen commune trained forty-two barefoot doctors who, with thirty-seven professional people and a central hospital, serve the commune's 28,000 people. All barefoot doctors are children of poor or lower-middle income peasants who spend a good part of their time in productive labor in the commune. They know how to use close to 100 drugs, diagnose diseases, administer acupuncture therapy, and give preventive injections. In case of serious illness or an emergency they take patients to the central hospital.

VI. Other

1959

Chu, F. T. "Accomplishments in Child Health Since Liberation." *Chinese Medical Journal* 79 (November): 384–97.

Li, H. H. "Studies on Filariasis in New China." *Chinese Medical Journal* 78 (February): 148–60.

Wang, C. F. "New China's Research Achievements in Nutrition in the Past Decade." *Jen-min Pao-Chien* (*People's Health*) 10 (October): 907–16.

Yeh, K. S. "Physical Growth of Chinese Children: A Summary of Work Done during the Past Half Century." *Chinese Medical Journal* 78–79 (May): 439–45.

From 1910 to 1926 the investigation of physical growth of children was mostly done by Christian missionaries such as Whyte, Scott, Stevenson, and Appleton. The work done was not valuable for the following reasons: (1) The number of subjects investigated was very small (ten for each age group) and not representative enough; and (2) there was no uniform standard for converting Chinese age into actual age.

Between 1922 and 1949, while the work improved, defects still existed: (1) The original data was accumulative and did not show the growth of the children during any given period; and (2) the divisions of age groups were varied and hence difficult for comparison purposes.

Since Liberation considerable improvements have been made, especially in planning, supervising, conversion of age, and accuracy of measurements.

Yen, C. C. et al. "Death Rates in the City Districts of Peking." *Chinese Medical Journal* 78 (January): 27–30.

From the study of the population of city districts in Peking from 1949 to 1957, the general death rate declined from 14.1 to 7.1, a reduction of 50.3 per cent. This decline is accounted for mostly by the fall in the infant death rate. Further analysis showed that the chief causes of infant mortality are prematurity, neonatal debility, pneumonia and other respiratory diseases, and congenital deformity. The neonatal death rate accounts for about half the total infant mortality.

1963

Tung, K. T. et al. "Studies on Immunity in Influenza I: Long-Term Observation on Virus Activity and Antibody Status in a City Population." *Chinese Medical Journal* 82 (January): 1–8.

Participants

E. RUSSELL ALEXANDER, M.D.
Professor and Chairman
Department of Epidemiology
  and International Health
School of Public Health
  and Community Medicine
University of Washington
Seattle, Washington

JOHN Z. BOWERS, M.D.
President
Josiah Macy, Jr. Foundation
New York, New York

R. F. BRIDGMAN, M.D.
Paris, France

PI-CHAO CHEN, Ph.D.
Assistant Professor
Department of Political Science
College of Liberal Arts
Wayne State University
Detroit, Michigan

CHU-YUAN CHENG, Ph.D.
Department of Economics
College of Business
Ball State University
Muncie, Indiana

TIEN-HSI CHENG, Ph.D.
Professor of Zoology
Department of Biology,
College of Science
The Pennsylvania State University
University Park, Pennsylvania

ROBERT CHIN, Ph.D.
Professor of Psychology
Boston University
Boston, Massachusetts

LESLIE CORSA, JR., M.D.
Professor and Chairman
Department of Population Planning
School of Public Health
University of Michigan
Ann Arbor, Michigan

E. GREY DIMOND, M.D.
Provost for the Health Sciences
School of Medicine
University of Missouri,
  Kansas City
Kansas City, Missouri

MARY CLARK DIMOND
Kansas City, Missouri

ALEXANDER ECKSTEIN, Ph.D.
Professor
Department of Economics
University of Michigan
Ann Arbor, Michigan

ROBERT N. GROSSE, Ph.D.
Professor and Director
Program in Health Planning
School of Public Health
University of Michigan
Ann Arbor, Michigan

341

PETER S. HELLER, Ph.D.
Assistant Professor
Department of Economics, and
Research Associate
Center for Research on
    Economic Development
University of Michigan
Ann Arbor, Michigan

ANNE KEATLEY
Executive Secretary
Committee on Scholarly
    Communication with the
    People's Republic of China
National Academy of Sciences
Washington, D. C.

ARTHUR M. KLEINMAN, M.D.
Department of the History of
    Science
Harvard University
Cambridge, Massachusetts

*TSUNG-YI LIN, M.D.
Professor of Mental Health
School of Public Health
University of Michigan
Ann Arbor, Michigan

OLIVER R. McCOY, M.D.
President
China Medical Board of
    New York, Inc.
New York, New York

A. MINKOWSKI, M.D.
Director
Centre de Recherches Biologiques
    Néonatales
Clinique Obstetricale Baudelocque
Hôpital Port-Royal
Paris, France

W. K. NG, M.D.
Professor
Department of Social Medicine
    and Public Health
Faculty of Medicine
University of Singapore
Republic of Singapore

LEO A. ORLEANS, Ph.D.
China Research Specialist
The Library of Congress
Washington, D. C.

JOSEPH R. QUINN, Ph.D.
Acting Director
Fogarty International Center
National Institutes of Health
Department of Health, Education,
    and Welfare
Bethesda, Maryland

SUSAN B. RIFKIN
Research Fellow
Science Policy Research Unit
University of Sussex
Sussex, England

MILTON I. ROEMER, M.D.
Professor of Health Administration
School of Public Health
University of California,
    Los Angeles
Los Angeles, California

RUTH SIDEL, M.S.W.
Bronx, New York

* Present affiliation: Professor of Psychiatry, Faculty of Medicine, University of British Columbia, Vancouver, Canada.

VICTOR W. SIDEL, M.D.
Chief
Department of Social Medicine
Montefiore Hospital and
   Medical Center
Bronx, New York

ROBERT B. WATSON, M.D., M.P.H.
Professor
Department of Parasitology and
   Laboratory Practice
School of Public Health
The University of North Carolina
Chapel Hill, North Carolina

IRENE B. TAEUBER, Ph.D.
Senior Research Demographer
Office of Population Research
Princeton University
Princeton, New Jersey

MYRON E. WEGMAN, M.D., M.P.H.
Dean
School of Public Health
University of Michigan
Ann Arbor, Michigan

ROBERT M. WORTH, M.D., Ph.D.
Professor of Public Health
School of Public Health
University of Hawaii
Honolulu, Hawaii

Index

Index

Index

347